CONQUER CANCER

and

LAUNCH THE TOTAL ATTACK TO CANCER

Cancer Prevention and Cancer Control and Cancer Treatment at the Same Attention and at the Same Time and at the Same Level

AUTHORS: Xu Ze (China) ; Xu Jie (China) ; Bin Wu (America)

Translators: Bin Wu ; Lily Xu ; Zihao Xu ; Bo Wu

Editors: Bin Wu ; Lily Xu ; Tao Wu

Illustrators: Lily Xu ; Bin Wu

authorHOUSE®

AuthorHouse™
1663 Liberty Drive
Bloomington, IN 47403
www.authorhouse.com
Phone: 1 (800) 839-8640

Published by AuthorHouse 11/29/2018

ISBN: 978-1-5462-6947-2 (sc)
ISBN: 978-1-5462-6946-5 (e)

Library of Congress Control Number: 2018913935

Print information available on the last page.

Conquer cancer and Launch the total attack to cancer cancer prevention and cancer control and cancer treatment at the same attention and at the same time and at the same level

- <u>Changed the mode of running a hospital</u>: reforming the current mode of hospitalization with attention of treatment and lightly prevention into the equal attention of cancer prevention, cancer control and cancer treatment
- <u>Changed the treatment model</u>: reforming the current treatment mode with emphasis on cancer middle stage and late stage treatment into <u>the early stage treatment</u>
- Change only treatment without the prevention into <u>the equal attention to cancer prevention, control and treatment</u>
- The way to cure cancer is "three early", early cancer treatment is good, and <u>it can be cured</u>.
- It is necessary to establish <u>a hospital for prevention, control and treatment</u> according to <u>the whole process of cancer occurrence and development</u>.
- The overall strategic reformation and shifting of cancer treatment in the globe world focusing on treatment <u>to cancer prevention and treatment.</u>
- <u>Proposed</u> the total attack design, blueprint and implementation rules and plans

TABLE OF CONTENTS

THE INTRODUCTION TO THIS BOOK

Bin Wu

Today is the voting day for our state in America. When I put my pen on the voting marks, my tears were full of both my eyes and I was very moved by this. How can I do more good things to benefit our society? Everyone wants to have the life with health. Now the technology develops rapidly and so advanced, why is the cancer incidence rising so fast and why are the patient's age getting younger? **Cancer is not terrible, but what is terrible is that we just have a small knowledge about cancer.** There are many excellent doctors who are working very hard to help the cancer patients, such as **that Dr. Xu Ze in China worked very hard to search the ways for conquering cancer. Everything in this book** is from his scientific research and from his hard work such as from making the tumor models to cancer micro circulation to tumor free surgery to cancer cell metastasis in the blood, etc to seek the new medications of metastasis and recurrence of cancer **and the complete theory of cancer treatment has been formed including the immune regulation and control; proposed the detail plans of cancer prevention; proposed the importance of cancer treatment and cancer prevention and cancer control at the same level and at the same attention and at the same time. No matter what methods the cancer cells be treated, what we should compare who lives longer and life qualities are better.** When we treat the cancer patient, it should never forget our body immune function and our body defense system and should try very hard to protect our immune function. **We should treat the cancer as the whole body disease and cancer is not just the single organ disease. Cancer is the whole body disease which the regulation and control function or the immune function of the whole body malfunctions or goes down and is not only the single organ or located disease such as when the patient has the stomach cancer, the whole body lost the balance and lost the defense against the disease.**

The key of conquering cancer is the good laboratory. In clinics the questions are found, then comes back to the experimental Lab to seek the method of solving these questions.

Cancer science is involved in multiple subjects such as immunology, endocrine, environmental science, etc Only the cancer can be understood completely, the cancer diagnosis and treatment can have the innovation breakthrough.

Along with the development of scientific technology, many concepts about cancer should be changed. In the past when people talked about cancer, their skin color changed; however, the fact is that cancer can be cured and can be prevented and be controlled if the correct things are done. We don't have to kill the last cancer cell during the treatment because the normal people have the cancer cells as well. People can live with cancer cells very well. Again Cancer is not terrible, what the terrible thing is that people just have a small of knowledge about cancer. In this book we summarized how to conquer cancer and how to prevent cancer and how to treat cancer. For example, our pancreatic cancer patients can live more than 15 years and they are still alive now while we publish this book. Our liver cancer patients live more than 28 year and the patients still alive while we publish this book. Cancer cell comes from the normal cell and grows from the normal cells so that cancer cells just have the subtle difference from the normal cell and no matter how treatment are, they often kill both the cancer cells and the normal cells.

In the body everyday there are many billions of cell proliferation and change, the old cell goes and the new cells will come and grow. Even If there is only one cell which has the gene mutation, the cancer cell will produce; almost all of our bodies have the cancer cells. **Everyone has cancer cell including the new born baby. Whether it develops into cancer or not, it depends on the cancer cell characteristics and mainly depend on the ability of the body control and regulating of cancer cell and depends on the balance. If the body immune function is strong, the cancer cells will be devoured in the organ microcirculation.** While the body immune function decreases, the cancer cell will survive in the organs. For example, when the doctor helps the patient to get the radiotherapy treatment and have to contact to radiation. After receiving the radiation one or two weeks, there will be the cancer cells which can exist in the doctor blood If the blood get check up. However why do these cancer cells not grow into cancer cells because our body can control and regulate all of these cancer cell growth. **Cancer is the issue of the body balance, it is the immune function malfunction of the regulation and control.** How do we correct this unbalance of our regulation and control? Dr. Xu Ze did the throughout research and found many medications to help with bringing back this unbalance.

Our goal of cancer treatment is that a third of cancer can be prevented before

it happens, a third of cancer can be cured completely and a third of cancer can be survived with living with cancer.

What is Cancer? Cancer cell comes from the normal cell and grows from the normal cells which have **subtle difference** from the normal cell so that when we kill the cancer cells with chemotherapy and radiotherapy, the normal cells are often be damaged too. The normal cells such as the wounded cell and embryo cells also proliferate and our body can control and stop this proliferation at the correct time, however when Our body lost the control and regulation of the cell proliferation or lost this kind of controlling or stopping the cell proliferation, the cancer cells will continue to grow and to damage our organ function. **Cancer is the disease of the whole body, which means cancer is the disease of the malfunction of the whole body balance on the regulation and control of cell proliferation**. It should be not only a single disease of that located the cancer sits or organs.

Cancer occurs when there is the gene mutation. The human body usually is designed perfectly : **there are two sets of balance gene: Proto-Oncogenes and Tumor-Suppressor Genes.** Normally the expression of these genes are controlled very well by the body. However what factor triggers proto-oncogenes to active into oncogenes and what factors cause the proto-oncogenes mutation into oncogenes then cause cancer occurenc and what factors cause all of these mutaton and what factor to promote all of these gene to express into RNA and protein; There should be some promoters there. **What are these promoters from?** Many cancers can be prevented before they happens if all of these promoters can be avoided. The environment of living and the lifestyle play a great role in the cancer occurrence. More than 90% of cancer can be prevented, which many cancer occurence is related to the environment, especially the lifestyle; lifestyle plays tremendous role in GI and GU cancers. **The prevention of cancer is the same important as the treatment of cancer.** Dr. Xu Ze always educates his patient and the patients' family to pay attention to the prevention cancer while he treats the patient. In this book we summarized all of our experimental results about how to prevent and how treat and how to conquer cancer and also **reflect the spirit and dedication of hard work from him and his team.** The three early" early detect and early treat and early diagnosis" is very important for cancer treatment and cancer can be cured completely. "The three early" is very important, early detect, early treat and early diagnosis, **the cancer can be cured completely.**

In brief, let us work together to keep the health body and conquer cancer and live longer and healthier.

The free-tumor surgery and the nutrition support after the surgery are tremendously important for completely curing the cancer. This month is November and my father passed away in November many years ago and I suddenly recall that he did many of esophagus cancers in my townhome. I never heard he told the cancer recurrence and metastasis after the surgery. A Long time ago that esophagus cancer operation was a huge and a long hour operation 12 hours. Also I still remember my father taught the patients how to eat and how to bring back the patients healthy condition back as soon as possible by the nutrition after the surgery. Many of his patients came back to appreciate my father for saving their life and the cancer was cured. **Dr. Xu Ze told me that: any procedure or operation even if the doctors had done this procedure more than thousands times, they should still treat them as this is the first time for them to do it. Review and recite each step before the operation carefully.** After the surgery, bringing back the patient immune function by nutrition is the same important as free-tumor surgery.

In addition, due to such a short time of finishing this book and there is huge information in this book and we work day and night. If there is any mistake, please forgive us and look forward to the feedback.

Bin Wu
11-06-2018
Timonium, MD 2108

A BRIEF INTRODUCTION
TO THE FIRST AUTHOR

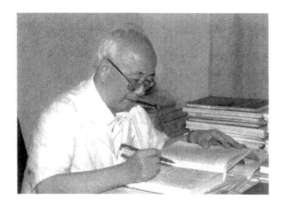

Xu Ze, male, born in Leping County of Jiangxi Province in Oct. 1933, gradated from Tongji Medical University in 1956, successively held the post of director of department of surgery of Affiliated Hospital of Hubei College of Traditional Chinese Medicine, professor, chief physician, tutor of postgraduate and doctoral student, President of Experimental Surgery Restitute Institute of Hubei College of Traditional Chinese Medicine, Director of Abdominal Tumor Surgery Research Room and Director of Anti Carcinomatous Metastasis and Reoccurrence Research Room. in addition, he held concurrent posts of Standing Director of China Medical Association Wuhan Branch, Vice President of Wuhan Micro-circulation Academy, Academic Member of International Liver Disease Research, Cooperation and Exchange Center, Member of International Surgeon Union, Standing Member of 1st, 2nd, 3rd and 4th Editorial Board of China Experimental Surgery Journal, Standing Member of 1st, 2dn and 3rd Editorial Board of Abdominal Surgery Journal. Enjoying Special Allowance of State Council.

He has been engaged in surgery work for 49 years and accumulated rich experience in radical operation of lung cancer, esophageal carcinoma, liver cancer, carcinoma of gallbladder, adenocarcinoma of pancreas, gastric carcinoma and intestinal cancer as well as in clinical therapy with Chinese Traditional Medicine combined with Western Medicine of prevention of reoccurrence and metastasis after operation.

He has been engaged in scientific research of surgery for 15 years and obtained many fruits, among which the task of Experimental Study and Clinical Application of Self-made Type Z-C1 Abdominal Cavity—Vein Flow Turning Unit in Therapy of Chronic Ascites of Hepatic Cirrhosis issued by Science Commission of Hubei Province was awarded Second Prize of Scientific Fruit by People's Government of Hubei Province and was popularized and applied in 38 hospitals in 12 provinces all over the country in 1982. The task "Experimental Study on Physiological Mechanism and Pathogenesis of Schistosome with Method of Experimental Surgery", issued by National Natural Fund Commission was awarded Second Prize of Scientific Fruit by People's Government of Hubei Province in 1986.

He began to study the tumor experience, established the tumor animal model and metastasis and reoccurrence animal model and probed into the mechanism and rules of carcinomatous metastasis and reoccurrence to find out the method to inhibit the metastasis. 48 kinds of Chinese traditional herbs that could counteract the intrusion, metastasis and reoccurrence were found and selected from a large number of natural herbs. Based on this, he invented and developed China Xu Ze (Z-C) Medicine Treating Malignancy, which had remarkable curative effects through over 10 years' clinical validation of many cases.

He has been engaged in teaching for 40 years and has cultivated many young doctors, 10 masters and 2 doctors. He has released 126 papers, published New Understanding and New Mode of Therapy of Cancer as the editor in charge, participate in writing 8 medical exclusive books including Therapeutics of Liver Disease, Surgery of Liver, Gallbladder and Pancreas and Surgical Operation of Abdomen.

A BRIEF INTRODUCTION TO THE SECOND AUTHOR

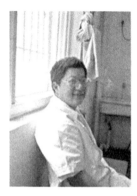

Xu Jie, male, graduated from Hubei College of Traditional Chinese Medicine in 1992, graduated from Hubei Medical University in 1996, Department of Clinical Medicine. Now He is chief physician in Hubei University of Traditional Chinese Medicine Hospital and Hubei Provincial Hospital of Surgery, engaged in experimental surgical tumor research and general surgery, urology clinical work.

Since 1992, he has been involved in the experimental tumor research of the Institute of Experimental Surgery of Hubei College of Traditional Chinese Medicine. He has carried out cancer cell transplantation and established a tumor animal model. He has carried out a series of experimental tumor research: exploring the mechanism of recurrence and metastasis of cancer and in vivo screening experiment of more than 200 kinds of Chinese herbal medicine in vivo tumor model of tumor inhibition s from a large number of natural medicine to find out, screening out of 48 kinds of anti-cancer invasion, metastasis, relapse traditional Chinese medicine

He participates in clinical validation and followed up for XZ - C immunoregulatory Chinese herbal medicine and completes the experimental research and clinical verification, data collection, collection and summary of this book.

A BRIEF INTRODUCTION TO THE THIRD AUTHOR AND THE MAIN TRANSLATOR AND ONE OF THE EDITORS

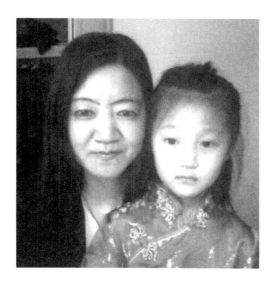

Bin Wu, MD, Ph.D., graduated from College of Yunyang of Tongji University of Medical Sciences for her MD degree; Studied her Master degree and her Ph. D degree in Sun Yat-Sen University of Medical Sciences. After she received her Ph.D., she worked as a Post-doctoral Follews in the Johns Hopkins Medical School and University of Maryland Medical School. She passed her USMLE tests and is going to do her residency training in America. She dedicated herself to oncology clinical and research. Her goal is to conquer cancer, which she believes this great contribution to our health. She has a daughter, named Lily Xu who drew all of the pictures in this book.

A BRIEF INTRODUCTION TO THE ILLUSTRATOR AND THE ADVISOR

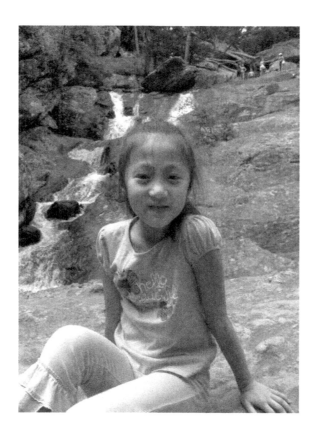

Lily Xu was born on November 17th 2006 and had an art presented in the Walter Art Museum in Baltimore at the age of 6; she got the fourth place trophy in the ES Double Digits or 24 and 24 games in the Baltimore County in Maryland; she got the first trophy in the BCPS STEM FAIR PHYSICS in Baltimore County; when she was in the sixth grade, she passed the advanced Math for 7th grade(which means the 8th grade math) test and moved the 8th grade math class; she loves the reading and the writing and she finished many seires of books. She got $3000 scholarship award for the Peabody music program in the Johns Hopkins University. She edits all of my books for the publishing and drew all of the pictures in this book.

FOREWORD(1)

XZ-C proposed "Walked out of a new road to overcome cancer 1- 8". <u>They are all proposed for the first time in the world, the first in the world, and the international leader.</u>

First, why do we propose to conquer cancer and need to launch a total attack?

<u>1. Because the goal of conquer cancer should be</u>:

(1) to reduce the incidence of cancer
To improve the rate of the cancer treatment cure, which significantly prolongs the survival of patients, to improve the quality of life, and to reduce the cancer mortality.
(2) To reach up to
1/3 can prevent
1/3 can be cured
1/3 can prolong life through treatment

<u>2, then, how can we reduce the incidence of cancer?</u>

It should be prevention-oriented, control-oriented, prevention-oriented
But for decades, the road we have traveled is to pay attention to treatment and to ignore the prevent, or only treatment without prevention.
As a result, the incidence of cancer is increasing, and the more patients are treated and the more the patients get cancer.

<u>3. What should I do? It should be prevention-oriented, control-oriented, and implement the prevention-oriented health work policy.</u>

<u>Only by paying attention to preventing cancer can we reduce the incidence of cancer.</u>
<u>Therefore, cancer prevention should be the most important</u>

4. Professor Xu Ze (XU ZE) proposed to launch the general attack. In fact, it is to put the prevention, control, and treatment at the same equal important attention. And put the prevention of cancer into an important part. In fact, it is to carry out and implement the "prevention-based" health work policy, <u>our medical seniors and the world's medical sages advocated "cancer prevention and anti-cancer" and is mainly based on the prevention of cancer</u>. This policy is very correct, but unfortunately our medical juniors have not paid attention to it.

Since the past century, the world has not paid attention to cancer prevention, it has led to such a high incidence of cancer today, and the more patients are treated and the more cancer patients we have. In 2015, the number of new cancer cases in China was about 4.292 million. There are 11,922 new cancers in our country every day, and 8 people are diagnosed with cancer every minute. Such amazing data should be a national event for the people and the people.

Second, under the guidance of Xi Jinping's new era of socialism with Chinese characteristics, we should strive to open up a new situation in scientific research in the new era, and the scientific research work to overcome cancer should be made forward and become a courageous struggle for this new era in this new era, a new journey, a new role, a new atmosphere.

Under the guidance of Xi Jinping's new era of socialism with Chinese characteristics, he strives to follow the path of independent innovation with Chinese characteristics and adheres to the road of independent innovation of Chinese and Western medicine combined with "Chinese-style anti-cancer". China will contribute more Chinese wisdom, China's programs, and China's power to the world, so that the sun of the humanity's destiny will shine in the world.

Third, disclaimer: This book is to guide and to be used to conquer cancer and launch the total attack on cancer and to create the Science City of conquer Cancer. XZ-C's overall design, planning, and blueprint for cancer research projects are the scientific thinking and theoretical innovation and experimental basis for conquer cancer. It is the overall strategic reform and development of cancer treatment. It is my 60 years of experience in medical work and 30 years of scientific research results, scientific and technological innovation, scientific thinking and scientific research wisdom to overcome cancer. It is planned to be located in the experimental area of Huangjiahu University City in Wuhan. The research project will be implemented by the experts and professors of the research team.

Internationally, the scientific research plan to overcome cancer is to focus on scientific research projects and is the frontier of science.

On January 12, 2016, US President Barack Obama proposed the National Cancer Program to "conquer cancer" in the State of the Union address, and named it as the Cancer Moon Shot, which was implemented by Vice President Biden. The specific plan is unknown.

FOREWORD(2)

This book is to guide and to be used to conquer cancer and to launch the total attack on cancer and to create the Science City of conquering Cancer. XZ-C's overall design, planning, and blueprint for cancer research projects are the scientific thinking and theoretical innovation and experimental basis for conquer cancer. It is the overall strategic reform and development of cancer treatment. It is my 60 years of experience in medical work and 30 years of scientific research results, scientific and technological innovation, scientific thinking and scientific research wisdom to overcome cancer. It is planned to be located in the experimental area of Huangjiahu University City in Wuhan. The research project will be implemented by the experts and professors of the research team.

Internationally, the scientific research plan to overcome cancer is to focus on scientific research projects and is the frontier of science.

On January 12, 2016, US President Barack Obama proposed the National Cancer Program to "conquer cancer" in the State of the Union address, and named it as the Cancer Moon Shot, which was implemented by Vice President Biden. The specific plan is unknown.

The disaster of cancer covers the whole world. People all over the world are eager to hope to overcome cancer one day. It is hoped that the country, government, experts, scholars, scientists and entrepreneurs can find out anti-cancer measures to keep people away from cancer.

According to the "2015 China Cancer Statistics" report published by the National Cancer Center and the National Cancer Registry, in 2015, the number of new cancer cases in China was about 4.292 million, and the number of deaths was about 2.814 million. With the continuous increase, cancer has become the "number one killer" threatening human health. It has brought great challenges to cancer prevention and control in China and the world, and has also caused enormous economic burden on society.

The way out for cancer treatment is "three early", and the way out for cancer is prevention. Coping with this challenge through cancer prevention and a combination of early diagnosis and early treatment can reduce the economic loss of cancer to a certain extent and save people's lives.

Therefore, XZ-C proposed to carry out the initiative of "conquering cancer, launching a general attack – to pay the equal attention to cancer prevention, cancer control, and cancer treatment."

Xu Ze
Prof. XU ZE
June 2018 in China • Hubei • Wuhan

ACKNOWLEDGEMENTS

This book is for all of people who concern human being health. We are deeply grateful to all of people who like our new ways to improve our human being health.

My daughter **Lily Xu** gave me many smart and creative ideas while we were finishing this book. Lily Xu drew all of the pictures such as the Thymus etc. **The characteristics of she loves the challenge** and **her judgment always encourages me to continue working hard to move on**.

I would like to express our sincere gratitude to the following:

1. All of Authorhouse staffs
2. Dr. Xu Ze's family and Dr. Xu Jie's family, especially his son **Zihao Xu**, who is the medical student in China
3. Mrs. Bo Wu's family and Mrs. Tao Wu's famly: espeicaly their daughters Chongshu Luo and Xunyue Wang

Bin Wu, M.D., Ph.D
11-06-2018 in Baltimore, Maryland in USA

Guidance : How to read this book in the details as the following:

The detail of Table of Contents

How to overcome cancer? How to prevent cancer? How to treat cancer?

1. In-depth study of the "Government Work Report"

- Must implement the research on strengthening smog control proposed in the report
- Advance the prevention and treatment of major diseases such as cancer, so that science and technology can better benefit the people.
- Resolutely fight to win the battle pollution prevention and pollution control and pollution treatment, to achieve the purpose of preventing cancer, anti-cancer research and effect
- The challenge of the times
- Post-guided review

2. Briefly describe the research process of anti-cancer research

- 4 stages of research
- New findings in experimental research
- Experimental screening, exclusive research and development products: XZ-C immune regulation and control anti-cancer Chinese medicine series $XZ-C_{1-10}$ indications
- Clinical validation: some typical cases
- Partial list
- Social benefit assessment

3. The report of carrying out " conquer cancer and launch the total attack to cancer, focusing on cancer prevention, control, and treatment"

- Reform the current building mode of hospitalization which attention the treatment and ignore prevention into attention the equal treatment and prevention of cancer.
- Reform the current treatment mode with emphasis on middle and late treatment into starting the early stage.
- Change the treatment of cancer only to prevent and control of cancer

- It is necessary to establish a hospital for prevention, control and treatment according to the whole process of cancer occurrence and development.
- The way out for cancer treatment is "three early", early cancer <u>treatment is effective and can be cured</u>

<u>The current is the best time to help with conquering cancer and launching the total attack to cancer.</u>

4. How to overcome cancer? How to prevent cancer?

XZ-C proposes to create the "Innovative Environmental Protection and Cancer Research Institute" and carry out preventing cancer system engineering

- XZ-C proposes:

Dawning A type cancer prevention plan

Dawning B type cancer prevention plan

Dawning D-type cancer prevention plan

Macro views, micro views, ultra-micro views

- Combine with the three major challenges, ride research, pollution prevention, pollution control, preventing cancer, anti-cancer

5. How to overcome cancer? How to treat cancer?

- XZ-C proposes: Dawning C-type plan No.1-6

Dawning C-type plan No. 1: "Conquer cancer and launch the total attack to cancer"

Dawning C-type plan No. 2: "Creating a full-scale prevention and treatment hospital"

Dawning C-type plan No. 3: "Building a science city to overcome cancer"

Dawning C-type Plan No. 4: "Building a Multidisciplinary and Cancer Research Group"

Dawning C-type plan No. 5: "The vaccine is human hope, immunological prevention"

Dawning C-type plan No. 6:

A "The prospect of immunomodulatory drugs is gratifying"

B The research group and Laboratory establishment "XZ-C immunomodulatory Chinese medicine active ingredient, molecular level analysis

6, " Walk out of a new way of immune regulation and control of Chinese and Western medicine combined with cancer treatment"

- navigate
- Pathfinding and footprinting (scientific footprints)
- Walking out of an XZ-C immune control and regulation on the molecular level, Western medicine combined with new cancer treatment
- XZ-C immune regulation and control anti-cancer Chinese medicine series products and adaptation range
- Has formed the theoretical system of XZ-C immune regulation and control and treatment of cancer, the theoretical basis and experimental basis for cancer immunotherapy
- XZ-C immunomodulation anticancer Chinese medications are the result of the modernization of traditional Chinese medications

7. "Our cancer prevention and treatment research has reached the world frontier"

- Over the past 30 years, we have focused on cancer research and scientific research. The Science and Technology Innovation Series has put forward 30 innovations in my series of monograph, <u>which are the first time in the world, all of which are original papers, international initiatives, and international leaders</u>. They have reached the world's leading position.
- Science – is the endless of the frontier. <u>The above 30 international proposals and international initiatives for the first time showed that our research work is at the forefront of the world</u>. Under the guidance of Xi Jinping's new era of socialism with Chinese characteristics, the scientific research work to overcome cancer should be striding forward, is the new era and new journey, and is New weather, new actions, and become the courager to fight for the new era.
- In short, if the above items can be achieved, of course the cancer can be overcome

(1).The goal of conquering cancer:
<u>reduce the incidence rate, improve the cure rate, reduce the mortality rate, significantly prolong the survival of patients, and improve the quality of life.</u>

(2).Achieve :
1/3 can be prevented, 13 can be cured, and 1/3 can prolong life by treatment.
It reports to the governments at all levels and requests leadership, guidance, and support for the benefit of the people. President Xi Jinping said that people's yearning for a better life is the goal of our struggle. People all over the country

and the world are eager to hope that one day they will be able to overcome cancer..., away from cancer.

8, "Condense Wisdom and Conquer Cancer" - for the benefit of mankind

- Guided materials
- preface

Volume: How to conquer cancer? How to prevent cancer?
[Has been published in December 2017 (published)]
Volume 2: How to conquer cancer? How to treat cancer?
[Published in February 2018 in U.S.A globally in English]

9. The initiative and academic report of carrying out "To conquer cancer and to launch the total attack of cancer"

10, XZ-C proposed: cancer prevention research work can not walk slowly and should run ahead to save the life and rescue the wounded.

The White Paper on the Status of Cancer Treatment
- (1) Cancer incidence worldwide
- (2) Cancer mortality worldwide
- (3) Status of 5-year survival rates of cancer worldwide

11, XZ-C proposed that research ethics should be advocated, medicine is benevolence, and ethics is the first

Research ethics: products should have ethical standards
Standard: the bottom line should not be harmful to human health
Basic ethics: All products should be harmless to human being and do not harm people's health, especially for children, not allowed to contain carcinogens

12. The past and future of oncology development

Next research prospects, vision predictive evaluation of cancer treatment
The prospect of immunomodulatory therapy is gratifying

13, how to overcome cancer? XZ-C proposes: Cancer is a disaster for all mankind. It is necessary for the people of the world to work together and China and USA should jointly tackle the problem.

A."Cancer moon shot" (US) and "Dawning C-type plan" (middle) – move forward together and head to the science hall to overcome cancer

B. Why do you want to move forward together? What are the common between them? China and the United States have their own advantages analysis and complementary advantages

- For the past 100 years, the history record of that internationally it was proposed of the "conquer cancer" program"
- Do an unprecedented event for the benefit of mankind
- Dawning C-type plan
- Situation analysis: (1), (2), (3), (4)

Our advantages are:

1. Traditional Chinese medications, anti-cancer traditional Chinese medications, immune-regulating traditional Chinese medications, activating blood circulation and removing blood stasis and anti- tumor thrombus Chinese medication, Soft firming and dissolving or dismissing nodule Chinese medications, heat-clearing and detoxifying to improve the microenvironment of cancer cells;
2. Combination of Chinese and Western medicine, combined with innovation

The advantages of the United States are:

Modern medicine, advanced diagnosis and treatment technology, targeted medicine

XZ-C believes that: **China's advantages and potentials should be exerted or bring into play. We should increase efforts to develop and explore the advantages of Chinese herbal medicine. Traditional Chinese medicine can improve symptoms, improve physical fitness, increase immunity, and prolong survival (the lesions generally do not shrink, but can survive with tumors and live a long time), can be used as an auxiliary treatment for surgery.**

14, pathfinding and footprint

- cause
- navigate
- Footprint (scientific footprints)
- Dawning research spirit
- Thinking in the morning

Note:

1. XZ-C is Xu Ze-China (Xu Ze - China), because science is borderless, but scientists have the nationalities and the intellectual property.
2. Cancer is a disaster for all mankind. It must evoke the struggle of the people all over the world. Therefore, there are 7 monographs in this series, which are all in English and distributed worldwide.

CHAPTER I

In-Depth Study of the "Government Work Report"

TABLE OF CONTENTS

1. It must implement the research on strengthening smog control proposed in the report

The report pointed out **the overall requirements and policy orientation of economic and social development in 2018;** and to accelerate the construction of an innovative country; and to grasp the world's new round of scientific and technological revolution and industrial transformation; to deepen the implementation of innovation-driven development strategy; and to continuously enhance economic innovation and competitiveness; to strengthen the construction of a national innovation system; to strengthen basic research; to apply research and original innovation; to launch a number of major projects for scientific and technological innovation; and to build national laboratories with high standards; to encourage enterprises to take the lead in implementing major science and technology projects; and to support research institutes, universities and enterprises to integrate innovation; to accelerate the transformation and application of innovation results. National science and technology investment must be tilted towards the people's livelihood; **to strengthen the research on smog or pollutin treatment, to promote the outbreak research of prevention and treatment for cancer major disease and make science and technology better for the benefit of the people;** to resolutely fight the three major battles; to make the significant progress in promoting major risk prevention and resolution; to increase the precision of poverty alleviation; to promote pollution prevention and control to achieve greater results, and to consolidate the achievements of the blue sky defense; to deepen the prevention and control of water and soil pollution; to strengthen the construction of sewage treatment facilities, and to improve the charging policy. It is strictly forbidden to enter foreign garbage, strict environmental law enforcement and accountability. We must work together to build a beautiful China and world with sky blue, green land and clear water.

In-depth study of the relevant part of the "Government Work Report", we must implement the requirements of the "Government Work Report"; strengthen research on smog governance, promote research on prevention and treatment of major cancer diseases, and make science and technology better for the benefit of the people. Resolutely fight to win the battle of pollution prevention and pollution control and treating pollution in order to achieve the purpose and effect of anti-cancer and cancer prevention research.

2. Promote or Advance the prevention and treatment of major diseases such as cancer so that science and technology can better benefit the people.

The more cancer patients are treated and the more and the more cancer patients occur, the incidence is rising, and 90% of them are related or closely related to environmental carcinogenic factors. Therefore, the target or "target" of cancer prevention should be researched and discussed in relation to the carcinogenic factors (external environment and internal environment) of the environment.

Therefore, we propose the cancer prevention general design and cancer prevention system engineering, and advocate the establishment of the "Innovative Environmental Protection and Cancer Research Institute" and the implementation of cancer prevention system engineering.

3. Resolutely fight to win the battle of pollution prevention and pollution control so as to achieve the purpose and effect of scientific research work of cancer prevention and anti-cancer

It is necessary to prevent and control the three major pollutions, and it is advisable to study the relationship between the environment and cancer.

In fact, pollution prevention and pollution control are cancer prevention and cancer detection; actually, it can get the first-level cancer prevention effect, we must prevent and control the three major pollutions, pollution prevention, pollution control, and overcome difficulties. We will certainly achieve the benefits of cancer prevention and cancer control and treating cancer, and reduce the incidence of cancer in China, our province, and our city and all of the world. Achievement is in the modern age and present time, Benefiting is in the future, it is seeking health benefits for future generations.

Under the guidance of Xi Jinping's new era of socialism with Chinese characteristics, **I will dedicate my scientific research ideas and scientific thinking and contribute my scientific wisdom of conquering cancer as the research direction which I have taken for 30 years to the people of my motherland and our province and our city**. I am 86 years old, a white-haired old man, from the age of 60 years old to the age of 70 years old to the age of 80 years old, is still perseverance and persevere in scientific research to overcome cancer, is adhere to the basic research of animal experiments and clinical validation research on anti-cancer, anti-cancer metastasis and recurrence, and have worked hard for 30 years, and have obtained a series of scientific and technological innovations and scientific research achievements. Because I am retired 20 years, no one cares a retired professor. I don't know who and where can manage these things, where and who can support me and where the scientific research results should be reported so that I have to publish the monographs to the benefit of mankind, and published a series of monographs. In the past 30 years, I have published ten medical monographs on cancer research, including three chinese versions with the national distribution, seven English versions with global distribution; setting up the theory in the book, passing on to the world, passing on to the future, passing on to the next generation.

Now it is a time of prosperity in China, the spring of science, and the innovation of science and technology. Under the guidance of Xi Jinping's new era of socialism with Chinese characteristics in this new era, the new journey and scientific research work should be advanced. I will work hard to dedicate this research result to the motherland and to the people of the motherland. Although I am a 86-year-old white-haired old man, I am still motivating me to make great efforts to overcome the cancer research work in this new era of scientific spring and become a In this new era, new journey, new action, new weather we still strive to be the courage of the new era.

老骥伏枥志未已，为控转移究歧黄（Meaning: **don't know the direction, still work hard to look for the Chinese medication to control cancer**）

老骥自知时日短，不用扬鞭自奋蹄（Meaing: **know there is not too much time, still work hard to control cancer** ）

(notes: these are the Chinese poems, which are interpreted as the following parts:

The old man knows that his time is short and he does not need to raise his own whip, however he works very hard to look for anti-cancer medication to conquer cancer)

<u>**Because I have made scientific research work to conquer cancer research as the research direction for 30 years, I have achieved a series of scientific research achievements, scientific and technological innovation series**</u>, and our cancer prevention and treatment research work has reached the world's leading edge, and has reached the forefront of the world, if it can be implemented. If it can achieve to the goal of conquering cancer, you can achieve the goal of conquering cancer.

__(1) The goal of conquering cancer is to reduce the incidence of cancer, improve the cure rate of cancer, reduce the cancer mortality, significantly prolong the survival of patients, and improve the quality of life.__

(2) reach:

1/3 can prevent, 1/3 can be cured, 1/3 can significantly prolong life through cleansing treatment

__Pathway:__ **the way out for cancer treatment is "three early", and the way out for anti-cancer is prevention.** It can push the research work of Hubei and Wuhan cancer prevention and treatment to the forefront of the country and push it to the forefront of the world.

I hope some universities can create this first-class discipline with conquer cancer as the research direction. It can establish the first batch of the first class of subject with conquer cancer as the research direction in the country and the world. __Under the guidance of Xi Jinping's new era of socialism with Chinese characteristics, we will strive to follow the road of anti-cancer transfer with Chinese characteristics, adhere to the road of independent innovation with Chinese characteristics, adhere to the combination of Chinese and Western medicine, and the road of independent innovation of "Chinese-style anti-cancer".__ **It is hoped that Hubei and Wuhan will first establish the first-class subject or discipline with conquer cancer as the research direction in the country and the world,** __promote cancer prevention research, make science and technology better for the benefit of the people, and make new achievements in conquering cancer, work in the present, and benefit in the future and generation.__

In order to In-depth study of the "Government Work Report" and to implement the "Government Work Report" requirements, we must conscientiously implement and accelerate the construction of innovative countries, promote the prevention and treatment of major cancer diseases, and make science and technology better for the benefit of the people and resolutely fight to win the battle against pollution and pollution prevention to anti cancer and cancer prevention.

__In-depth study of the "Government Work Report" and resolutely implement the "Government Work Report"; and now suggest and advice and contribute "scientific anti-pollution, pollution control, anti-cancer, cancer prevention, promoting the prevention and treatment of major cancer diseases so that science and technology can better benefit the people" to Hubei Provincial Committee, Wuhan The municipal party committee.__

4. The challenge of the times

The development of medicine in the 21ˢᵗ century should be the century of conquering cancer.

Cancer is now not only a household name, but also a problem that is often encountered in life. When it comes to cancer or it is talked of the cancer, it is always that the emotion is in a heavy burden, even while talking of cancer, the skin color changes or discoloration. In the long years, mankind has fought against disease and won one victory after another. The plague, typhoid fever, cholera, smallpox, and plague that have seriously threatened human life in the past have caused humans to die in batches. Before the 19ᵗʰ century, when the smallpox was in a hurry, the smallpox won the alias of "God of Death."

In the Song Dynasty of China, vaccination was carried out with vaccinia, and later spread to Europe. Since then, the smallpox has been conquered. Tuberculosis was considered "incurable disease" decades ago, invented streptomycin in 1944, invented in 1945 Remy wind, it is not terrible. In short, the diseases that once caused people to die in batches were eliminated and controlled one by one. Today's cancer has risen to become a major disease endangering human health. Coupled with the rapid development of modern industry, the three wastes are increasing, and cancer poses more and more serious challenges to human life.

Therefore, it should be proposed to conquer cancer and launch a general attack.

Anti-pollution and pollution prevention and control can achieve the effect of first-class anti-cancer and anti-cancer.

XZ-C proposed an initiative to establish the "Innovative Environmental Protection and Cancer Research Institute" and carry out anti-cancer system engineering.

5. Review after Reading Guidance

"Condense wisdom and conquer cancer – for the benefit of mankind" is a medical monograph with the relatively complete, systematic, comprehensive design, more specific planning of how to conquer cancer. The book is divided into two parts: 1. How to conquer cancer? How can I prevent cancer by I see? 2. How to conquer cancer? how to treat cancer by I see.

1. **This book discusses how to prevent cancer specific plans, programs, and blueprints in 4/10 pages. It is put forward that how to conquer cancer? how can I prevent cancer?**

It positioned or set up the research goals or "targets" on how to reduce the incidence of cancer.

The current status quo is: the more treatment of cancer patients and the more cancer patients, the incidence rate continues to rise, the mortality rate remains high. The road that has passed in a century is to attention the treatment of cancer with lightly prevention, or only treatment without the prevention. In the cancer prevention work, it has done very little, almost nothing has been done, cancer prevention has not been taken seriously, prevention has not been taken seriously, and the incidence of cancer has been rising.

How to prevent cancer? Where is the target or "target" of cancer prevention? There must be specific cancer prevention targets, clear goals, and operability.

Professor Xu Ze proposed how to prevent cancer. I (1), (2), (3), and (4) propose that it should be analyzed what are the causes or factors that causes cancer to increase the incidence of cancer. The more patients are treated, the more and more of the cancer patients, the incidence rate is rising, and 90% of them are related to the environment. Research and discussion should be conducted on environmental carcinogenic factors (external environment and internal environment).

The cause of cancer is related to the carcinogenic factors of the external environment and the internal environment.

If we have a deeper understanding of the causes of cancer, then in the future we can ask: how to prevent cancer-causing factors, how to monitor which carcinogenic factors, and which to eliminate cancer-causing factors, so that we can stay away from cancer and prevent cancer.

Therefore, Professor Xu Ze proposed that: from the big environment, small environment to prevent cancer, should be from clothing, food, shelter, and anti-cancer.

2. **This book discusses how to treat cancer with 6/10 pages. Positioning the research target or "target" on how to improve the cure rate of cancer, prolong the survival of cancer patients, improve the quality of life, and propose how to treat cancer by I see.**

What we are taking in cancer treatment is a new way of combining Chinese and Western medicine at the molecular level, which is a new way for our laboratory to find immunomodulatory methods and drugs based on the new findings of animal experiments. After years of animal experiment screening and clinical verification, we finally found a new way of immunomodulating and treating cancer by a series of XZ-C$_{1-10}$ immunomodulation anti-cancer Chinese medications series.

- From our laboratory experiments, it was found that the host's thymus was acutely progressively atrophied after being inoculated with cancer cells, and the volume was significantly reduced.

- From the above experimental results, thymus atrophy, immune function is low, may be one of the etiology and pathogenesis of the tumor, therefore, its treatment principles must try to prevent thymus atrophy, promote thymocyte proliferation, increase immune functions.

- In order to prevent thymus atrophy, promote thymocyte proliferation, and increase immune functions, we look for both Chinese medication and western medication. The existing medications of western medications which can improve immune function and promote the proliferation of thymocytes are few or a little so that we went or change to the Chinese medications to find, because traditional Chinese medication with tonic medication has a general immunomodulatory effect.

- After 7 years of laboratory research, we have screened XZ-C$_{1-10}$ immune function control and regulation anti-cancer and anti-metastatic Chinese medications from natural medications to protect Thymus and to increase immune functions and to protect bone marrow hematopoietic function. Clinical validation work was carried out on the basis of the success of animal experiments. After 30 years of more than 12,000 clinical applications of oncology clinics it has achieved the good results.

- After the experimental research and anti-cancer research of Chinese medications immunopharmacology and the combination of Chinese and Western medication at the molecular level, walked out of a new way with XZ-C immune regulation and control combined with Chinese and Western medications at the molecular level, which regulate immune activities, prevent thymic atrophy, promote thymocyte proliferation, protect bone marrow hematopoietic function, improve immune surveillance.

3. **This medical monograph is practical, applied, research-oriented, is the outline of the implementation of how to conquer cancer. This scientific research program, scientific research design, scientific research plan, and blueprint can be used by countries, provinces and states to implement the macro of conquering cancer and to benefit humanity.**

The main project of this medical monograph implementation outline is:

Structural work {
a. Conquer cancer and launch the total attack to cancer, prevention + control + treatment at the same time and the same attention

b. Create a scientific research base for multidisciplinary and cancer- related research - Science City

Two-wing projects:

A wing - how to prevent cancer - to reduce the incidence of cancer
B wing - how to treat cancer - to improve cancer cure rate

Aims:

A: Reduce the incidence of cancer
B: Improve cancer cure rate, prolong patient survival and improve quality of life

If this overall design and the planning blueprint can be implemented and achieved, it is possible or likely to conquer cancer.

4. **The next step of the job is how to implement and how to achieve this overall design and this program and this plan and this blueprint for conquering cancer.**

1. It should set up a team "conquer cancer and launch the general attack; in order to overcome the general attack on cancer, talent is the key, and the first thing which should be done is to set up a research team. The conditions of the research team and academic committee are the really academic and academic achievements and academic results in cancer research, basic research or clinical work, monographs, editors, special issues, international papers, and having the practical clinical experience and the experimental research results which the direction of the research and academic research is to conquer cancer.

Leading and organizing cancer leaders, supporting cancer research, supporting cancer research, supporting scientists, entrepreneurs, leaders, and volunteers who have overcome cancer must have both ability and political integrity, medical skills, and morality first.

2. In order to conquer cancer and launch the general attack to cancer, talent is the key. First, the organization should organize a research team and issue an invitation to form:

1). The Wuhan Anti-Cancer Research Society of conquering cancer and launching the general attack to cancer was established on December 26, 2017.

2). Invite domestic colleagues to participate in the research team to conquer cancer and launch the general attack of cancer

3). Inviting international fellows to participate in the research team to conquer cancer and launch the general attack to cancer.

2. The Invitation letter:

Invitation from the chief designer of the "Science City for the General Attack on Cancer and the Establishment of a Multidisciplinary and Cancer-Related Research Base"
Invite famous experts, professors, academic leaders or leading scientists to support scientists, entrepreneurs, leaders and volunteers who have overcome the general attack on cancer.

Drafting
Within the province: Invitation to the team
Domestic: Invitation to the team
International: Invitation to the team
Invite:

"Overcoming the general attack of cancer and creating a science city for cancer research base" Chinese and Western medicine combined academic leader: Academician Wu Xianzhong (Tianjin)

Academician Tang Wei (Shanghai)
Professor Xu Ze (Wuhan)

Professor Xu Ze (Wuhan) $\Big\{$ Chief designer of "Overcoming the General Attack of Cancer and Creating a Scientific Research Base for Cancer Research - Science City"

Project Leader of "Overcoming the General Attack of Cancer"

CHAPTER 2

Brief Description of the Course of Anti-Cancer Scientific Research

TABLE OF CONTENTS

1. Briefly describe the research process of anti-cancer research

In 1985, I conducted a petition with more than 3,000 patients who underwent radical resection of various extra-thoracic and general surgery. The results showed that most patients relapsed and metastasized about 2-3 years after surgery, and some even metastasized several months after surgery. I realized that the operation was successful and the long-term effect was not satisfactory. Postoperative recurrence and metastasis are the key factors affecting the long-term efficacy of surgery. Therefore, it also raises a question: Studying prevention and treatment of postoperative recurrence and metastasis is the key to improving postoperative survival.

Therefore, clinical basic research must be carried out, and without breakthroughs in basic research, clinical efficacy is difficult to improve. So we established the Institute of Experimental Surgery and spent 15 years conducting a series of experimental research and clinical validation work from the following three aspects:

(1).Exploring pathogenesis, invasion mechanism and mechanism of recurrence and metastasis of cancer, looking for experimental research on effective measures to control invasion, recurrence and metastasis.

My colleagues and I have been conducting experimental tumor research in our laboratory for 4 years. The research topics are all raised from the clinical point of view, trying to explain some clinical problems through experimental research, or solve some clinical problems. Both are clinical basic research.

(2) The experimental research of looking for the new drug for anti-cancer, anti-metastatic, anti-recurrence from natural medicine Chinese herbal medicine. The existing anticancer drugs not only kill cancer cells but also kill normal cells, and have toxic side effects. Our laboratory uses a tumor suppressor test in cancer-bearing mice to find new drugs that inhibit cancer cells without affecting normal cells from natural Chinese herbal medicines. Our laboratory spent three years on the traditional anti-cancer prescriptions and 200 kinds of Chinese herbal medicines commonly used in anti-cancer prescriptions reported in various places for the tumor-inhibiting screening experiment in cancer-bearing animals carried out one by one

RESULTS: 48 kinds of traditional Chinese medicines with good tumor inhibition rate were screened out, and at the same time, there was a good effect of increasing immune function and so on, and the traditional Chinese medicine TG which can inhibit the new microvessels was found out.

(3) Clinical verification work: Through the above four years to explore the basic experimental research on the mechanism of recurrence and metastasis, and after three or three years of experimental research on the screening of natural Chinese herbal medicines. A batch of XZ-C1-10 anti-cancer immune regulation Chinese medication was found. Through the clinical verification of more than 12,000 patients with advanced or postoperative metastatic cancer in 30 years, XZ-C immunomodulation of traditional Chinese medicine has achieved good results, improved quality of life, improved symptoms and significantly prolonged survival.

Recently, I have reviewed, analyzed, reflected, and experienced and the results and findings of my clinical research on clinical practice for more than 60 years, from experiment to clinical, from clinical to experimental, experimental research and clinical verification data. After the summary and collection, three monographs were published:

1. "New understanding and new model of cancer treatment", published by Hubei Science and Technology Press, Xu Ze, January 2001.
2. "New Concepts and New Methods for Cancer Metastais Treatment", Beijing People's Military Medical Press, Xu Ze, January 2006. In April 2007, the General Administration of the People's Republic of China issued the "Three One Hundred" original book certificate.
3. "New Concepts and New Methods for Cancer Treatment", published by Beijing People's Military Medical Press, Xu Ze, October 2011. Later, the American medical doctor Dr. Bin Wu and others translated into English. The English version was published in Washington, DC on March 26, 2013, and is distributed internationally.

2. Four stages of scientific research

1). Our thought and understanding and scientific thinking of Cancer research Journey can be divided into four stages in the past 28 years:

(1) The first stage 1985—1999
- **Identify problems** from follow-up results → ask questions → study questions;
- Review, analyze, reflect, and discover the problems of current cancer traditional therapies, which need further research and improvement;

- Recognize that there are problems, change your mindset, and change your mindset;
- Summarize the materials, collate, collect and publish the first monograph "New Understanding and New Model of Cancer Treatment" published by Hubei Science and Technology Press in January 2001.

(2) The second stage After 2001 -

- Positioning the goals of the study and the "target" of cancer treatment on anti-metastatic, pointing out that the key to cancer treatment is anti-metastasis;
- Conducted a series of anti-cancer metastasis, recurrence experimental research and clinical basis and clinical validation research, and rose to theoretical innovation, and proposed new ideas and methods for anti-metastasis;
- Summarize the materials, collate, collect and publish the second monograph "New Concepts and New Methods for Cancer Metastasis Treatment" published by People's Military Medical Press in January 2006, published by Xinhua Bookstore, and published in the People's Republic of China in April 2007. The "Three One Hundred" Original Book Awards issued by the General Administration.

(3) The third stage After 2006 -

- Study the goals and priorities of the research on the prevention and treatment of the whole process of cancer occurrence and development;
- Closely combined with clinical practice, propose reforms and innovations, research and development in response to the problems and shortcomings of current clinical traditional therapies;
- Recognize that the strategy of cancer prevention and treatment must move forward, the way out for cancer treatment is "three early", and the way out for cancer is prevention;
- I have been engaged in oncology surgery for 60 years. There are more and more patients, the incidence of cancer is rising, and the mortality rate is high. I deeply understand that cancer should not only pay attention to treatment, but also pay attention to prevention, so as to stop at the source. He conducted a series of related research, summary materials, collation, collection and publication of the third monograph "New Concepts and New Methods for Cancer Treatment", published by People's Military Medical Press in October 2011, and published by Xinhua Bookstore. Later, the American medical doctor Dr. Bin Wu and others translated into English. The English version was published in Washington, DC on March 26, 2013.

(4) The fourth stage After 2011 -

- **Now it is the fourth stage of our research work, which is being carried out and carried out, research work, step by step, positioning the research target or "target" to reduce the incidence of cancer, improve the cure rate and prolong the survival period.**

- **Our 28 years of cancer research work: the first three stages of experimental research and clinical research work, mainly in the treatment of new drugs, new methods of diagnosis, new technologies, new concepts and new methods of treatment.**

- However, the second 10 years of cancer in the 21st century is still very rampant. The more patients are treated, the higher the incidence rate and the higher the mortality rate. I am deeply aware that cancer should not only pay attention to treatment, but also pay attention to prevention, in order to stop at the source.

- **The current tumor hospital or oncology hospital model is fully focused on treatment. For the patients in the middle and late stages, the curative effect is poor, the human and financial resources are exhausted, and the incidence rate is not reduced. The more patients are treated and the more and more patients. <u>The status quo is: the road that has passed in a century is to attention treatment with light prevention, or only treatment without prevention. For many years we have only been working on cancer treatment. However, work on cancer prevention has been done very little and almost nothing has been done. As a result, the incidence of cancer continues to rise.</u>**

Looking back, reflecting, and talking about anti-cancer and anti-cancer work, what research or work did we do in anti-cancer for a century? What has been achieved?

Medical school textbook teaching content does not pay attention to cancer prevention knowledge;

The hospital model did not pay attention to the setting up of cancer prevention science;

Medical research projects in medical schools or hospitals have not paid attention to cancer prevention research projects;

The Journal of Oncology Medicine does not pay attention to cancer prevention work papers.

In short, cancer prevention has not been taken seriously, and prevention has not been taken seriously. The prevention of the old-fashioned talks is mainly based on failure to pay attention.

How to do? How to reduce the incidence of cancer? How to improve the cure rate of cancer? How to reduce cancer mortality? How to prolong the survival period? How to improve the quality of life? **It should launched the general attack to conquer cancer with cancer prevention and treatment at the same attention and level and the same time.**

The goal of conquering cancer should be: reduce morbidity, increase cure rate, reduce mortality, prolong survival, improve quality of life, and reduce complications.

- At present, global hospitals and hospitals in China are all devoted to treatment, attention to treatment with light prevention, or only treatment.

XZ-C believes that this mode of hospitalization or cancer treatment is unlikely to overcome cancer and it is impossible to reduce the incidence. Global hospitals and hospitals in China must carry out overall strategic reforms focusing on treatment into focusing on prevention and treatment at the same time and at the same attention and at the same level.

- Therefore, we propose to launch a general attack plan and design to overcome cancer. XZ-C (Xu Ze-China) proposed to launch a general attack, which is to carry out the three-stage work of anti-cancer, cancer control and cancer treatment.

Proposing the "Necessity and Feasibility Report for Overcoming the General Attack of Cancer Attack"

Proposed "XZ-C Scientific Research Plan for Overcoming the General Attack of Cancer"

2) Briefly describe the research process of anti-cancer research

In 1985, I conducted a petition with more than 3,000 patients who underwent radical resection of various extra-thoracic and general surgery. The results showed that most patients relapsed and metastasized about 2-3 years after surgery, and some even metastasized several months after surgery. I realized that the operation was successful, and the long-term efficacy was unsatisfactory. Postoperative recurrence and metastasis were the key factors affecting the long-term efficacy of the operation. Therefore, it also raises a question: Studying prevention and treatment of postoperative recurrence and metastasis is the key to improving postoperative survival. Therefore, clinical basic research must be carried out, and without breakthroughs in basic research, clinical efficacy is difficult to improve. So we established the Institute of Experimental Surgery and spent 15 years conducting a series of experimental research and clinical validation work from the following three aspects:

(1) Exploring the pathogenesis of cancer, the mechanism of invasion and the mechanism of recurrence and metastasis, and looking for experimental research on effective measures to control invasion, recurrence and metastasis.

My colleagues and I have been conducting experimental tumor research in our laboratory for 4 years. The research topics are all raised from the clinical point of view, trying to explain some clinical problems through experimental research, or solve some clinical problems. Both are clinical basic research.

(2) Looking for new anti-cancer, anti-metastatic, anti-recurrence new drug experimental research from natural medicine Chinese herbal medicine.

The existing anticancer drugs not only kill cancer cells but also kill normal cells, and have toxic side effects. Our laboratory uses a tumor suppressor test in cancer-bearing mice to find new drugs that inhibit cancer cells without affecting normal cells from natural Chinese herbal medicines. Our laboratory spent three years on the traditional anti-cancer prescriptions and 200 kinds of Chinese herbal medicines commonly used in anti-cancer prescriptions reported in various places. RESULTS: 48 kinds of traditional Chinese medicines with good tumor inhibition rate were screened out, and at the same time, there was a good effect of lifting and so on, and the traditional Chinese medicine TG which can inhibit the new microvessels was found out.

(3) Clinical verification work: Through the above four years to explore the basic experimental research on the mechanism of recurrence and metastasis, and after three or three years of experimental research on natural medicine herbal extracts, we found a batch of XZ-C1-10 anti-cancer immunity. Regulating traditional Chinese medicine, and then through the clinical verification of more than 12,000 patients with advanced or post-transfer cancer in 20 years, XZ-C immunomodulation of traditional Chinese medicine has achieved good results, improved quality of life, improved symptoms and significantly prolonged survival. period.

Recently, I have reviewed, analyzed, reflected, and experienced the results and findings of my clinical research on clinical practice for more than 60 years, from experiment to clinical, from clinical to experimental, experimental research and clinical verification data. Summary collection, published three monographs: 1, "new understanding and new model of cancer treatment", published by Hubei Science and Technology Press, Xu Ze, January 2001.

2. "New Concepts and New Methods for Cancer Metastasis Treatment", Beijing People's Military Medical Press, Xu Ze, January 2006. In April 2007, the General Administration of the People's Republic of China issued the "Three One Hundred" original book certificate. 3. "New Concepts and New Methods for Cancer Treatment", published by Beijing People's Military Medical Press, Xu Ze, October 2011. Later, the American medical doctor Dr. Bin Wu and others translated into English. The English version was published in Washington, DC on March 26, 2013, and is distributed internationally.

3.) Why do I study cancer? Proposed to launch a general attack and prepare for the "Science City to Conquer Cancer" because:

(1). In 1985, I made a petition to more than 3,000 patients who had undergone chest and abdominal cancer surgery. I found that most patients relapsed or metastasized within 2-3 years after surgery. Therefore, it is necessary to study methods to prevent postoperative recurrence and metastasis in order to improve long-term postoperative efficacy.

2. I suddenly had an acute myocardial infarction in 1991. After the treatment was improved and recovered, it was not advisable to go to the operating table again. It was quiet and I went to the small building to concentrate on scientific research.

3. Through experimental research, it was found that thymus atrophy and immune function are low, which is one of the causes and pathogenesis of cancer, and it is expanded and studied in depth.

4. Through experimental research and clinical verification, after more than 12,000 clinical verification observations in 28 years, I initially found the modernization of traditional Chinese medicine, and at the molecular level, Western medicine combined with innovation, this new way of "Chinese-style anti-cancer" has initially entered a use. The immune regulation of traditional Chinese medicine prevents thymus atrophy, promotes thymic hyperplasia, protects bone marrow hematopoietic function, enhances immune surveillance, and combines Western medicine at the molecular level to overcome the new path of cancer, so it persists and perseveres. Therefore, it is proposed to overcome the general attack of cancer and to build a "science city" to overcome cancer, in an attempt to achieve: reduce

the incidence of cancer; improve the cure rate of cancer; prolong the survival of cancer patients; achieve "three early" (early detection, early diagnosis, early Treatment), can be cured in the early stage. To achieve prevention, control, and treatment. Prevention and treatment can only overcome cancer and reduce the incidence of cancer.

All basic research must be for the clinical, to improve the patient's efficacy and benefit patients. The evaluation criteria for the efficacy of cancer patients should be: prolonged survival, good quality of life, and fewer complications.

I came to Wuhan in 1951 and entered the Central South Tongji Medical College. I graduated from Tongji Medical College in 1956 and was assigned to the Affiliated Hospital of Hubei College of Traditional Chinese Medicine. She was the director of surgery and the director of the Institute of Experimental Surgery of Hubei College of Traditional Chinese Medicine.

In 1991, due to sudden acute myocardial infarction, he was rescued by emergency department and recovered after hospitalization for half a year. Because I can no longer go to the stage for surgery, I calm down to hide in the small building to carry out basic and clinical research on cancer. Because of the good equipment conditions in my experimental surgical laboratory, a large number of experimental studies on the etiology, pathology, pathogenesis, cancer metastasis mechanism of cancer, and experimental screening of anti-cancer Chinese herbal cancer by cancer-bearing animal model mice.

I was 63 years old in 1996 and applied for retirement. After retirement, research will continue, and Science will not stop. I have been living in a small building for 30 years, fighting alone (no one cares after retirement, no one knows in the unit and organization, no one asks, no one supports), single-handedly, self-reliant, from the year of the flower to the age of the ancient, in the year of more than 80 years continued to carry out a series of experimental studies and clinical verification observations. Finally, a series of scientific research achievements and technological innovation series were obtained. The experimental and clinical data, data, conclusions, and conclusions were compiled, and more than 100 scientific research papers were written and published in a new book. He has published 7 series of monographs that focus on cancer research. Three of them are in Chinese and sevens are in English. The English version is published in Washington and distributed worldwide. **The book proposes a series of new concepts and new methods to overcome cancer, puts forward the theory of cancer treatment innovation, proposes the road to overcome cancer, and initially forms the theoretical system of immune regulation and treatment. It is the theoretical basis and experimental basis for cancer** immunotherapy. Clinical application observation and verification, initially out of a new path to overcome cancer. Why is the English version? Because cancer is a disaster for all mankind, the people of the world must work together for it. I will take my 60 years of medical practice, 30 years of scientific research and clinical verification work to overcome cancer research, scientific understanding, experience, experience, lessons, wisdom to contribute to the people, for the benefit of mankind.

I am 86 years old this year. I am the chief designer of the XZ-C research project "conquer cancer and launch the General Attack on Cancer and Building a Science City for Cancer Research." I will use my academic, knowledge, wisdom and strength. Fully participate in the preparation of the "conquering the Cancer Science City" practice, to build a "global demonstration of prevention and treatment of hospitals", prevention and control + treatment, and the establishment of a good laboratory and multidisciplinary and cancer research group.

Change the mode of running a hospital, from attention of treatment with light defense into prevention, control, and treatment at the same level and at the same attention and at the same time; Change the treatment mode from the emphasis on the treatment of severe disease in the middle and later stages into the "three early" (early detection, early diagnosis, early treatment) precancerous lesions, early carcinoma in situ. This will benefit mankind and will open up a new era of anti-cancer research, making China's prevention and treatment of cancer and medical care into the forefront of the world.

4) After 30 years of basic and clinical research on cancer to overcome cancer, we deeply understand that we want to achieve the purpose of cancer prevention and control:

(1). It must launch the general attack. That is to say, the three stages of cancer prevention, cancer control and cancer treatment at the same time and at the same attention, the three carriages, go hand in hand, in order to reduce the incidence of cancer, improve cancer cure rate, reduce cancer mortality, and prolong the survival of cancer patients. If you only treatment without prevention, or you attention to treatment with light prevention, you can never overcome cancer because it can't reduce the incidence, and the more patients be treated, the more and more patients come.

How to launch a general attack, implement cancer prevention + cancer control + cancer treatment? It is necessary to establish a hospital with the cancer prevention and control and treatment during the whole process of cancer occurrence, and change the current hospitalization mode with only treatment and no prevention; Change the current treatment model for advanced cancer.

(2). It must be led by the government, experts and scholars work hard, the masses participation, and thousands of households can participate in it. At present, China is building an innovative country. It is the government-led, mass participation, national mobilization, and the work of thousands of households. This is great timing, if it can carry out medical scientific research on conquering cancer, cancer prevention and cancer control, it will definitely improve the awareness of cancer prevention among the whole people, and achieve the cancer prevention and cancer-control effects. It will reach the effects of significantly reducing the incidence of cancer in China, our province and our city.

(3). Why do you want to launch a general attack? Because the status quo is:

a. The current mode of running a hospital is to heavy treatment with light prevention, or only treatment without prevention; the more treatment, the more the patients.
b. The current treatment mode is mainly in the middle, late stage and late metastasis of cancer, and the curative effect is very poor.
c. The current radiotherapy and chemotherapy cannot be cured, and can only be alleviated. The slow-release period can still progress in 4 weeks, and the curative effect is very poor. There are still problems and drawbacks.

It is necessary to emphasize early diagnosis, early treatment, early rehabilitation, and insist on prevention as the main parts:

a. Change the mode of running or building hospital into for prevention, control, and treatment at the same attention.
b. change the treatment mode into "three early", precancerous lesions.
c. The way out for cancer is on cancer prevention and on scientific research and research on cancer prevention.

5) I have been conducting experimental basic research and clinical validation for the purpose of conquering cancer for 30 years, all in laboratories and hospitals. Why do you want to apply for government support now?

Because 90% of cancers are related to the environment, the occurrence of cancer is closely related to people's clothing, food, housing, travel and living habits. Therefore, I deeply think that cancer prevention and cancer control work cannot be done only by medical personnel, experts and scholars, but it must rely on the government's major policy. The current serious environmental pollution and the ecosystem degradation may be closely related to the rise in cancer incidence.

The treatment of cancer depends on medical personnel and researchers to study new drugs and new treatment techniques.

Cancer prevention and control, how to reduce the incidence of cancer, cancer prevention work only can be carried out through relying on the government's major policy, relying on government leadership and leadership, experts, scholars and efforts, and the masses participation.

3. The New findings in the experimental research

1. Our laboratory removes Thymus (TH) from mice (30) to produce a model of cancer-bearing animals. Injection of immunosuppressive drugs can also help establish animal models of cancer. The conclusion of the study proves that the occurrence and development of cancer have obvious relationship with the thymus and its function of the host immune organs.

2. whether it is immune first low and then easy to get cancer, or get cancer first and then low immunity, the experimental results are: first immunological low and then the occurrence and development of cancer, if no immune function decline, it is not easy to vaccinate successfully. The results of this experiment suggest that improving and maintaining good immune function is one of the important measures to prevent cancer.

3. When we studied the relationship between cancer metastasis and immunity, we established 60 animal models of liver metastases, and divided them into groups A and B with immunosuppressive drugs in group A, and group B did not. RESULTS: The number of intrahepatic metastases in group A was significantly higher than that in group B. The results of this experiment suggest: Metastasis is associated with immunity, low immune function or the use of immunosuppressive drugs may promote tumor metastasis.

4. When we explored the effect of tumor on the immune organs of the body, we found that with the progress of cancer, the thymus is progressively atrophied (600 mice bearing cancer model mice), and the host thymus is acute after inoculation of cancer cells. Progressive atrophy.

5. through experiments also found: some experimental mice did not vaccinate successfully, or the tumor grows very small, the thymus does not significantly shrink.

   In order to understand the relationship between tumor and thymus atrophy, we removed a group of experimental mice when the transplanted solid tumor grew to the size of the thumb. After 1 month, the thymus was found to have no progressive atrophy. Therefore, we speculate that a solid tumor may produce a factor that is not known to inhibit the thymus, which needs further study.

6. The above experimental results prove that the progression of the tumor can cause progressive atrophy of the thymus. Then, can we adopt some methods to prevent the atrophy of the host thymus? Therefore, we further design and want to find the stopping tumor mouse thymus atrophy or drug through animal experiments. Therefore, we used this immune organ cell transplantation to restore the experimental function of the immune organ.

While we were doing the experiments of investigating the atrophy of the thymus gland during suppressing tumor progression and looking for ways to restore the function of the thymus and reconstituting the immune system, the mice were transplanted with fetal liver, fetal spleen and fetal thymus cells, and the immune function of the immune system was re-established.

The Results: S, T, L three groups of cells (200 rats), the recent-term complete tumor regression rate was 40%, the long-term tumor complete regression rate was 46.67% and the tumor completely disappeared and received the long-term survival.

4. The experimental screening:

Our laboratory conducted the following experimental studies to screen new anticancer and anti-metastatic drugs from traditional Chinese medicine:

1). In vitro screening test: In vitro culture of cancer cells was used to observe direct damage of cancer cells to cancer cells. In the test tube for culturing cancer cells, the crude drug product (500 ug/ml) was separately placed to observe whether it inhibited the cancer cells and inhibited the tumor rate.

2), in vivo anti-tumor screening test: the production of cancer-bearing animal models, the Chinese herbal medicine on the cancer screening rate of cancer-bearing animals in the experimental screening study, each batch of experiments with 240 mice, divided into 8 experimental groups, 30 per group, the first Group 7 was a blank control group, and group 8 was treated with 5-Fu or CTX as a control group. The whole group of mice were inoculated with EAC or S_{180} or H_{22} cancer cells. After inoculation for 24 hours, each rat was orally fed with crude drug powder, and the traditional Chinese medicine was screened for a long time. The survival time was observed and the tumor inhibition rate was calculated.

In this way, we conducted a four-year experimental study. More than 1,000 tumor-bearing animal models were used each year. A total of nearly 6,000 tumor-bearing animal models were made in 4 years. Each rat died after liver, spleen, lung, and thymus. The pathological anatomy of the kidney was performed in more than 20,000 sections.

3). Experimental results: Among the 200 kinds of Chinese herbal medicines screened by animal experiments in our laboratory, 48 kinds of positive and even excellent inhibitory effects on cancer cells were screened, and the tumor inhibition rate was above 75-90%. In this group, 152 species were eliminated from animal experiments and had no obvious anticancer effect.

5. Clinical verification:

1) The detail of methods
It was based on the success of animal experiments and clinical validation

(1).Method:

Establishing a combination of oncology clinic and integrated Chinese and Western medicine for anti-cancer, anti-metastasis and recurrence research, retain the outpatient medical record, establish a perfect follow-up observation system, observe the long-term efficacy, from experimental research to clinical verification, in the clinical verification process. Discover new problems and return to the laboratory for basic research, and then apply new experimental results to the clinic. Thus, the experiment - clinical - re-experiment - re-clinical. Experimental studies must be clinically validated and observed in a large number of patients for 3-5 years or even 8-10 years, according to evidence-based medicine, with long-term follow-up and evaluable data.

The standard of efficacy is: good quality of life and long survival.

RESULTS: XZ-C immunomodulatory anticancer traditional Chinese medicine preparations have achieved remarkable effects after being used in a large number of patients with advanced cancer.

(2). Clinical data:

Chinese and Western medicine combined with anti-cancer research collaboration group and Shuguang oncology clinic, XZ-C immunomodulation of anti-cancer Chinese medicine combined with Western medicine for treatment of stage III, IV or metastatic and recurrent cancer 4698 cases, including 3,051 males and females 1647 cases, the youngest 11 years old, the largest 86 years old, all patients were diagnosed by pathological section or CT, MRI, B-ultrasound imaging, according to the International Anti-Cancer Alliance staging criteria, all cases were intermediate stage III or higher patients, Among them, there were 1021 cases of liver cancer, 752 cases of lung cancer, 694 cases of gastric cancer, 624 cases of esophagus and cardia cancer, 328 cases of rectal cancer, 442 cases of colon cancer, 368 cases of breast cancer, 74 cases of pancreatic cancer, 30 cases of cholangiocarcinoma and 43 cases of retroperitoneal tumor. 38 cases of ovarian cancer, 9 cases of cervical cancer, 11 cases of brain tumor, 34 cases of thyroid cancer, 38 cases of nasopharyngeal carcinoma, 9 cases of melanoma, 27 cases of renal cell carcinoma, 48 cases of bladder cancer, 13 cases of leukemia, 47 cases of supraclavicular transfer For example, 35 cases of various sarcomas and 39 cases of other malignant tumors.

(3). The drugs and methods of administration:

The treatment is to protect the chest from lifting, protect the marrow from blood, thereby improving the host's immune surveillance, control the immune escape of cancer cells, from the perspective of Chinese medicine is to correct the evil, soft and loose, blood Double supplement, the drugs are XZ-C1, XZ-C2, XZ-C3, XZ-C4, XZ-C5, XZ-C6, XZ-C7, XZ-C8, ... XZ-C10, depending on the cancer, condition, The situation of the transfer, according to the condition of dialectic, the use of the above drugs. Solid tumors or metastatic masses are all taken internally for anti-cancer powder and topical anti-cancer swelling cream. For pain, external application of anti-cancer painkiller cream, astragalus and ascites plus anti-cancer soup or water-removing soup.

(4). The treatment results:

Improved symptoms, improved quality of life, prolonged survival.

(1) Among the 4277 patients with advanced cancer who have been treated with XZ-C1-10 immunomodulation for more than 3 months, the medical records have detailed observation records, see the table below.

Observation of curative effect on 4 277 patients: fully improving the quality of life of the carcinoma patients in medium and advanced stage

Improvement	Vigor	Appetite	Reinforcement of physical force	Improvement in generalized case	Increase of body weight	Improvement of sleep	The restriction of improvement activity and capability released activity	self servicing normal walking	Resumption of work Engaged in light work
No. of cases (%)	4071	3986	2450	479	2938	1005	1038	3220	479
	95.2	93.2	57.3	11.2	68.7	23.5	24.3	75.3	11.2

This group is a middle-late stage patient, with varying degrees of symptom improvement after taking the drug, the effective rate is 93.2%. In terms of improving the quality of life (according to the Kasper's scoring standard), the average score was 50 points before the drug administration, and after the drug was increased to an average of 80 points. The patients in this group had metastasis and dysfunction of different tissues and organs in the third stage or above. For the kinds of the patients, it was reported that the median survival time is about 6 months. The maximum length of this group of patients has reached **18 years(while we gathered this data, the patient was still alive),** and the average survival time of the remaining cases is more than 1 year. 1 case of primary hepatic lobe of hepatic lobe, recurrence of right liver after resection, only treatment with XZ-C for 18 years; another case of XZ-C for 10 and a half years; 2 cases of hepatocellular carcinoma with multiple liver cancer, after taking XZ-C medicine for half a year, after 2 CT examinations, the cancer lesion completely subsided and it has been stable for half a year. One case of double renal cell carcinoma, extensively transferred to the abdominal cavity after one side resection, was completely restored to work after taking XZ-C medicine. 3 cases of lung cancer open chest exploration cannot be cut, long-term use of XZ-C medicine has been 3 and a half years. Two cases of residual gastric cancer were treated with XZ-C for 8 years. Three cases of rectal cancer had been treated with XZ-C for 3 years. 1 case of breast cancer metastasis of liver and ribs has been taken for 8 years. One female patient had a walnut-sized lymph node mass in both the groin and the neck. The pathological diagnosis was non-Hodgkin's lymphoma. Due to economic difficulties, chemotherapy could not be performed, the patient has been long-term taking XZ-Cl+XZ-C4+XZ-C2 for 4 years and comes to our outpatient clinic every month to refill the medications, which the patient's general condition is good. One case of recurrent bladder cancer after renal cell carcinoma, XZ-C drug has been used for 9 and a half years. The above cases are all of the cancer patient cases who can not have surgery, can not do radiotherapy, chemotherapy, and the advanced patients, and the patients only take XZ-C drugs with no other drug treatment. So far, the patients still come to the clinic every month to follow-up and to review and to refill medications. After long-term medication, the condition is controlled in a stable state, so that the body and the tumor remain in a balanced state for a long time, and obtain the better survival life living with tumors, the patient's condition is improved, the quality of life is improved, and the survival period is prolonged.

(2) For 84 patients with solid tumors and 56 patients with metastatic supraclavicular lymphadenopathy, XZ-C series and external XZ-C3 anti-cancer light firming cream were obtained by internal administration, and the results were as follows.

Changes of 84 cases of solid tumors and 56 cases of metastatic nodules after XZ-C cream externally

	Solid tumor				Enlargement of upper lymph node of metastatic compact bone			
	Disappearance	Shrinkage 1/2	Softening	No change	Disappearance	Shrinkage 1/2	Softening	No change
No. of cases (%)	12	28	32	12	12	22	14	8
	14.2	33.3	38.0	14.2	21.4	39.2	25.0	14.2
Total effective rate (%)	85.7				85.7			

298 patients with cancer pain were treated with XZ-C orally, and XZ-C anti-cancer analgesic cream was applied to achieve significant analgesic effect. See the table below.

Analgesic condition after oral administration of XZ-C and external XZ-C anti-cancer analgesic cream in 298 patients

Clinical Symptoms	Pain			
	Light alleviation	Obvious alleviation	Disappearance	Avoidance
No of cases	52	139	93	14
(%)	17.3	46.8	31.2	4.7
Total effective rate (%)		95.3		

2).The summary of clinical validation

XZ-C immunomodulation Chinese medications are applied to clinical research on the basis of experimental research or based on the success of animal experiments and clinical validation:

so it can be applied to clinic to verify its curative effects.

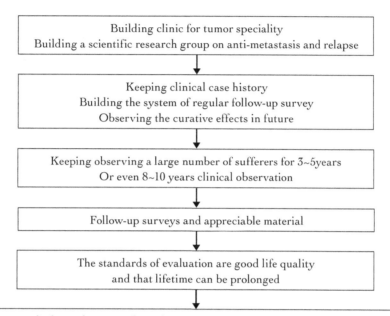

Building clinic for tumor speciality
Building a scientific research group on anti-metastasis and relapse

↓

Keeping clinical case history
Building the system of regular follow-up survey
Observing the curative effects in future

↓

Keeping observing a large number of sufferers for 3~5years
Or even 8~10 years clinical observation

↓

Follow-up surveys and appreciable material

↓

The standards of evaluation are good life quality
and that lifetime can be prolonged

↓

After having been applied to a large number of cancer sufferers of intermediate and advanced stages for 12 years, it has achieved significant curative effects. XZ-C immunological regulation and control can be used to kill cancer cells on the way of metastasis and improve immune surveillance, which opens up the third area of anti-cancerometastasis treatment

↓

It can improve the life quality of the sufferers with intermediate and advanced stages and strengthen immunity. It can also improve the ability to regulate and control and the ability to resist cancer. By increasing appetite and physical strengthen, it can protect marrow and reinforce hematopiesis.

↓

For those who have taken this medicine for a long period, the rates of postoperative relapse and metastasis is very low. For those who have suffered relapse and metastasis, most of them can keep stable with no further metastasis. For those who experienced several organ transplantations, it can help them stabilize the state of an illness, control metastasis and prolong lifetime.

A. Clinical information

From 1994 to Nov. 2002, XZ-C traditional Chinese medicine has been used in 4698 cases of III stage, IV stage, relapse and metastasis, in which 3051 cases are male and 1647 cases are female with the oldest being 86 years old and the youngest being 11 years old. All these have been above III stage according to TNM of International Union against Cancer by histopathology diagnosis or type-B ultrasonic, CT or MRI.

B. **Curative effects**

Symptoms can be alleviated and life quality has been improved and lifetime has been prolonged. Among those 4277 cases of these middle and later stages of the cancer patients who have taken XZ-C traditional Chinese medicine for more than three months, all of these cancer patients with advanced cancer have had improvement of symptoms in different degree. The effective rate has researched 93.2% with general information in table A, the improvement of life quality is seen in table B as the followings:

Table A Overall Health information about 4277 cases of relapse and metastasis

		Liver cancer	Lung cancer	Gastric cancer	Cardia Cancer	Rectal and anal cancer	Colon cancer	Breast cancer	Cancer of pancreas
Cases		1021	752	668	624	328	442	368	74
Male: Female		4:1	4.4:1	2.25:1	3.1:1	1:1	2.1:1	All female	3.2:1
Focus	primary	694(68.8%)	699(93.9%)	-	-	-	-	-	-
	metastatic	327(31.2%)	53(6.1%)	-	-	-	-	-	-
General parts of metastasis		from lung (2%) from gorge (27.2%)	lymph nodes metastasis in clavicle (11.6%)	from liver (23.8%) from lung (3%)	from clavicle (13.1%)	rate of relapse (14.8%)	from liver (16.0%)	lymph nodes metastasis in clavicle (17.5%)	from liver (11.7%)
		from cardia (19.5%) from recta (31.2%)	from brain (3.1%) from marrow (4.6%)	from peritoneum(29.1%) from clavicle (6.1%)	from liver (8.3%)	from liver (7.0%)	from peritoneum (6.0%)	lymph nodes metastasis in armpit (15.0%) from bone (5.0%)	behind peritoneum (39.1%)
Age (year)	popular (%)	30-39 (76.2)	50-69 (71.6)	40-49 (73.4)	40-69 (80.4)	40-49 (75.2)	30-69 (88.0)	40-59 (65.9)	40-59 (70.0)
	youngest	11	20	17	30	27	27	29	34
	oldest	86	80	77	77	78	76	80	68

Table B the life qualities of the sufferers with advanced cancer among the 4277 cases with comprehensive improvement in observation of curative effects

	Spirit	Appetite	Physical strengthen	Improvement of general situation	Gain in weight	Improvement of sleep	Improvement of mobility and alleviation of movement restriction	Living by oneself and ambulating normally	Recovery of the ability to do light muscular work
Cases with improvement	4071	3986	2450	479	2938	1005	1038	3220	479
Percentage (%)	95.2	93.2	57.3	11.2	68.7	23.5	24.3	75.3	11.2

6. Assessment of social benefits:

Cancer is a common disease that threatens human life, and it is the first and second cause of death among urban residents in China. It goes without saying that cancer is still one of the medical problems. At the beginning of the 21st century, the most important problem in cancer treatment is the shift. The most urgent problem to be solved is how to resist metastasis, but the transfer is only a phenomenon, an understanding, and a target. Invisible, intangible, how to be specific, how to clearly understand the specific process, steps and mechanisms of cancer cell transfer, we propose anti-cancer transfer as the target of the goal, in order to achieve this goal, the goal of anti-metastasis, measures must be specific, otherwise The purpose of the anti-transfer can not be achieved. The contents of this book propose 14 new discoveries, new theories, new concepts, and the process of cancer metastasis. The countermeasures are embodied: for example, the current cancer research is proposed in this book. Where? Anti-metastasis, found and proposed cancer in human form in three forms, this third form is the cancer cells on the way to transfer: this new understanding, the new doctrine initiative will cause the chain reaction The reform and update of the series of treatments, found that the goal of cancer treatment should be directed to these three forms: discover and propose a two-point line theory of the whole process of cancer development, that cancer treatment should not only pay attention to two points, but also pay attention to cut off the front line; The specific measures against metastasis should be to carry out the tracking and interception of cancer cells on the way of transfer; discover and advocate new concepts and new models of cancer treatment - should be carried out A new mode of immunochemotherapy; discovering and proposing a new model of cancer metastasis treatment, and proposing a "three-step" of anti-cancer metastasis treatment. Some of the above new understandings, new theoretical insights, new concepts, important academic significance and important academic value, The development of oncology medical science will have an important impact, which may benefit the patients with millions of cancer metastases and embark on a new path to overcome cancer. How to find measures to prevent cancer cell metastasis, and how to explore it, in the research of anti-cancer, Chinese medicine is China's advantage, develop the role of this advantage in anti-metastasis research, give play to China's advantages, and catch up with the international advanced level - In this book, Zc immunomodulation anti-cancer anti-metastatic Chinese medicine, after 3 years of experimental screening of tumor-inhibiting rate in cancer-bearing animal models, and 30 years of clinical verification application, not only for the benefit of millions of cancer metastasis patients, but also for the country to obtain Billions of economic benefits.

C H A P T E R   3

Carrying out the report "Conquer cancer and Launch the total attack to cancer — Prevention and Control and Treatment at the same attention"

The Main Topics and Concepts of the Report

1. Reform the current mode of setting up the hospitalization
2. Reform the current treatment model of focusing on the middle and late stages of treatment into "three early : early detect, early treatment
3. Change only treatment without prevention into prevention, control, and treatment at the same attention
4. It is necessary to establish a hospital with prevention and control and treatment according to the whole process of cancer occurrence and development.
5. The way out for cancer treatment is "three early", the effect of the early cancer treatment is good and cancer can be cured

TABLE OF CONTENTS

1. What is the report of carrying out the report of "conquer cancer and launch the total attack to cancer — pay the equal attention to the prevention and control and treatment"

1. Carry out the project:

"To conquer cancer and launch the total attack to cancer—pay the **equal attention** to **cancer prevention** and **cancer control** and **cancer treatment**"

2.The project name:

"Conquer cancer and launch the total attack to cancer and to build a science city to overcome cancer"

3. Significance of the project:

Why did I propose to launch a general attack? As the current incidence of cancer in China has increased and the mortality rate remains high, the current status quo is:

(1) The current situation of cancer incidence: **The more patients are treated, the more cancer patients.** 8550 new cancer patients are born every day in China, and 6 people diagnosed with cancer every minute in the country.

(2) The status of cancer mortality: stay high and does not decrease, and stay the first cause of death in urban and rural areas in China, an average of 7,500 people die of cancer every day.

(3) The status quo of treatment: Although the application of traditional three major treatments has been nearly a hundred years, thousands of cancer patients have been exposed to radiotherapy and chemotherapy, **but what is the result? Cancer is still the leading cause of death so far.**

(4) The current status of the current tumor hospital or oncology hospital model: pay attention to treatment with little prevention or treatment alone without prevention, **the more treatment and the more cancer patients.**

Therefore, the significance of the project is **to change the above status quo**, and must turn only focusing on treatment into prevention and treatment at the same attention level.

<u>4: The goal of the project or the goal of the total attack:</u>

Reduce the incidence of cancer, reduce cancer mortality, improve cancer cure rate, and prolong survival.

<u>5. Project content:</u>

(1) "conquer cancer and launch the total attack to cancer"

1) What is called as "conquer cancer and launch the total attack on cancer?

The total attack is to prevent cancer, cancer control, and to treat cancer at the same attention level and the same attention and the same time.

The general attack is to carry out the three-stage work of cancer prevention, cancer control and cancer treatment in the whole process of cancer occurrence and development, and carry out simultaneously. Cancer prevention and cancer control and cancer treatment are the same important.

What is called as cancer prevention and cancer control and cancer treatment? Namely:

<u>cancer prevention</u> - before cancer formation

<u>Cancer control</u> - precancerous lesions with malignant tendencies

<u>Treating cancer</u> - has formed a cancerous foci or metastasis

2). What is called as "conquer cancer and launch the total attack to cancer?

a. **Conquer cancer and launch the general attack is that cancer prevention + cancer control + cancer treatment, three-stage work, simultaneous moving forward**, three carriages, go hand in hand, drive together, change the current hospital mode, change the current treatment mode.

<u>Namely:</u> change the current mode of hospitalization with a focus on treatment, and change the current treatment mode focusing on the treatment for the patients in the middle and late stages.

Change the only cancer treatment into putting the cancer prevention, cancer control, and cancer treatment at the same attention level.

b. **How to implement this new mode of running a hospital?**

It is necessary to establish a hospital for prevention, control and treatment according to the whole process of cancer occurrence and development.

Content:

A. To Establish cancer prevention department, cancer control department, "three early outpatient clinic", "three early ward" (three early: early detection, early diagnosis, early treatment), and precancerous lesions outpatient and ward...

B. To Establish multidisciplinary research groups (immunity, virus, endocrine, fungi...) and laboratories, and create the **"Three Early" research laboratory**:

——Research "three early" treatment, new reagents, new technologies, new methods, new drug;

——Research on effective measures for treating, preventing and reversing precancerous lesions, and setting up a cancer transfer research laboratory;

——Research on anti-metastatic, recurrent intravascular "target" organ treatment research laboratory, cancer prevention research laboratory

——**Set up anti-cancer, anti-metastasis research laboratory at the Molecular level and the combination of Chinese and Western medications.**

The way out of treatment of cancer is in the "three early " - in this way, most patients can be stopped in the "three early", the early stage of precancerous lesions will be cured, and it will not be allowed to develop into the middle and late stages. It is reducing the incidence rate.

The way out for cancer treatment is "three early" (early detection, early diagnosis, early treatment), the effect of early cancer treatment is good, can be cured, **especially precancerous lesions, while well treated, can be completely cured**.

How to implement it? As shown in the figure, to build an innovative molecular tumor full process with cancer prevention + control + treatment hospital.

1	
2	
3	

4	
5	
6	

Rent two buildings on the 6th floor(first rent and build) for early development

then choose a new hospital, there must be enough parking spaces.

(first rent and then build) to start 500-1000 beds early

(The hospital itself has income, self-accumulation, diligently building hospitality)

First floor clinic for high risk population group inspection

Second floor clinic for renting for three years, pay one year's rent each year

Third floor, three mornings

Fourth floor, three mornings

Fifth floor, early morning, precancerous lesions. Figure 1 and Figure 2

Sixth floor office, school group, research room, laboratory

(2) "Building a science city to overcome cancer"

We have proposed a "science city" as the following basic design, planning, blueprints, and the establishment to overcome cancer.

Figure:

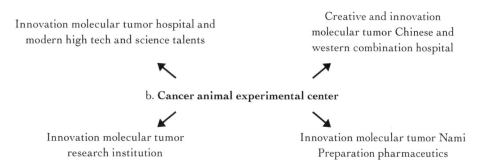

Figure. The medical education research and development science city or science base

1 How to overcome cancer? The Cancer Animal Experimental Center must be established.

If you want to overcome cancer → conquer cancer → overcome cancer, you must first understand the understanding of cancer: the etiology, pathogenesis, pathophysiology, immunopharmacology, immunopathology, cancer cell biological behavior of cancer? Transfer mechanism? Why is implant? Pathogenesis?

A series of oncology and tumor-related problems have not been clearly understood. Oncology is still a scientific virgin for scientific research, and it needs a lot of basic science and clinical basic research. Carrying out basic research in cancer science is an urgent need of the current oncology discipline.

Therefore, it is necessary to establish a cancer animal laboratory with good experimental equipment and establish a cancer experimental research center.

2 How to overcome cancer? It must establish the medical school of Innovative Molecular Oncology.

Talents must have multidisciplinary knowledge such as Chinese medicine, western medicine, pharmacy, life sciences, molecular biology, genetic engineering, environmental science, medical multidisciplinary knowledge, immunology, virology, endocrinology, mycology, immunopharmacology, etc, can participate in the relevant talents to overcome cancer and to launch the general attack on cancer.

Nowadays, the current status of oncology talents are mainly professionals such as radiotherapy and chemotherapy.

To overcome cancer, talent is the key. How to train talent is the key. Researching cancer requires multidisciplinary knowledge and technology. It

must be truly practical, have theory, have technology, must have both ability and political integrity, medicine is benevolence, ethics first.

3 How to overcome cancer? The Institute of Innovative Molecular Oncology must be established

Oncology research is the most complex, difficult, esoteric, and difficult subject in medical research. It involves multidisciplinary knowledge and theory, including pathology, cytology, immunology, virology, endocrinology, medical genetics, Immunopharmacology, molecular oncology, study the pathogenesis of tumors at the molecular level, understand the causes of diseases, and provide preventive and therapeutic measures for cancer prevention and treatment.

Establish anti-cancer research, anti-cancer theoretical knowledge, technology, drugs, methods to study anti-cancer measures, from **clothing, food, housing, anti-cancer, from the big environment and small environment to prevent cancer, from living habits, life hobbies to prevent cancer. The following specialist groups closely related to cancer should be established to specialize in molecular level and clinical research to find theoretical knowledge, techniques, drugs, methods and measures related to cancer prevention and cancer prevention.**

(1) Immunization and cancer research groups and laboratories - **there is a positive relationship between immunity and cancer**, and theories, techniques, drugs, and methods for prevention and treatment should be sought from this;

(2) **Virus and** cancer research groups and laboratories - **some cancers and viruses have a positive relationship,** and should look for theories, techniques, drugs, and methods of prevention and treatment;

(3) Endocrine hormones and cancer research groups and laboratories, some cancers **and hormones** have a positive relationship, should look for the theory, technology, drugs, methods of prevention and treatment;

(4) Mycotoxin and cancer research groups and laboratories - **some cancers and fungi have a positive relationship**, should look for the theory, technology, drugs, methods of prevention and treatment;

(5) Environmental and Cancer Research Groups and Laboratories - **90% of cancers are related to the environmen**t. It is necessary to increase and strengthen the macroscopic, microscopic and ultra-microscopic anti-cancer research of the environment and cancer, and establish a good laboratory;

(6) Chinese medicine and cancer research groups and laboratories - **should strengthen the traditional Chinese medicine immunopharmacology, active ingredient analysis, molecular structure, immune regulation, molecular level of immune mechanism experimental research, gene level experimental research, establish a good equipment experiment Room, Chinese medicine is the key research of immune regulation treatment.**

It starts to build the above groups → research institutes → joint research institute and it develops while it sets up.

4. How to overcome cancer? It must establish the "Cell Cancer, Development and Prevention of the Hospital" and "Innovative Molecular Tumors in Combination with Western Medicine and Prevention and Treatment Hospital"

How can we reduce the incidence of cancer? How can we improve the cure rate of cancer?

It is necessary to carry out prevention, control, and treatment, and change the mode of running a hospital.

So how to prevent it? How to control? How to cure?

How to improve the cure rate?

——The way out for cancer treatment is "three early"

How to reduce the incidence rate?

——The way out of fighting cancer is prevention

In summary, we propose that the basic design of the Science City to build a general attack on cancer is:

(1) Establishing the School of Innovative Molecular Oncology and Graduate Schools - Training Advanced Tumor Subjects for the Country

(2) Establishing an innovative molecular tumor in the combination of Chinese and Western prevention and treatment hospitals

(3) Establishing the Institute of Innovative Molecular Oncology and the Institute of Cancer Prevention and carrying out anti-cancer system engineering

(4) Establishing a cancer animal experiment center

(5) Establishing an innovative molecular tumor nano-preparation pharmaceutical factory

5 What is the area required for the construction of the Science City to overcome the cancer attack? How much is it?

☐

☐

☐

It is planned to rent first and then build. According to the current international scientific research situation, the situation is compelling, and it must start in the morning. Rent two buildings on the 6th floor and start work early. First, establish a defense, control, and treatment hospital. At the same time, establish a cancer research group → research institute → research institute in the hospital. The oncology medical school can start a class first.

(The hospital itself has income, self-accumulation, diligent entrepreneurship, diligent hospitality)

6. How to achieve this unprecedented event in human history?

Do a big thing, do an unprecedented event, for the benefit of mankind, cancer is a disaster for all mankind, we must fight with the world, and the people of the world work together.

(1) Report to the government, to the provinces and cities, and request instructions:

It is planned to be established in Wuhan: "The first science city in the country to overcome cancer" and "The world's first science city to overcome cancer".
Site selection: planned to be in the university town of Huangjiahu
Abbreviation: "Huangjiahu Science City" Cancer Medical Research Center
It requires leadership support because Conquering the general attack of cancer is an unprecedented work of mankind. It is necessary to personally create experience and must practice it personally. This is a new cement road. Every step will leave an eternal scientific research footprint.
Conquering cancer and launching a general attack is an unprecedented event

in human history. It is the forefront of science and can revitalize China and benefit mankind.

Human beings should move forward to overcome the difficulty of cancer. Technically, curing cancer is even harder than going to the moon. Based on these new scientific discoveries, we should put the general attack on cancer on the agenda, work hard, and start.

How to overcome cancer? We believe that a pilot should be set up in the University City (Huangjiahu) to change the current mode of hospitalization, change the current treatment model, launch a general attack and create a science city to overcome cancer. This is the only way to overcome cancer.

How to implement this plan to overcome cancer?

I have elaborated the overall design, master plan, specific plans, talents of the team, etc. Planning, blueprint; put forward the general design, blueprint, and the "Science City for the Attack of Cancer Attack"; t he overall design and preparation work of Science City. Now I AApply to establish a test area for the cancer research team (station) in Hubei and Wuhan

Now it is designed as the followings:

1. Conquer the Cancer Academic Committee
2. Science City (conquering the medical, teaching, research, and science cities that attacked the cancer attack) to prepare a working group.

It applys and suggests the provincial government and the Wuhan municipal government to Established in Wuhan: "The first science city in the country to overcome the general attack on cancer", namely: "The world's first science city to overcome the general attack of cancer"

It Requests leadership support:

1)It needs leadership support (policy support, agree to prepare)

Because "to overcome the general attack of cancer and to build a science city to overcome cancer" is an unprecedented work of mankind. It must be supported by the leaders and agree to prepare for construction.

Don't approve the funds, don't approve the land, because the Science City has established the "Danger Prevention and Treatment Hospital for Cancer Development and Development". The hospital itself has income and can self-accumulate and raise itself. Only hope to get leadership support, agree to prepare for construction, in order to organize a meeting, in order to formally carry out the work of establishing a science city to overcome the general attack of cancer, and to prepare for the construction according to the general design and blueprint of "Collecting the Cancer Attack General Science City". Work hard, start off, no matter how far the road to conquer cancer, you should start.

<u>2) Conquering cancer and launching the general attack is an unprecedented event. It is the frontier of science and can revitalize China and benefit mankind.</u>

President Xi Jinping said that people's longing for a better life is the goal of our struggle. The disaster of cancer covers the whole world, the people of the whole country, and the urgent hope of the people all over the world will one day overcome cancer. I hope that the state, government, experts, scholars and scientists can find out the anti-cancer measures. Keep away from cancer.

I read the "Government Work Report" mentioned in the article... Strengthening the research on smog control, promoting the prevention and treatment of major diseases such as cancer, making science and technology better for the benefit of the people, and resolutely fighting the three major battles. We must implement the requirements of the "Government Work Report", strengthen research on smog governance, promote research on prevention and treatment of major cancer diseases, and make science and technology better for the benefit of the people. Resolutely fight well to win the anti-pollution and pollution control battles to achieve the purpose and effect of anti-cancer and anti-cancer research.

After 30 years of basic and clinical research in cancer research to overcome cancer, we have achieved a series of scientific research and technology innovation series to propose how to overcome cancer? How to prevent cancer? And how to overcome cancer? How to treat a series of general designs, plans, plans, blueprints, and proposed and developed the Dawning C-type plan and the Dawning A, B, and D anti-cancer plans, and published a series of monographs.

Under the guidance of Xi Jinping's new era of socialism with Chinese characteristics, I will dedicate my scientific research ideas and scientific thinking. For 30 years, I have contributed to the scientific wisdom of cancer research, and contributed to my motherland, our province, and the people of our city. Although I am a 86-year-old white-haired man, I am still motivating me to make great efforts to overcome the scientific research work of cancer in this new era of scientific spring. I hope to report to the provincial and municipal leaders in detail, and please Leadership, guidance, and support.

Dr. Xu Ze is : 1.The chief designer of "To overcome the general attack on cancer and to create a science city to overcome cancer";2.Project leader of the project "Collecting the general attack on cancer"3.Honorary President of Wuhan Anticancer Research Association

<u>"Conquer Cancer Science City" to establish the following genetic testing research groups:</u>

(1) Establish genetic testing and cancer research groups and laboratories

(2) Establish HPV anti-cancer research group and laboratory

(3) Establish genetic testing and immunology and cancer research groups and laboratories

(4) Establish genetic testing and endocrine hormone and cancer research groups and laboratories

(5) Establish genetic testing and pathological sections, and related studies on immunohistochemistry

(6) Establish correlation analysis and research on gene detection and tumor markers

(7) Establish HPV treatment, exploration research groups and laboratories

2. The basic idea and design of the total attack which XZ-C launches

Professor Xu Ze (XU ZE) proposed to build the following general plan to overcome cancer and the basic design of Science City.

a. Dawning scientific research spirit

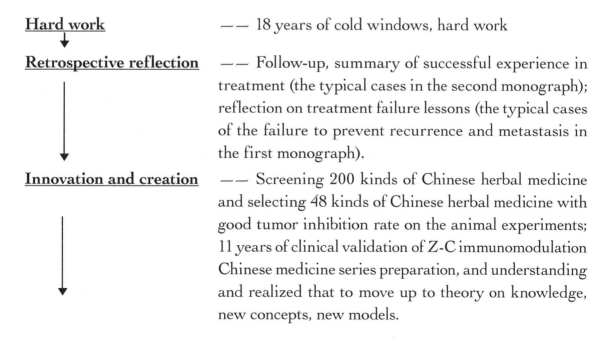

<u>Hard work</u> —— 18 years of cold windows, hard work

<u>Retrospective reflection</u> —— Follow-up, summary of successful experience in treatment (the typical cases in the second monograph); reflection on treatment failure lessons (the typical cases of the failure to prevent recurrence and metastasis in the first monograph).

<u>Innovation and creation</u> —— Screening 200 kinds of Chinese herbal medicine and selecting 48 kinds of Chinese herbal medicine with good tumor inhibition rate on the animal experiments; 11 years of clinical validation of Z-C immunomodulation Chinese medicine series preparation, and understanding and realized that to move up to theory on knowledge, new concepts, new models.

<u>Face the future medicine</u> ——Recognizing some of the shortcomings of traditional therapy in the 20th century There are problems that recognize the direction of the 21st century.

↓

<u>Look forward to the future</u> ——Recommendations:

- Establish a School of Innovative Molecular Oncology – for The state trains senior oncology research talents.
- Establish an innovative molecular tumor hospital (in the molecule Level Chinese and Western medicine combined) - make more Cancer patients benefit for more cancer patients service.
- Established the Institute of Innovative Molecular Oncology Study cells begin to malignant - to CT can be between now and for a long time, to reach three early target, "target" metastasis, cancer lesions, Precancerous condition.
- Establish an innovative molecular oncology drug factory – walk out of a new way of conquering cancer with Chinese characteristics.

The scientific base of conquering cancer and launching the general attack to cancer(the scientific city) including :

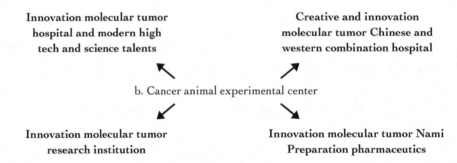

Medical education research and development science city or science base

c. What is the general attack on cancer?

The general attack is to carry out the three-stage work of anti-cancer, cancer control and cancer treatment in the whole process of cancer occurrence and development.

<u>That is</u>:

<u>Cancer prevention</u> - before the formation of cancer

<u>Cancer control</u> - precancerous lesions with malignant tendencies

<u>Treat cancer</u> - has formed a cancerous foci or metastasis

<u>The goal of the total attack</u>: reduce the incidence of cancer, reduce cancer death, improve cure rate, prolong survival, improve quality of life, and reduce complications.

d. Professor Xu Ze (XU ZE) proposed the idea, strategy, and planning sketch for conquering cancer and launching the general attack as the following:

How to overcome cancer?

Where is the way?
↓
Our thought, strategy and experience should be divided into three parts
↓
Before the formation of cancer——prevention part——**anti- mutation**
↓
Precancerous lesion with possible tendency of malignant change——**intervention part**
↓
The therapeutic part of primary cancer with the formation of focus and anti-metastasis
↓

Stage of preventing susceptibility	precancerous lesion	cancer and metastasis

Early ↙   ↓   ↘ transferred
not transferred

⇑ | ⇑ | ⇑

Cancer prevention   cancer control   Cancer treatment

e. The brief graph of the basic design and plan of XZ-C (Xu Ze-China)'s launching the general attack

Dawning scientific research spirit

<u>**Hard work**</u>	—— 18 years of cold windows, hard work
Retrospective reflection	—— Follow-up, reflection on treatment failure lessons and summary of successful experience in treatment
<u>**Innovation and creation**</u>	—— Screening 200 kinds of Chinese herbal medicine and selecting 48 kinds of Chinese herbal medicine with good tumor inhibition rate on the animal experiments; 11 years of clinical validation of Z-C immunomodulation Chinese medicine series preparation, and understanding and realized that to move up to theory on knowledge, new concepts, new models.
<u>**Face the future medicine**</u>	——Recognizing some of the shortcomings of traditional therapy in the 20th century There are problems that recognize the direction of the 21st century.

Look forward to the future ——Recommendations:

- Establish a School of Innovative Molecular Oncology
- Establish an innovative molecular tumor hospitalne combined
- Established the Institute of Innovative Molecular Oncology
- Establish an innovative molecular oncology drug factory

The scientific base of conquering cancer and launching the general attack to cancer(the scientific city) including :

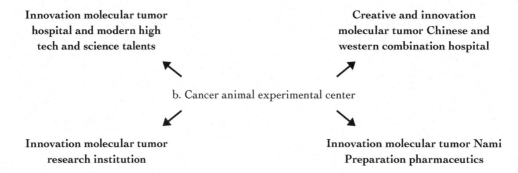

Innovation molecular tumor hospital and modern high tech and science talents

Creative and innovation molecular tumor Chinese and western combination hospital

b. Cancer animal experimental center

Innovation molecular tumor research institution

Innovation molecular tumor Nami Preparation pharmaceutics

Medical education research and development science city or science base

F. The program and steps of conquering cancer and launching the total attack to cancer are shown in the following schematic drawing.

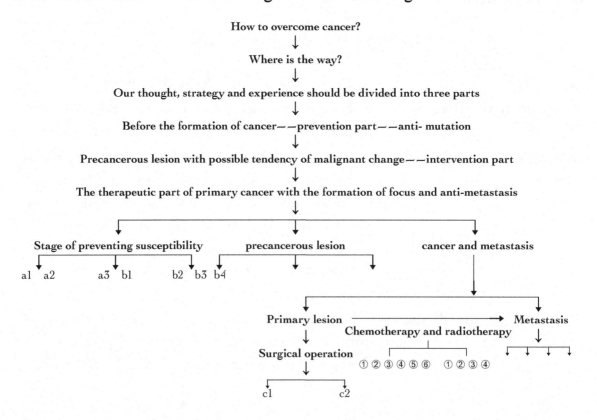

How to overcome cancer?

↓

Where is the way?

↓

Our thought, strategy and experience should be divided into three parts

↓

Before the formation of cancer——prevention part——anti- mutation

↓

Precancerous lesion with possible tendency of malignant change——intervention part

↓

The therapeutic part of primary cancer with the formation of focus and anti-metastasis

↓

Stage of preventing susceptibility   precancerous lesion   cancer and metastasis

a1   a2   a3 b1   b2 b3 b4

Primary lesion ——————→ Metastasis

Chemotherapy and radiotherapy

↓

Surgical operation   ① ② ③ ④ ⑤ ⑥   ① ② ③ ④

↓

c1   c2

a1. "Two-oriented society" contains essences and measures

a2. "Lift scientific research" makes plans and measures of cancer control

a3. Propaganda, education and study of popular science

b1. General investigation of physical examination

b2. Selective examination of high risk group

b3. Outpatient service of "early detection, early diagnosis and early treatment"

b4. Induced differentiation

c1. Improve free-tumor technique

c2. Prevent intraoperative implantation of cast-off cells

① with indication

② individuation

③ scientization

④ drug sensitive test

⑤ try to reduce untoward reaction

⑥ "intelligent resistance to cancer" of target administration

① targeted therapy

② anti-metastasis and anti-relapse therapies

③ BRM biological therapy

④ immunoregulation therapy

Win Cancer, and Focus on action

What should I do next? Now it is proposed to overcome cancer and launch a general attack. I hope to get support from leaders at all levels. We must work hard to make progress in cancer prevention and control. We must do so by government leaders, government leaders, experts, scholars, people, mobilization, and participation of thousands of households.

No matter how long and how long the road to conquer cancer is, we must avoid talks, work hard, and should start. The journey of a thousand miles begins with a single step. As long as we move forward, we will always walk out a new way, avoid talk, work hard, and start to go.

3. The theoretical system of XZ-C immunomodulation and cancer treatment has been formed.

1). In the book "New Concepts and New Methods of Cancer Treatment", Professor Xu Ze published a series of research papers on basic and clinical research results with 60 years of self-reliance and hard work.

This book has initially formed the theoretical system of XZ-C immune regulation and treatment of cancer, and the clinical basis and experimental basis for cancer treatment are undergoing clinical application observation and verification.

The Clinical Verification for XZ-C immune regulation and control medication:

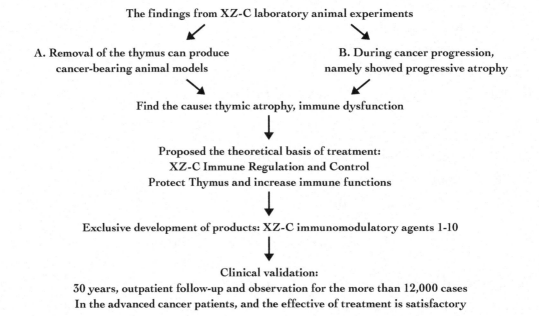

The findings from XZ-C laboratory animal experiments

A. Removal of the thymus can produce cancer-bearing animal models

B. During cancer progression, namely showed progressive atrophy

Find the cause: thymic atrophy, immune dysfunction

Proposed the theoretical basis of treatment:
XZ-C Immune Regulation and Control
Protect Thymus and increase immune functions

Exclusive development of products: XZ-C immunomodulatory agents 1-10

Clinical validation:
30 years, outpatient follow-up and observation for the more than 12,000 cases
In the advanced cancer patients, and the effective of treatment is satisfactory

<u>Theoretical System of XZ-C immune regulate and control of cancer therapy</u>

2). At the age of 85, he published the medical monograph "Condense Wisdom and conquer cancer — for Benefiting Mankind", XZ-C proposed that "How to overcome cancer? How can I prevent cancer? I see; how to treat cancer? By my opinion."

Professor Xu Ze proposed the engineering planning diagram of how to conquer cancer.

This medical monograph is a practical, applied, research-oriented, implementation of how to overcome the outline of cancer. This set of scientific research programs, scientific research design, scientific research planning, and blueprints can be used by countries, provinces, and states to implement the vision of conquering cancer and benefit humanity.

This implementation outline of the main project is:

1. Conquer cancer and launch the total attack ; Put the equal attention to cancer prevention and cancer control and cancer treatment
2. Create a scientific research base for multidisciplinary and cancer-related research – The Science City.

The two-wing project is:

A wing - how to prevent cancer? To reduce the incidence of cancer
B wing - how to treat cancer? To improve cancer cure rate

Aims:

A: Reduce the incidence of cancer
B: Improve cancer cure rate, prolong patient survival and improve quality of life

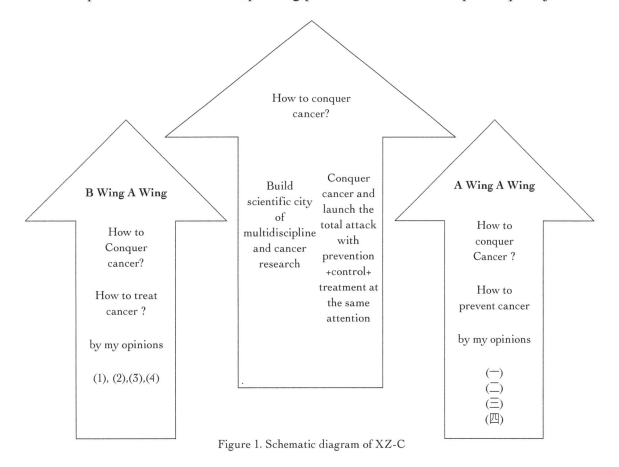

Figure 1. Schematic diagram of XZ-C

4.Proposed to conquer cancer and launch the total attack of cancer, this is unprecedented work

(1) For the first time in the world, the "XZ-C Scientific Research Plan for Overcoming the General Attack of Cancer"

——The overall strategic reform and development of cancer treatment in China
- Avoid talk, work hard, start off
No matter how far the road to cancer is, you should always start.
——Proposed to overcome the general attack of cancer, this is unprecedented work

(2) For the first time in the world, the "Necessity and Feasibility Report on Overcoming the General Attack of Cancer"

——The overall strategic reform of cancer treatment in China will focus on treatment and turn to prevention and treatment.
——XZ-C proposes the general idea and design of conquering cancer
- What is the total attack on cancer and the goal of the total attack?
——XU ZE proposes ideas, strategies, plans, blueprints to overcome cancer and launch a general attack

(3) For the first time in the world, "Providing the construction of cancer prevention and development, prevention and treatment of hospitals"

(Global demonstration cancer prevention and treatment hospital)
——The current problems in the hospital hospital hospital model
——How to overcome the road of cancer is to study the establishment of prevention and treatment hospitals for the whole process of cancer occurrence and development, and reform the current mode of hospitalization for re-treatment and light defense.
——XU ZE's strategic thinking, planning sketch, prevention and treatment of cancer occurrence and development

(4) For the first time in the world, the "General Plan for Overcoming Cancer and the Basic Design of Science City"

- Equivalent to designing an overall framework for Chinese characteristics to overcome cancer design

——How to set up the basic idea and design to overcome the general attack of cancer

- How to overcome cancer? The Cancer Animal Experimental Center must be established.

Innovative Molecular Oncology Medical College

Cancer and Multidisciplinary Research Institute

- How to overcome cancer? It is necessary to "prepare a medical, teaching, research, and science base to overcome the general attack of cancer - Science City"

5. Exclusive research and development products: XZ-C immune regulation anti-cancer Chinese medicine series products (introduction)

The self-developed XZ-C (Xu Ze China) immune regulation anti-cancer series of traditional Chinese medicine preparations, from experimental research to clinical verification, applied to clinical practice on the basis of the success of animal experiments, after more than 12,000 clinical cases in 20 years, Significant effect. Clinical application can improve symptoms, good spirits, good appetite, significantly improve the quality of life, and significantly prolong the survival period. It is independent innovation and independent intellectual property rights.

To search for and screen new anti-cancer and anti-metastatic drugs from traditional Chinese medicine:

The purpose is to screen out the anti-cancer, anti-metastatic and anti-recurrent immunomodulatory Chinese medicine XZ-C1-10 which has no drug resistance, no toxic side effects, high selectivity and long-term oral administration. (XZ-C immunomodulation series of Chinese medicine products, see the first volume, the eighth volume)

(1) The 83-year-old year (April 2016) proposes to advance together with the "Cancer Moon Shot", because since 2013, Xu Ze has proposed the necessity and feasibility of conquering the general attack of cancer. The Sexual Report and the report "Collecting the General Attack on Cancer and Preparing to Conquer the Cancer Science City" are being planned and designed.

"New Moon Plan" (US) and Dawning C Plan (middle)

- Moving forward together, heading for the science hall to overcome cancer

1. "Introduction to the Cancer Moon Shot"
On January 12, 2016, US President Barack Obama announced a national plan to overcome cancer in his State of the Union address:
Plan Name: "New Moon Plan"
Goal: Conquer cancer
Nature: National plan to overcome cancer
Announcer: President Obama
The person in charge of the plan: Vice President Biden
Announced: January 12, 2016
The specific plan of the plan: unknown

2. Shuguang C-type plan introduction

a. Before January 12, 2016, the progress of the XZ-C Scientific Research Plan for Overcoming the General Attack of Cancer Attack was put forward.
b. Before January 12, 2016, we have carried out research results in the field of cancer research, technology innovation series
c. Dawning C-type plan (developed in July 2015)

I "Overcome the general attack of cancer"
II "Preparation of the whole process of prevention and treatment of hospitals"
III "Preparing to build a cancer science city"
IV "Forming a Multidisciplinary Research Group"
V "The vaccine is the hope of mankind"
VI "The prospect of immunomodulatory drugs is gratifying"

3. The situation analysis

a. analyze their respective technological advantages
b. Analyze the current status quo
c. Analyze the next research prospects
d. "Dawning C-type plan" technology innovation realization outline
e. How to implement this unprecedented event in human history?
f. expected results

(2) Conducting anti-cancer metastasis research is an urgent need

1. Conducting anti-cancer and anti-cancer metastasis research is an urgent need for the development of oncology. "Oncology" is one of the most backward disciplines in medical science. Its "name" is not yet unified. Some people write it as "tumor" and " Cancer, "cancer", "malignant tumor", "new organism". Because a disease name is defined, its cause and pathogenesis must be clarified. Because the etiology, pathogenesis, and pathophysiology of oncology are not well understood, the oncology discipline is still a scientific virgin for scientific research, and it needs a lot of basic scientific research.

2. Anti-cancer metastasis, recurrence, basic research must be carried out on animal models of cancer-bearing animals. Currently, many large hospitals have not established laboratories and cannot conduct basic research on cancer. It is necessary to establish various cancer metastasis animal models in nude mice to study cancer cell metastasis. The law and mechanism (the author's laboratory uses pure Kunming mice to make cancer-bearing animal models about 10,000 times), because without the breakthrough of basic research, the clinical efficacy is difficult to improve.

3. Research on anti-cancer and anti-cancer metastasis focuses on the study of unknown knowledge. Researchers should look ahead and face the science of the future. Science is the end of the world. Researchers must surpass the old knowledge and constantly update with a developmental perspective. Constantly surpassing, constantly developing and moving forward.

(3) How to innovate in science and technology? How to leave a scientific research footprint?

An old cement road, with hundreds of people walking every day, will not leave footprints, only a new cement road, every step will leave eternal footprints, so scientific research must have innovative thinking, must be innovative Results.

In the past 30 years (1985-), our research history, cancer research work, scientific research series of scientific research achievements in animal experiments, clinical basic research and clinical verification work, only the results catalogue (scientific research footprint) is listed here, and each research result is Belonging to original innovation or independent innovation, it is every eternal scientific research footprint.

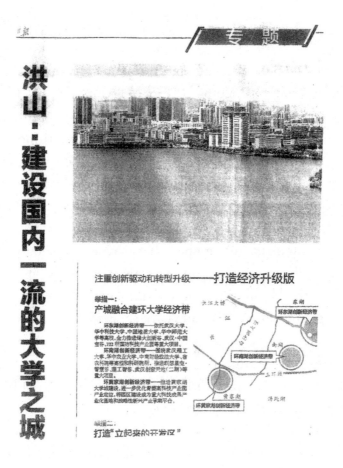

6. Professor Xu Ze (XZ-C) proposed: How to overcome cancer (1-6)

A. The introduction (1-6) of how to conquer cancer

How to overcome cancer I see one:

1. How to overcome cancer? In order to overcome cancer, we must create the "Innovative Molecular Oncology School"
——To conquer cancer, one of the scientific research bases for multidisciplinary and cancer-related research that overcomes the general attack of cancer

(1) Why did you want to start the "Innovative Molecular Oncology Medical School"?

because:

1. To overcome cancer, talent is the key. Cultivate relevant talents who can participate in the fight against cancer and launch the general attack. Talents must be truly practical. There are techniques and theories, and both must be both ethical and moral, medical is benevolence, and ethics is the first.
   Talents must have knowledge of medical school undergraduate knowledge, life science knowledge, Chinese medicine knowledge, molecular biology, genetic engineering, environmental science, environmental science, medical multidisciplinary knowledge, immunology, virology, endocrinology, immunopharmacology, etc.

2. to overcome cancer, talent is the key, how to train talent is the key. The research of cancer requires multidisciplinary knowledge and technology. It requires genetic engineering, molecular biological immunology, and virological experimental talents. Knowledge must also have technology, hands-on ability, and technology needs knowledge. Under the guidance of theory, The development of high-end technology, the first-class talents that need to tackle the problem, must concentrate and calm down and concentrate on this work. Where do talents come from, based on their own training, they create their own work machine to hatch talents.

3. overcome cancer, launch a general attack, prevent cancer + control cancer + cure cancer, the three go hand in hand, so the teaching plan must cultivate cancer prevention science talents, cancer disease control personnel and related cancer prevention, preventive medicine teaching content, knowledge, courses. At present, there are a shortage of talents for cancer prevention and cancer control, and there is an urgent need to speed up training to meet the urgent needs of launching a general attack.
   Since more than 90% of cancers are caused or closely related to environmental factors, we are currently working on energy conservation, pollution prevention and pollution control. This policy has a great correlation with work and cancer prevention and cancer control. This related talent.

4. The current educational content cannot keep up with the development of the times. In order to overcome the general attack of cancer, it is necessary to develop modern high-tech disciplines, all of which must have good laboratories,

but the current laboratory talents are scarce. It has a general attack on cancer prevention, anti-cancer and cancer control, lack of laboratory-experimental modern high-tech talents, and intermediate-level specialists who can go deep into the community to prevent cancer and control cancer.

Laboratory talents should be established for colleges and universities. Modern life science and technology is progressing rapidly, and genetic engineering, molecular biology, and cytogenetics are developing at a rapid pace.

Because Professor Xu Ze (XZ) proposed to overcome the general attack of cancer, it is an unprecedented work of humanity. It is necessary to train high-tech talents and technologies with basic medicine, clinical medicine, life sciences, Chinese and Western medicine, and molecular level to practice and create experience. Develop medicine. Therefore, at the same time, the graduate school was established to cultivate senior scientific and technological talents who have overcome the general attack of cancer.

(2) How to create the "Innovative Molecular Oncology Cancer School"?

Apply for the leadership and leadership of the Provincial Department of Education
XZ-C proposes how to overcome cancer. I see two:
2. How to overcome cancer? In order to overcome cancer, we must create the Innovative Molecular Oncology Institute.
——To conquer cancer, one of the scientific research bases for multidisciplinary and cancer-related research that overcomes the general attack of cancer

(1) Why did you want to start the "Innovative Molecular Oncology Research Institute"?

because:

1. "Oncology" is still the most backward discipline in the current medical sciences. why? Because the etiology, pathogenesis, pathophysiology of "oncology" have not been clearly understood, there are a large number of basic theoretical problems that have not been clearly understood, and there is still insufficient understanding of the biological characteristics of cancer cells and the molecular mechanism of cancer cell metastasis. Multi-disciplinary research must be carried out in relation to carcinogenic factors such as viruses, immunity, fungi, endocrine hormones, and the environment.

Oncology research is the most complex subject in medical research. It involves multidisciplinary knowledge and theory. It is necessary to form a specialist group closely related to cancer and conduct in-depth research to help overcome the general attack of cancer.

2. Therefore, the creation of the "Innovative Molecular Oncology Research Institute" is to further conquer cancer, launch a general attack to explore the cause of cancer, pathogenesis, cancer cell metastasis mechanism, immune mechanism, conduct in-depth research, and organize a scientific research group closely related to cancer to further study Based on the knowledge and theory of the discipline, known medicine, research and exploration of the unknown knowledge of the discipline, future medicine, marginal disciplines, interdisciplinary, understanding the causes and mechanisms of cancer, thereby providing intervention for effective prevention and treatment of tumors. And treatment measures to help overcome cancer.

(2) How to create the "Innovative Molecular Level Oncology Institute"? How to implement and create?

Apply for the leadership and leadership of the Provincial Science and Technology Department

XZ-C proposes how to overcome cancer. I see three:

3. How to overcome cancer? In order to overcome cancer, we must create an "innovative molecular tumor prevention, control, and treatment hospital" (global demonstration of cancer occurrence, development, prevention, control, treatment of hospitals)
——To conquer cancer, one of the scientific research bases for multidisciplinary and cancer-related research that overcomes the general attack of cancer

(1) Why should we create "innovative molecular tumor occurrence, development, and prevention and treatment of hospitals"?

because:

1. The current problems in the hospital model of the global, Chinese cancer hospital or hospital oncology department

a. go all out, the focus of treatment, for advanced cancer patients with middle, late, metastasis, recurrence, poor efficacy, exhausted human and financial resources, and failed to achieve lower mortality, improve cure rate, reduce morbidity, death The rate is still the first cause of death for urban and rural residents.

b. Only cure, or re-treatment, the more the patient is treated.

2. The current global and Chinese oncology hospitals or hospital oncology departments, their hospital models are treatment hospitals, the treatment of patients are in the advanced stage, metastatic period, the efficacy is very poor.

Its mode of hospitalization: all treatment hospitals, re-treatment and light prevention, or only cure.

The treatment mode: all for advanced patients with advanced cancer metastasis. Should (required) reform:

Reform of the school mode: should be changed to prevention, control, and treatment

Treatment model reform: should focus on early, precancerous lesions, etc., the way out for cancer treatment in the "three early", must study the "three early" diagnosis of new technologies, new methods, new reagents, early cancer can be cured.

3 Therefore, the creation of "innovative molecular tumor occurrence, development of the whole process of prevention and treatment of hospitals" in order to overcome cancer, should reform the hospital model, change the treatment model, XZ-C proposed to overcome cancer, launch a general attack - prevention, control, and treatment, The troika is carried out at the same time and goes hand in hand.

What is the general attack on cancer?

The general attack is to comprehensively carry out the three stages of cancer prevention, cancer control and cancer treatment in the whole process of cancer development, and carry out simultaneously, troika, go hand in hand, drive together, reform the current hospital mode, and change the current treatment mode.

Namely: reform the current mode of hospitalization with emphasis on treatment. Change the current treatment model focusing on the middle and late stages of treatment. Only cure and prevent, reform as prevention, control, and governance.

How to implement this new mode of running a hospital?

It is necessary to establish a hospital for prevention, control and treatment according to the whole process of cancer occurrence and development.

(2) How to create the "Innovative Molecular Level Full-Defense Prevention, Control and Treatment Cancer Hospital"? How to implement and create?

Apply for the leadership and leadership of the Provincial Health and Safety Committee

XZ-C proposes how to overcome cancer. I see four:

4. How to overcome cancer? In order to overcome cancer, the Experimental Medicine Cancer Animal Experimental Center must be created.
——To conquer cancer, one of the scientific research bases for multidisciplinary and cancer-related research that overcomes the general attack of cancer

(1) Why create an "Experimental Medical Cancer Animal Experimental Center"?

1. In order to overcome cancer → conquer cancer → overcome cancer, we must first understand the understanding of cancer: the cause, pathogenesis, pathophysiology, immunopathology, biological behavior of cancer cells? Transfer mechanism? Why plant? Recurrence mechanism? A series of oncology and tumor-related problems have not yet been clearly understood. Oncology is still a scientific virgin for scientific research, and it needs a lot of basic scientific research and clinical basic research. Carrying out basic research in cancer science is an urgent need of the current oncology discipline. Therefore, the Experimental Medicine Cancer Animal Experimental Center must be established.

2. Carry out basic research on oncology. A good laboratory is the key. Scientific design and scientific assumptions must be studied through laboratory experiments in order to draw conclusions and produce results.
   We believe that the establishment of a scientific research base (Science City) to overcome the general attack on cancer, we must first vigorously build a laboratory, so that many basic problems have experimental research, open up research on the basic issues of oncology, should encourage the opening of new research areas, talents Out of the results to help cancer.

3. In order to overcome cancer, launch a general attack, and build an experimental medical cancer animal experiment center, a laboratory with good equipment is the key.

In order to study new anti-cancer and anti-metastatic drugs, it is necessary to conduct experimental research on nude mouse models. Experimental surgery is extremely important in the development of medicine. It is a key to opening the medical exclusion zone. Many disease prevention and treatment methods have been studied in many animal experiments, and the stability results have been applied to the clinic to promote the development of the medical cause.

How can technology innovation? How can we overcome cancer? A laboratory with good equipment should be built.

Therefore, the development of science, technological innovation, results, patents, laboratories are the key conditions.

How to carry out basic research on cancer? How to develop new areas of cancer research?

How can I get the original innovations in cancer research? A good laboratory should be established.

(2) How to establish the "Experimental Medicine Cancer Animal Experimental Center"?

Experimental animal experiment center, not suitable for downtown, downtown
Can be located in the suburbs of the city, university city
Site selection: planned to be in the university town of Huangjiahu
Animal buildings should be enclosed terraces, isolated
Managed according to national laboratory requirements.

XZ-C proposes how to overcome cancer. I see five:

5. How to overcome cancer? In order to overcome cancer, we must create the "Innovative Environmental Protection Cancer Research Institute" and carry out anti-cancer system engineering.
- one of the science cities to overcome cancer
(1) Why should we create an innovative environmental protection and cancer prevention research institute?

Because: the current cancer incidence is on the rise, 90% is related to the environment.

The occurrence of cancer is closely related to people's clothing, food, housing, travel and living habits.

The current environmental pollution is serious and the ecosystem is degraded, which may be related to the rising cancer cancer rate.

After 28 years of research and clinical work on cancer research, we have deeply realized that cancer should not only pay attention to treatment, but also pay attention to prevention, in order to be at the source, must be prevention and treatment, and the way to prevent cancer is in prevention. Mainly for prevention.

So how to prevent it? What to prevent? It is necessary to measure, characterize, locate, and quantify various environmental carcinogens and try to remove them.

Therefore, it is necessary to establish an anti-cancer research institute, which should conduct anti-cancer research from clothing, food, housing, and transportation, and conduct microscopic and ultra-microscopic anti-cancer research from the big environment and small environment.

How to prevent cancer from clothing, food, shelter, and cancer? First of all, you should master the situation of clothing, food, shelter, and other carcinogens, whether it contains carcinogens, qualitative and quantitative monitoring, and then set standards and set the bottom line, in order to discuss and propose prevention and control measures.

(2) How to create the "Innovative Environmental Protection and Cancer Research Institute"?

XZ-C proposed to overcome the general attack on cancer, and must establish the Cancer Research Institute and the anti-cancer system project, which was first proposed internationally.

Conduct anti-cancer research, find carcinogenic factors, detect the source of carcinogens or carcinogenic factors, and try to prevent these carcinogens from harming the human body. The Cancer Research Institute should conduct anti-cancer research, trace the source of carcinogens or carcinogenic factors, and try to remove them.

Because cancer patients cover the whole world, industrial and agricultural wastewater, waste residue, and waste gas also cover the whole world, it is necessary to launch a general attack globally.

Anti-cancer research is a major event. At present, there is no anti-cancer research institute in the world. We will apply to capture the Cancer Science City and create the world's first environmental protection and cancer prevention research institute to monitor macroscopic, microscopic and ultra-micro environmentally friendly carcinogens.,analysis.

Apply for the leadership and leadership of the Provincial Department of Ecological Environment

XZ-C proposes how to overcome cancer. I see six:

1). How to overcome cancer? In order to overcome cancer, we must create "Innovative Molecular Tumor Nano-Pharmaceuticals" and "Building Anti-Cancer, Anti-Cancer Metabolic Traditional Chinese Medicine Active Components,

Molecular Weight, Structural Formula, Immunopharmacology, Molecular Level Analysis Research Group and Laboratory"

(1) Why should we set up an innovative molecular tumor nano-preparation pharmaceutical factory and an effective component of anti-cancer and anti-cancer metastatic traditional Chinese medicine, and a Chinese medicine immunopharmacological analysis research group?

Because it is necessary to research and develop effective drugs for anti-cancer and anti-cancer metastasis, XZ-C believes that it is necessary to have two wheels for cancer, one is life science, biomedicine (modern medicine) A wheel, one is clinical basis, immune Regulatory, anti-cancer (Chinese herbal medicine) B wheel.

Its purpose is to further develop the anti-cancer and anti-cancer metastasis of Chinese herbal medicines, and to use it as a resource for natural medicine and natural medicine, so as to become a precise medicine.

Further study on the molecular level of immunomodulatory anti-cancer Chinese medicine cells.

Further explore the effects of anti-cancer and anti-cancer Chinese herbal medicines on early carcinoma in situ and precancerous lesions.

2). How to create innovative tumor nano-preparation pharmaceutical factory and Chinese herbal active ingredient analysis group and laboratory as one of the cancer research and medical centers

7. How does a country carry out a "science city" to overcome the general attack on cancer? XZ-C initial vision and design:

A. The Suggestion is to set up the "Conquer Cancer Working Group"

Each professional working group is set up as the following:
Ministry of Science and Technology - Guidance Department of Science and Technology of the Province - responsible for the establishment of "Innovative Molecular Oncology Research Institute"

National Ministry of Education - Guidance Provincial Department of Education - responsible for the establishment of "Innovative Molecular Oncology Medical School"

National Health and Health Commission - Guidance Provincial Health and

Health Commission - responsible for the establishment of "innovative molecular level Chinese and Western medicine combination

Prevention and treatment of cancer in the whole process of cancer occurrence and development

(Cancer prevention and treatment hospital)

Ministry of Ecology and Environment - Guiding the Provincial Department of Ecology and Environment - responsible for the establishment of the "Environmental Protection and Health Cancer Research Institute", New areas, new technologies and new industries for environmental protection and cancer research should be developed. Because 90% of cancers occur closely related to the environment. It is necessary to establish multi-project laboratories from the clothing, food, housing, and anti-cancer, from the big environment, small environment to prevent cancer, first monitoring, qualitative, quantitative, and standard, to conduct macroscopic, microscopic, and ultra-microscopic research to study the specificity of anti-cancer Methods and measures.

National Association for Science and Technology - Guidance Provincial and Municipal Science Association - Association of Science and Technology Associations, multidisciplinary associations and associations organized Contact, easy to handle multi-disciplinary research groups to prevent cancer and cancer. If you collaborate with the Society of Viruses, establish a research group on viruses and cancer;Collaborate with the Society for Immunology to establish an immunology and cancer related research group;Collaborate with the Endocrine Hormone Society to establish endocrine hormones and cancer-related research groups... and other research groups should establish laboratories. In this way, the cancer research teams in various countries will inevitably bloom, the results will be beneficial to the people, benefit the well-off society, everyone's health, and stay away from cancer.

All provinces can set up a cancer prevention working group (station), or "provincial cancer work office", have full-time staff to work, should be diligent and thrifty, do everything for the people, do good things, do good things for future generations, and seek health and welfare for future generations. In the contemporary, it is beneficial to the future.

B. How to carry out "to overcome the general attack of cancer" in Hubei and Wuhan?

1.It should propose:

1) Conducted an academic report on "Proposal to Overcome the General Attack of Cancer Attack"

2) set up and formed a team of "conquer cancer and launch the general attack on cancer", and on December 26, 2017, the Wuhan Anti-cancer Research Society was established to tackle the general attack on cancer.

3) To formulate the tasks and achievements of each team member, not to name but to seek truth, to strive to achieve results, must be truly practical, must have both ability and political integrity, medical is benevolence, ethics first.

The contribution of each team member, the tasks and indicators of each member, the tasks and indicators of the team, must clearly define the goals and objectives, and strive for innovation.

2. Can cancer be conquered?

It should be able to overcome because 90% of cancer is caused or led by the environment.

Environmental factors lead to genetic mutations that lead to chromosomal deletions and abnormalities.

Environmental factors are possible or can be managed to find ways to solve them.

"condense wisdom and conquer cancer — for benefiting mankind" is a comprehensive design, specifically planning how to overcome cancer medical monographs, is the outline of how to overcome cancer, this set of scientific research plans, scientific research plans, blue maps, available everywhere Reference application.

3. Do cancers need to be conquered?

It must be and urgently overcome, because the incidence rate is rising and the mortality rate is high. The number of cancer deaths worldwide is 8.18 million. About 8550 people in China are diagnosed with cancer every day, and 6 people are confirmed to be cancer every minute. Therefore, research to overcome the scientific research work of cancer attack, can not walk slowly, should run forward, save the wounded. Because people all over the world are eager to hope that one day they will be able to overcome cancer and stay away from cancer for the benefit of mankind.

4. How should I conquer cancer?

(1) it should conquer cancer and launch the general attack of cancer and put cancer prevention + control + treatment at the same importance level and the same attention and at the same time.

(Change the current mode of hospitalization for attention of treatment and light prevention, and change the current treatment mode that focuses on the middle and late stages of treatment)

(2) It should be implemented and realized in accordance with the report on "conquer cancer and launch the general attack on cancer" and the proposal book.

The next step is how to implement, how to achieve this overall design and scheme and plan and blueprint for cancer.

C H A P T E R 4

How to conquer cancer? How to prevent cancer?

XZ-C proposed: To build "Innovative Environmental
Protection Cancer Prevention Research Institute" and to
Carry Out Cancer Prevention System Engineering

TABLE OF CONTENTS

Combine with the three major challenges, ride research, anti-pollution, pollution control, anti-cancer, anti-cancer

Declaration

The core design of the cancer research plan, the core content of the plan with the general attack on cancer and XZ-C proposed Sun-up or Dawn-A, B, D-type plan for conquering cancer are the international key points and are kept the serious attitude to carry out so that the cancer can be controlled and prevented and cured. It is only for reporting to senior leaders to help decision-making. The research project is implemented by my team experts, professors, etc., and its intellectual property belongs to XZ-C.

The next step is how to implement, how to achieve this master plan, scheme, programme, blueprint for the general attack of cancer. First, to set up : "Wuhan Anti-cancer Research Society and team to conquer cancer and to tackle the general attack". Under the guidance of the city leadership, state leadership, the provincial government and the municipal government, it will be gradually implemented and realized.

The Wuhan Anti-Cancer Research Society and team which conquer cancer and launch the general attack was established on December 26, 2017.

1. XZ-C proposes to create the "Innovative prevention cancer research institute of the Environmental Protection" and to carry out anti-cancer system engineering

1). XZ-C proposes "in order to conquer cancer and to launch the general attack, it must build the "Innovative prevention cancer research institute of the Environmental Protection" and cancer prevention system **engineering, which is the first time in the world**

In order to conduct cancer prevention research, find cancer-causing factors, detect the source of carcinogens or carcinogenic factors, and try to stop or prevent these carcinogenic factors from harming the human body, the Cancer Research Institute should conduct cancer prevention research, and there are a lot of contents which are in need for research.

Track the source of carcinogens or carcinogenic factors.

In the search for the cause and condition of cancer, the most prominent thing is the factor that more than 90% of cancers are caused by environmental factors.

(1) Relationship between air pollution and cancer

Humans have developed tens of millions of tons of coal, oil and natural gas as fuel and energy. In the production and life processes such as thermal power generation, smelting steel, automobiles, airplanes, and household fuels, **a large amount of tar, bituminous coal, dust and other harmful substances staying up all night are discharged into the atmosphere around the clock, causing air pollution.**

Air pollution can cause many diseases, especially respiratory diseases, the most serious is lung cancer.

(2) Water pollution and cancer

The pollution of water quality is mainly caused by industrial and agricultural production and urban sewage. There are many types of pollutants in water. **Pesticides and insecticides are one of the important pollutants in water. Surfactants in neutral detergents also have cancer-promoting effects.**

(3) Soil pollution and cancer

A large amount of industrial waste water residue and pesticides and fertilizers are injected into the soil, **which deteriorates soil quality and accumulates poisons, posing a threat to human health and a carcinogenic factor.**

(4) Chemistry and cancer

(5) Physical factors and cancer

(6) Biological factors and cancer

(7) Diet and cancer

(8) Lifestyle and cancer

(9) clothing, food, housing, transportation, house decoration, etc. and cancer

It should be studied of the action method in which so many carcinogens or carcinogenic factors
To study these sources of pollution and try to stop at the source
To study these carcinogenic mechanisms and their carcinogenic effects
To study how to reduce or prevent these carcinogens

2. Internationally it is proposed for the first time: XZ-C proposed Dawning cancer prevention program A, B, D for pollution prevention, pollution control and pollution treatment and cancer prevention and anti-cancer

Dawning Type A Plan: Goal: Prevention and treatment of Air Pollution
Dawning B-type plan: goal: prevention and treatment of water pollution
Dawning D-type plan: goal: prevention and control of soil pollution

How to overcome cancer? How to prevent cancer? I see:

Professor Xu Ze proposed that the "Innovative Environmental Protection and Cancer Prevention Research Institute" should be established and the cancer prevention system project should be carried out.

Where is the target or "target" of cancer prevention? How to prevent?

The more cancer patients are treated and the more and more cancer patients occur, the incidence is rising, and 90% of them are related or closely related to environmental carcinogenic factors. **Therefore, the target or "target" of cancer prevention should be to study, explore and take scientific prevention and treatment measures against the carcinogenic factors (external environment, internal environment) of the environment.**

XZ-C proposed cancer prevention general design and cancer prevention system engineering:

Since the disaster of cancer covers the whole world, industrial and agricultural waste gas, waste water and waste residue also cover the whole world. Therefore, it is necessary to establish "Innovative Environmental Protection and Cancer Prevention Research Institute" and carry out cancer prevention system engineering.

It must prevent and control the three major pollutions, the first thing it should study the relationship between the environment and cancer.

There are many examples in history, such as ensuring the relationship between environmental pollution and cancer. In particular, environmental pollution such as air pollution, water pollution, and soil pollution has a serious impact on human carcinogenesis.

1. **Air pollution and cancer in environmental pollution**:

Human beings cannot be separated from air every minute of their lives. Air pollution can cause many respiratory diseases, the most serious of which is lung cancer.

(2) <u>Water</u> pollution and cancer in environmental pollution:

Human beings can't live without water every time they are in production activities and life. Water pollution is mainly caused by industrial and agricultural production and urban sewage. In China, industrial pollution has intensified due to the rapid development of township and village enterprises. Water pollution is related to the high incidence of <u>lung cancer</u>, and it is related to the occurrence of <u>gastric cancer, intestinal cancer and esophageal cancer.</u> Drinking water that does not meet the standard is not able to induce or promote cancer.

<u>(3) Soil</u> pollution and cancer in environmental pollution:

Fertilizers, pesticides and pesticides in agricultural production can cause soil water quality in farmland, soil pollution is serious, agricultural workers are exposed to a variety of pesticides, herbicides and fertilizers, and some are known human carcinogens.

In fact, Pollution prevention and pollution control are cancer prevention and cancer control. It can receive the effect of first-class anti-cancer, and it must prevent and control the three major pollutions, pollution prevention, pollution control, and overcome difficulties, can certainly achieve the benefits of cancer prevention, cancer control, reduce the incidence of cancer.

3. XZ-C proposed and formulated four Dawning cancer prevention plans, which was first proposed internationally.

The Cancer Prevention Research Institute will carry out cancer prevention system engineering and conduct microscopic view, ultra-micro view, high-tech research, monitor and analyze carcinogenic factors, and try to eliminate it. We have developed four Sun-up or Dawning Cancer Prevention Programs:

1).Dawning A-type plan:

<u>The Goal:</u> Try to study the microscopic study of air pollution caused by air pollution, and try to remove it to prevent air pollution leading to lung cancer.

Why is the anti-cancer system project the first to solve air pollution? Because the current global respiratory cancer has the highest incidence rate, 1.295 million /

8.18 million, both male and female are the first, therefore, how to solve the problem of preventing lung cancer is a top priority.

The Ways and methods: Through the microscopic view, ultra-micro view, high-tech monitoring and analysis of carcinogenic factors, try to detect, monitor, and try to remove it.

2).Dawning B plan

The Objective: To study the microscopic study of carcinogenic factors of environmental pollution caused by water pollution, and to eliminate cancers such as liver cancer, stomach cancer, and intestinal cancer caused by waterproof pollution.

Why do you currently have to pay attention to water pollution and cause cancer? Because the mother rivers of the whole country and the world are all polluted by industrial and agricultural sewage, urban sewage, river water pollution, carcinogens have increased significantly. Professor Xu Ze (XZ-C) suggested that efforts should be made to save the nation and the global mother river from being seriously polluted.

The ways and methods: "target"

To Solve the pollution of industrial and agricultural sewage, the first should try to reduce fertilizer
To solve urban and rural drinking water, it must be purified
To Resolve drinking water and drink standard water

(3) Dawning C-type plan

Already mentioned in Chapter 3 which **mainly is how to treat cancer.**

(4) Dawning D plan

Objective: To study the microscopic study of the carcinogenic factors of soil pollution to the environment
Try to solve the problem of chemical fertilizers, pesticides, genetic modification and cancer
Try to detect the presence or absence of carcinogenic factors from clothing, food, housing, and samples, and take samples of carcinogens from microscopic monitoring.
Ways and methods: Conduct microscopic detection and monitoring of cancer prevention, and put forward ethical standards for cancer prevention.
Through the above-mentioned Dawning A, B, and D-type plans, the pollution prevention and pollution control of the atmosphere, water, and soil are actually

<u>the first-class cancer prevention</u>, which can reduce the incidence of cancer, and can reach the green hills, the green water, and the mountains and rivers and the ecological environment of birds and flowers and Human living environment.

Because cancer patients cover the whole world, industrial and agricultural wastewater, waste residue, and exhaust gas pollution also cover the whole world. Therefore, it is necessary to globally attack the cancer attack.

Professor Xu Ze suggested:

1) All countries, provinces and states should establish anti-cancer research institutes (or institutions), carry out anti-cancer system projects, and carry out anti-cancer work for their own country, province and city.

2) Countries establish anti-cancer regulations and carry out comprehensively (some should be legislated)

3) I will use this project to recommend the World Health Organization to hold an anti-cancer campaign, with the goal of reducing the incidence of cancer. Conquering cancer is a frontier of science and a worldwide problem. Cancer is a human disaster. It covers the whole world. People all over the world are eager to hope that one day they can overcome cancer and benefit humanity.

C H A P T E R 5

XZ-C proposed Dawning C-type plan No.1-6

How to conquer cancer? How to treat cancer?

TABLE OF CONTENTS

1. What is Dawning C-type plan No.1-6?

A. There are the following 6 plans:

Dawning C-type plan No. 1: "conquer cancer and launch the total attack to cancer"
Dawning C-type plan No. 2: "Create the hospital with the whole process of prevention and treatment"
Dawning C-type plan No. 3: "Building a science city to overcome cancer"
Dawning C-type plan No. 4: "Building a multidisciplinary research group"
Dawning C-type plan No. 5: "The vaccine is human hope and immunological prevention"
Dawning C-type plan No. 6: "The prospect of immunomodulatory drugs is gratifying"

B. The detail Plans are the followings:

(1) Dawning C-type plan No. 1: "Conquer cancer and launch the total attack"

——The overall strategic reform and development of cancer treatment in China

a. Proposed a general plan and program and design and blueprint and accurate rules for conquering cancer
b. Avoid talk and attention to work hard, start to go
c. **No matter how far the road of conquering cancer is, you should always start to go**.
(see separate article)

(2) Dawning C-type plan No. 2: "Building the hospitals with the whole process of prevention and treatment"

(Global Demonstration Prevention and Treatment Hospital)
——Strategic reform, changing the mode of running a hospital and reforming treatment mode

(3) Dawning C-type plan No. 3: "Building a science city to overcome cancer"

——XZ-C proposes the overall design, planning and blueprint of Science City to overcome cancer and launch the general attack to cancer ; this is the only

91

way to overcome cancer; this is the "high-speed rail" and "high-speed" channel to overcome cancer)

(see separate article)

(4) Dawning C-type plan No. 4: "Building a multidisciplinary research group and laboratory"

- for the cause, pathogenesis, pathophysiology, metastasis, recurrence mechanism of cancer...

Study anti-cancer, anti-recurrence, anti-metastatic measures to improve the overall level of medical care

and benefit the patients.

——**The standard of efficacy evaluation is: long life expectancy, good quality of life, no complications or less, each school group is a provincial key or important laboratory.**

(see separate article)

(5) Dawning C-type plan No. 5: "The vaccine is human hope, immunological prevention"

—— Today's immunology prevention and treatment have become an extremely important in clinical medicine and preventive medicine

Required field

——△△group+△△group+△△group→Scientific Alliance, Joint Group

(see separate article)

(6) Dawning C-type plan No. 6:

A. "The prospect of immunomodulatory drugs is gratifying"

- Regardless of the complexity of the mechanisms behind cancer, immune suppression is the essence or key of the progression of cancer

——From the analysis of experimental results, obtaining the new discoveries and the new inspirations:

Thymus atrophy, immune function, immune surveillance ability and immune escape are one of the causes and pathogenesis of cancer, so the treatment principle should be to prevent thymus atrophy, promote thymic hyperplasia, and improve immune surveillance.

——XZ-C immune regulation and control Chinese medication is 48 kinds of Chinese herbal medicines with good cancer suppression rate in which there are 26 of them had better immune regulation and control selected and screened from 200 kinds of the traditional Chinese traditional Chinese herbal medications in vivo anti-tumor experiments In the animal model of cancer mice. (see separate article)

B. "The research group and laboratory of XZ-C immunomodulation anti-cancer Chinese medication active ingredient and the molecular level analysis"

—— Further research and development of XZ-C immunomodulation anti-cancer Chinese medicine active ingredients, molecular weight, structural formula and the molecular level analysis

——**Methods and steps:** animal experiment, molecular level experiment; gene level experiment, first

Separating the active ingredients makes the precious heritage of traditional Chinese medication modernization and scientific. (see separate article)

2. Dawning C-type plan in China

Hope: Apply to incorporate the "Dawning C-type plan" into the National Cancer Program

To Apply and report to *the Party Central Committee and the State Council* and *Hubei Provincial Party Committee and Provincial Government* and *Wuhan Municipal Party Committee and Municipal Government*

Goal: Conquer cancer

Mission: Prepare or set up a science city of conquering cancer and launching the general attack on cancer

The President of Science City, General Director, President of the General Academic Committee is **Professor Xu Ze** (Previous Director of Institute of Experimental Surgery, Hubei College of Traditional Chinese Medicine)

Science City Innovative Oncology Medical College
Innovative Cancer Research Institute:
Innovative Tumor hospital combined with Chinese and Western Medicine: } Chief Dean
General Secretary of Science City: } Hospital Leadership Team
Dean of the Graduate School of Science City:
The chief scientist team of Wuhan Anticancer Research Association:

The chief designer of "conquer cancer and launch the general attack
on cancer and to create a science city to overcome cancer"
Project Leader of "Overcoming the General Attack of Cancer"

} **Professor Dr Xu Ze**

"The Science City of Conquer Cancer" to establish the following genetic testing research groups:

(1) Establish genetic testing and cancer research groups and laboratories

(2) Establish HPV anti-cancer research group and laboratory

(3) Establish genetic testing and immunology and cancer research groups and laboratories

(4) Establish genetic testing and endocrine hormone and cancer research groups and laboratories

(5) Establish genetic testing and pathological sections, and related studies on immunohistochemistry

(6) Establish correlation analysis and research on gene detection and tumor markers

(7) Establish HPV treatment, exploration research groups and laboratories

The Expected results:

It is to use modern science and technology and analytical testing methods to study the traditional Chinese medication; the material basis of the efficacy of traditional Chinese medication in clinical practice is the chemical composition contained therein; to study the anticancer effect and mechanism of traditional Chinese medication, it is necessary to conduct in-depth research and analysis. The active ingredients in it make the precious heritage of traditional Chinese medication more modern and scientific.

After 28 years of experimental research, basic research and clinical verification, a series of "protecting Thymus and increase immune function" immunomodulatory anticancer Chinese medications XZ-Cl-10 had been screened. After 30 years of clinical observation, more than 12,000 cases have been verified, and the outpatient medical records have been saved, and **has a list of disease analysis; these medications can prolong life, improve symptoms, improve the quality of life, how to know and evaluate that the medications can extend the survival period? After the patients** <u>**who some surgical explorations can not be cut down (all pathological sections confirmed diagnosis), or have been widely transferred, it is estimated that only can be alive for 3-6 months, or 6-12 months**</u> **used XZ-C immune regulation and control anti-cancer medications of anti-metastasis and recurrence, some patients can still survive for 4 years - 5 years - 8 years - 10 years - 15 years with original data and complete data as well as follow-up data.**

After the recovery from heart attack, a retired professor calm down and hide in a small building, self-reliance, hard work, adhere to anti-cancer, anti-cancer metastasis, recurrence of animal experiment basic research and outpatient clinical validation research, from the year of the flower (60 years old)→To the age of the ancients (70s)→To the age of (80s), still perseverance, persevere in scientific research to overcome cancer, because he has retired, he failed to apply for projects and programs, so no research Funding is to fight alone, to fight alone, to be self-reliant, to work hard, no one cares, no one knows, nowhere to report, no support, **hard work for more than 30 years, has achieved a series of scientific and technological innovations, scientific research results, due to retirement In the past 20 years, no one cares, no one supports, retired professors, I don't know where and who will take care or manage, where and who can support and where the scientific research results are reported, I have to make a "monograph" for the benefit of mankind,** but published a series of monographs, and then Report to the Provincial Department of Science and Technology and the Provincial Department of Education: 1 hope to open an international high-end academic forum; 2 report to the government to apply for cancer, launch a general attack; 3 report to the province and the government. Hope: Apply to establish the "National Science City to overcome the general attack of cancer" in Hubei and Wuhan, which is the "World's first science city to overcome the general attack of cancer."

How to implement this unprecedented event in human history?

(1) Reporting to the government, requesting instructions
(2) Report to the province and city, request instructions
(3) Make recommendations to the city to build in Wuhan: "The first national cancer science city"
"The world's first to overcome Cancer Science City"

3. "Cancer moon shot" (US) and "Dawning C-type plan" (middle

How to overcome cancer? XZ-C proposes that cancer is a disaster for all mankind and must be fought together by the people of the world.
- Moving forward together, heading for the science hall to overcome cancer
Why do you want to move forward together? What are you together?

(1) Introduction to "Cancer Moon Shot"

On January 12, 2016, US President Barack Obama announced in his last State of the Union address during his term of office a national plan to overcome cancer, the "Cancer Moon Shot", which will be under the responsibility of Biden.

Biden will visit the Abramson Cancer Center at the University of Pennsylvania School of Medicine next week to discuss the plan. He said that the "new moon landing plan" is a commitment to overcome cancer in the world and will inspire a new generation of scientists to explore the scientific world.

Obama did not mention the specific plan of the plan in his speech, but he mentioned that the expenditure and tax bill passed by Congress in December 2015 has raised the financial budget of the National Institutes of Health (NIH).

The United States has just recently established a national immunotherapy alliance consisting of pharmaceutical companies, biotechnology companies and academic medical organizations. The alliance is trying to develop a vaccine immunotherapy by 2020 to overcome cancer and complete cancer. Monthly plan."

The American Society of Clinical Oncology (ASCO) issued a statement on its website to welcome Obama's "New Moon Plan" and support Biden's leadership, arguing that the "New Moon Plan" will reduce the pain and reduce the risk of cancer for humans. Death caused by cancer. The statement mentions that "all effective treatments should be transformed from the laboratory to the clinic"; the application of "big data" technology, such as ASCO's "CancerLinQ" rapid learning system, can accelerate the pace of cancer. Enable physicians to better develop individualized treatment options for each patient and understand which areas are urgently needed to invest more research (Liu Quan).

(January 21, 2016, China Medical Tribune)

(2) Introduction to the Dawning C plan

1). Before January 12, 2016, the progress of the scientific research plan "to overcome the general attack on cancer"

2). Before January 12, 2016, we have carried out scientific research and scientific innovation series with the research direction of cancer.

3 Dawning C plan

4. XZ-C first proposed "Dawning C-type plan" No.1-6 internationally

a. Why use "Dawning "?

The dawning or Sunrise is the morning light, it is the dawn, it is the morning sun.
Vigorous, vigorous, original innovation, independent innovation
C=China
Type C = Chinese mode
About 8550 people in China are diagnosed with cancer every day, and 6 people are diagnosed with cancer every minute. Therefore, the research work of conquering cancer and launching the general attack to cancer can not walk slowly and should run forward to save the wounded.
Time is money, time is money = one inch of time, one inch of gold
Time is life, time is life
Time flies, time flies
Empty talking will make mistakes; It should do hard work; It avoids talk and it should work hard and should start to go. No matter how far the road to cancer is, you should always start.
This research plan is the original innovation, it is time to declare war on cancer, and the general attack should be launched. Our dreams are to conquer cancer, build a well-off society, everyone is healthy, away from cancer

b. Dawning C plan

1. Dawning C-type plan No. 1: "Collecting cancer, launching the general attack"
Anti-control + treatment and treatment, and drive together, put forward the general idea and design of conquering cancer
——The overall strategic reform and development of cancer treatment in China
Turn treatment-oriented to focus on prevention and treatment (see separate article)
Avoid talk, work hard, start off
No matter how far the road to cancer is, you should always start.

2. Shuguang C-type plan No. 2: "Preparation of the whole process of prevention and treatment of hospitals"
(Global Demonstration Prevention and Treatment Hospital)
Strategic reform, changing the mode of running a hospital
Reforming treatment mode

Target: three early, precancerous lesions, carcinoma in situ
Research early diagnostic methods, reagents, techniques, theory
Research on early methods, techniques, and theories
Study chemical anti-cancer, endocrine and cancer prevention
Research to promote cancer prevention, "hold your mouth" to prevent cancer
(see separate article)

3. Dawning C-type plan No. 3: "Building a science city to overcome cancer"
Preparing an innovative molecular tumor medical school
Innovative molecular level integrated Chinese and Western medicine hospital
Innovative Molecular Oncology Institute
Innovative Environmental Protection and Health Cancer Research Institute
Innovative molecular tumor nano preparations
Cancer Animal Experimental Center
This is the only way to overcome cancer
This is the "high-speed rail" and "high-speed" channel for cancer (see separate article)

4. Shuguang C-type plan No. 4 "Building a multi-disciplinary research group"
(For the cause, pathogenesis, pathophysiology, metastasis, recurrence mechanism of cancer...
Anti-cancer, anti-metastasis, recurrence measures)
Form:
A, Immunology and Cancer Research Group and Laboratory
B, virus and cancer research groups and laboratories
C, (endocrine) hormone and cancer research groups and laboratories
D. Environmental and Cancer Research Group and Laboratory
E, fungal and cancer research groups and laboratories
F, Molecular Biology and Cancer Research Group and Laboratory
G, Genetic Engineering and Cancer Research Group and Laboratory
H, Chinese Medicine and Cancer Research Group and Laboratory
I, Three Early and Cancer Research Groups and Laboratories
J, precancerous lesions and cancer research groups and laboratories

The objectives, tasks, planning, implementation, coordination of projects, projects, and goals of the above research groups, research institutes, and research institutes; scientific research achievements, scientific and technological innovation. To overcome the cancer research direction, to benefit patients with the overall level of medical treatment, the criteria for efficacy evaluation are: long survival time, good quality of life, and no or no complications. Each school group is a provincial key laboratory.

(see separate article)

5. Dawning C-type plan No. 5 "vaccine is the hope of human beings Immunological prevention"

With the development of immunology theory and technology, human application of immunological control methods has successfully eliminated smallpox and effectively controlled the spread of many infectious diseases. Immunology prevention has made tremendous contributions in the history of medical development. (A case of rabies, whooping cough, tetanus, influenza, hepatitis B, measles, water beans, etc.), today's immunological prevention has become an extremely important field in clinical medicine and preventive medicine.

Form:

Immunology group + virology group + △ △ group + △ △ group → scientific alliance, science conquer cancer group, alliance

A, anti-hepatitis B vaccine → further suppression of cirrhosis → anti-hepatocellular vaccine

B. Development of EB virus vaccine for prevention and treatment of nasopharyngeal carcinoma

C, research and treatment of viral lymphoma

D. Studying virus particles in breast milk to prevent breast cancer vaccine

E. Studying herpes simplex type 2 virus to prevent cervical cancer vaccine

F. Study on the relationship between type C virus and leukemia, sarcoma and sputum gold lymphoma

Study vaccines to prevent their occurrence and control their prevalence

composition:

Immunization and Cancer Research Group

Virus and Cancer Research Group

Goal: Immunization prevention

Specific immunization target (target): development of cancer vaccine

Possibility: Hepatitis B vaccine + Dawning C plan → Liver cancer vaccine

Milk Ca vaccine

Ovarian Ca vaccine

Prostate Ca vaccine

Lymphoma vaccine

Leukemia vaccine

The experimental center is located in Huangjiahu, Science City, Cancer Experimental Animal Center.

It is required to start from the city, the municipal science association, and the Wuhan University, accelerate the formation, and implement the plan.

Implementation and completion methods:

1 graduate student 100; 2 city and province combination

3 Wuhan Anti-Ca Research Association collaborates with universities and research institutes

The chief conductor and chief designer are Professor Xu Ze, Professor Gong Feili, and academic committee members:

a laboratory building, a single column, and the United States

Hurry: than: super

Experiment first - you can get a batch of papers, results

Post-clinical - based on the above success

Establishing an immunology laboratory

Immunological test

Immunomolecular detection: complement determination

Immunoglobulin assay

Cytokine detection

Immune cells and their function tests

Basic technology of immunology experiment

Research and prospects of new vaccines

(see separate article)

6. Sunrise C-type plan No. 6 "Immune regulation drug prospects gratifying"

Defects in abnormal immune function can lead to a variety of diseases, such as autoimmune diseases, immunodeficiency diseases and tumors.

Immunotherapy consists of two aspects: immune regulation and immune reconstitution.

Immunomodulators can be divided into synthetic drugs, microbial preparations, immune molecules, immune cells and Chinese herbal medicines according to their sources.

With the development of immunology and penetration with other disciplines, a large class of biologically active substances with immunomodulatory effects have been discovered. They have a wide range of biological activities and anti-tumor activities, collectively referred to as biological response modifiers (BRM). The research and application of BRM is an important advancement in modern immunotherapy.

Regardless of the complexity of the mechanisms behind cancer, immune suppression is the key to cancer progression. By removing immunosuppressive factors and restoring the recognition of cancer cells by systemic cells, it is effective against cancer.

In order to explore the etiology, pathogenesis and pathophysiology of cancer, we conducted a series of animal experiments. From the analysis of experimental results, we obtained new findings and new enlightenments: thymus atrophy and low immune function are one of the causes and pathogenesis of cancer. Therefore, Professor Xu Ze proposed one of the causes and pathogenesis of cancer at international academic conferences, which may be thymus atrophy, central immune organ damage, immune dysfunction, decreased immune surveillance, and immune escape.

As a result of the above laboratory experiments, it was found that the cancer-bearing animal model had progressive thymus atrophy and low immune function. Therefore, the treatment principle must be to prevent progressive atrophy of the thymus, promote thymic hyperplasia, protect bone marrow hematopoietic function, improve immune surveillance, and provide theoretical basis and experimental basis for immune regulation and treatment of cancer.

XZ-C immunomodulatory Chinese medicine is a traditional Chinese herbal medicine from China. It has screened 48 kinds of Chinese herbal medicines with good cancer suppression rate in mice with cancer-bearing mice. After compounding, it inhibits tumor growth in mice. The compound tumor inhibition rate is much higher than that of single drug inhibition. Among them, XZ-C1100% inhibits cancer cells from killing 100% of normal cells, XZ-C4 promotes lymphocyte transformation, enhances cellular immune function, inhibits cancer cells, and prevents thymus atrophy. It promotes thymic hyperplasia and is a promising immunomodulatory anticancer drug in clinical practice. It should be further researched and developed to benefit the majority of cancer patients.

c. Shuguang C-type plan No. 6

① **To build anti-cancer, anti-cancer metastatic active ingredients, analytical research groups and laboratories**

The goals :

(1) Further research and clinical application and clinical application of XZ-C immunomodulation anti-cancer Chinese medicine cell molecular and molecular levels.

(2) Further research on the prevention and treatment of early cancer in situ and precancerous lesions by anti-cancer and anti-cancer Chinese herbal medicines and its clinical application.

(3) Further research and development of the effective components, molecular weight and structural formula of XZ-C immunomodulation anticancer Chinese medicine.

(4) Further research and development of the XZ-C1-10 series of drugs to carry out the following studies one by one:

1)Z-CA→Z-CB→Z-CC→......→Z-CZ

A total of 26 kinds, divided into 6 batches, 4 in each batch, each batch takes 4 months

2) For example, Z-CA steps and content:

A, Z-CA phytochemical study: extraction and identification

B, Z-CA immunopharmacology:

a. toxicity
b. Changes in immune organs in mice (thymus, spleen, brain, liver, kidney)
c. the effect on the peripheral cells of mice
d. the effect of mouse peritoneal autophagic cells (MΦ) function
e. the effect on mouse T lymphocytes

C, main components, chemical structure
D, pharmacological effects
E, preparation of preparation

Purpose:

In-depth development of Chinese herbal medicine anti-cancer, anti-cancer metastasis is indeed an effective drug, to crude storage, to the false truth, natural medicine Chinese herbal medicine as a resource, modern research, so that become a precise medicine.

Method steps:

(1) Animal experiment: a, in vitro experiment screening

b, in vivo experimental screening
c, experimental tumor model

(2) Experimental study at the molecular level: screening of Chinese herbal medicine for anti-cancer and anti-cancer metastasis

Induction of differentiation of precancerous lesions

(3) Gene level experimental study of anti-cancer, anti-cancer transfer Chinese herbal medicine screening

Topic selection and selection: Firstly, the Chinese herbal medicine which is effective in clinical application will be further studied, and the active ingredients will be separated first.

The laboratory:

(1) Equipment: equipment for pharmaceutical composition analysis
(2) Personnel: Scientific and technical personnel who can conduct drug composition analysis
(3) Topic selection and material selection

The Expected results:

Using modern science and technology and analytical testing methods, the research on traditional Chinese medicine, the material basis of the efficacy of traditional Chinese medicine in clinical practice is the chemical composition contained therein. To study the anticancer effect and mechanism of traditional Chinese medicine, it is necessary to conduct in-depth research and analysis. The active ingredients in it make the precious heritage of traditional Chinese medicine more modern and scientific.

After 7 years and 28 years of experimental research, basic research and clinical verification, the series of "Chest Enhancement" immune regulation anti-cancer Chinese medicine XZ-C1-10 has been screened. After 20 years of clinical observation, more than 12,000 cases have been verified. Can prolong life, improve symptoms, improve quality of life, how to know, evaluate can prolong survival? Some surgical explorations can not be cut down (all pathological sections confirmed diagnosis), or have been widely transferred, it is estimated that only 3-6 months, or 6-12 months of cases, XZ-C immune regulation and anti-cancer, For patients with anti-metastasis and recurrence, some patients can still survive for 4 to 5 years to 8 years, with original data and complete data as well as follow-up data.

A retired professor, after rehabilitation of the heart attack, calm down, hide in a small building, self-reliance, hard work, adhere to the basic research of animal experiments and clinical validation of anti-cancer, anti-cancer metastasis, recurrence, by the flower Year → to the age of ancient times → to the year of ages, still perseverance, persevere in scientific research, because he has retired, failed to apply for projects, projects, so no research funding, is alone, fighting alone, no one cares, hard work For more than 20 years, he has obtained a series of scientific and technological innovations and scientific research achievements, published a series of monographs, and then reported to the Provincial Science and Technology Department and the Provincial Department of Education: 1 hope to open an academic council or high-end academic forum; 2 report to the government to apply for cancer And launch the general attack; 3 report to the provinces and departments to set up the province and the city to overcome the cancer test area (station), and try first.

② The Preparation for publishing work: cancer prevention, anti-cancer

Wuhan Anti-Cancer Research Society will publish the following publications and monographs

1. Popularize anti-Ca scientific research and popular science maps
2. the publication of anti-Ca, anti-Ca science reading "People's Medicine" quarterly
3. published magazine publication "Clinical recurrence, metastasis based and clinical" bimonthly
4. Publish the monograph on "The Road to Conquer Cancer"
5. the publication of "tumor-free technology" - how to do a good radical cancer surgery, intraoperative anti-recurrence, anti-metastasis monograph
6. Publication of "Three Early" and "Precancerous Lesions" publications
7. Publication of the journal "From clothing, food, housing, and anti-cancer knowledge", quarterly

CHAPTER 6

"Walked out of a new way of cancer treatment with immune regulation and control combined with Chinese and Western medications"

The main points of "Walking out of a new road to conquer cancer"

The Experimental research: **Anti-cancer research of Chinese medication immunopharmacology and the combination of Chinese medicine with Western medications at the molecular level**

——Step out of a new way of conquer cancer with XZ-C immune regulation and control combined Chinese medication with Western medication at the molecular level

——Step out of a new road of conquering cancer with traditional Chinese medication immune regulation and control, regulate immune activity, prevent thymus atrophy, promote Thymic hyperplasia, protect bone marrow hematopoietic function, improves immune surveillance combined Chinese medicine and Western medicine at the molecular level

- navigate
- Path finding and footprint
- Walking out of a new way of cancer treatment with XZ-C immune regulation and control combining Western medication and Chinese medication at the molecular level
- Has formed the theory basic and experimental basis of cancer immune treatment and theoretical system of cancer treatment of XZ-C immune regulation and control

- A series of products of XZ-C immune regulation and control anti-cancer Chinese medicine and adaptation range
- XZ-C immunomodulation anticancer Chinese medicine is the result of the modernization of traditional Chinese medication

TABLE OF CONTENTS

Foreword (1)

Why did I take the title of the book as: "Getting out of a new road to overcome cancer", the title of the book is due to the guidance and inspiration from several experts, scholars, predecessors, and teachers.

On July 2, 2001, Academician Wu Wei mentioned in his letter: "The overall impression is: from clinical to experimental, from experimental to clinical mode is very good, the road of combining Chinese and Western is also very correct, I sincerely wish you Keep moving forward and get out of a new path to overcome cancer."

On February 22, 2006, Academician Tang Yu mentioned in his letter: "... Chinese medicine and biological therapy are the two most promising ways to resist metastasis, especially Chinese medicine. I hope that you will get out of the anti-metastasis road with Chinese characteristics."

On March 22, 2006, Academician Liu Yunyi mentioned in his letter: "...I agree with your concept and thinking about cancer in your book... I hope that you can make a breakthrough contribution to traditional Chinese medicine to make the majority of patients Benefiting, the traditional Chinese medicine can be further developed, and my medical career will reach a world status."

On January 9, 2006, Academician Wu Xianzhong mentioned in his letter: "... the tumor is a difficult bone, but it should continue to be continued. Fortunately, everyone is very objective, only if it is effective, whether it is treating the tumor or the body. In the letter of April 10, 2012, "We think that the road you have traveled is very special. Methods, drug combinations, and the development of XZ-C series of drugs have all innovated and formed their own patents. This road should continue."

Thanks for their guidance, guidance, and assistance in our research work, research thinking, research direction, research routes, research goals, and research methods. Our research work has been working in the direction of its guidance. I would like to express my gratitude to the academicians Wu Hao, Tang Wei, Wu Xianzhong and Liu Yunyi.

In the past 28 years (1985-present), cancer research has achieved a series of scientific and technological innovations and scientific research achievements in animal experimental research, clinical basic research and clinical verification. After 20 years of hard work, XZ-C immune regulation has been initially formed. Anti-cancer treatment. In the past 20 years, a new road to cancer has been taken out.

In the past 20 years, this series of experimental and clinical research work has received enthusiastic support and cordial guidance from internationally renowned foreign scientists and Chinese general practitioners. In 1990, when the author submitted the "Eighth Five-Year Plan" key scientific and technological research project to the State Science and Technology Commission (to further explore the anti-cancer and anti-metastasis experimental and clinical studies of cancer and anti-cancer Chinese herbal medicine for precancerous lesions of liver cancer and gastrointestinal cancer), Academician Yan said in an expert opinion: "It is a very important topic to study cancer metastasis and how to prevent metastasis. It is feasible to explore clinical prevention methods through experimental research and it is beneficial to people's work." Under the guidance of my teacher, rigorous academics, and scientific study, we have initially completed the above projects, and I would like to thank you.

Scientific research must have nutritional feeding of the literature. In 1986, we just established an experimental surgical animal laboratory to make an animal model of cancer metastasis and conduct experimental research. We saw Professor Gao Jin's book "Invasion and Metastasis of Cancer - Basic Research and Clinical Medicine", and saw the monograph of Academician Tang Wei, "Basic and Clinical Metastasis and Recurrence of Liver Cancer". The theories in the two books make us suddenly clear. It also encourages and promotes our experimental work and clinical validation work from another aspect. Professor Tang Wei proposed in his monograph: "The next important goal of primary liver cancer research - prevention and treatment of recurrence and metastasis", and said: "Transfer recurrence has become a bottleneck to further improve the survival rate of liver cancer, and it is also the most important to overcome cancer. One of the difficulties." These theoretical documents have given us the wisdom and courage to update our thinking and be brave in innovation, and have also strengthened the confidence and determination of our experimental team. I would like to express my gratitude to Academician Tang Wei and Professor Gao Jin.

In the past 7 years, we have used more than 6,000 tumor-bearing animal models to explore one basic problem after another. The screening of 200 kinds of Chinese herbal medicines in the tumor-bearing animal model in vivo was carried out by several graduate students. Master Zhu Siping, Dr. Zou Shaomin, Master Li Zhengxun, Master of Liu Wei, etc., they carried out and completed a lot of hard work. The experimental work, hard work, day and night, contributed to the development of experimental oncology medicine for anti-cancer and anti-cancer. I sincerely thank you all.

Foreword (2)

Experimental surgery is extremely important in the development of medicine. It is a key to opening the medical exclusion zone. Many disease prevention methods have been studied in many animal experiments, and the stability results have been applied to the clinic to promote the development of the medical cause.

Developing science and technological innovation, the laboratory is the key condition. I deeply understand the importance of the laboratory. I am the first batch of college students in the post-liberation college entrance examination. I have not studied or studied abroad, but I have achieved many international achievements. The key is that I have a good laboratory. In the 1960s, I participated in the open heart surgery laboratory for cardiopulmonary bypass. In the 1980s, I established a cirrhosis ascites laboratory. In the 1990s, I established the Institute of Experimental Surgery to focus on cancer. My animal laboratory has good equipment conditions, including white mice, white rats, Dutch pigs, rabbits, dogs, monkeys and other animal experiments. It has a good sterilization operating room and can be used for major surgery and animals in the chest and abdomen. After the postoperative observation room, various designs, ideas, and experimental operations can be used to achieve results or conclusions.

Therefore, the laboratory is the key condition, and the key is to build a good equipment laboratory.

University teachers should have dual tasks on their shoulders. One is to do a good job of teaching; the other is to develop science.

University teachers should have good laboratories for scientific research, follow the scientific development concept, base on known science, explore unknown science, face the future science, emerging disciplines, marginal disciplines, interdisciplinary, face the frontiers of science, strive for innovation, advancement, The hall of science, adding bricks and tiles.

In summary, experimental research and basic research are very important. Without experimental research and breakthroughs in basic research, clinical efficacy is difficult to improve, and it is difficult to propose new understandings, new concepts, and new theoretical insights. Among them, the experiment is the key. I have a good laboratory. I am the director of the Institute of Experimental Surgery and the director of clinical surgery. The experimental research, basic research and clinical verification are easy to take care of.

Basic research in medicine is very important for achieving progress in combating diseases. Experimental oncology is the basic science of cancer prevention research and has promoted the continuous development of cancer research in China.

Our Experimental Surgery Institute conducted a series of experimental studies to explore the mechanisms of cancer onset, invasion and recurrence and metastasis. We conducted a full-scale experimental study of tumors in the laboratory for 4 years. From experimental tumor research, we found that thymus atrophy and immune function are low. May be the cause of the tumor, one of the pathogenesis, how to prevent thymus atrophy? How to regulate immune function is low? How to promote immunity? How to "protect the chest"? Immune regulation should be carried out, and Western medicine should be combined at the molecular level to embark on a new path of Chinese characteristics to overcome cancer.

Facing the future of medicine, we will look forward to the future. After 20 years of hard work, we will practice the scientific development concept and face the frontier of science, striving for innovation and progress. To overcome cancer, we must come from the clinical, through experimental research, to the clinical, to solve the actual problems of patients; must seek truth from facts, use facts, use data to speak; must constantly self-transcend, self-advance; in scientific research should emancipate the mind, Breaking away the traditional old ideas, based on independent innovation and original innovation; our research route for decades is to find problems → ask questions → study problems → solve problems or explain problems, the road is like this, step by step, difficult trek, we hope Stepping out of an innovative road of anti-cancer and anti-transfer with Chinese characteristics and independent intellectual property rights.

Our research on oncology medical research is based on patients, discovering and asking questions from clinical work, conducting in-depth basic research on animal experiments, and then turning basic research results into clinical applications to improve the overall level of medical care and ultimately benefit patients.

1. Walked out of a new road of conquering cancer

The Experimental research, Chinese medicine immunopharmacology and molecular level Chinese and Western medicine combined with anti-cancer research

1).The New findings in anti-cancer and anti-cancer metastasis research

Implications of anti-cancer metastasis research:
I am a clinical surgeon. Why do you study cancer? This is due to the results of a patient interview with a group of cancer patients.
In 1985, I conducted more than 5000 cancer patients operation and did a survey

to all of my patient. There were more than 3,000 patients with postoperative chest and abdominal cancer who gave me reply. The results showed that most of the patients relapsed or metastasized 2-3 years after surgery, and some even after several months and one year after surgery. Recurrence and metastasis.

From the follow-up results, it was found that postoperative recurrence and metastasis were the key factors affecting the long-term efficacy of surgery.

Therefore, we also raised an important issue: **clinicians must pay attention to and study the prevention and treatment of postoperative recurrence and metastasis, in order to improve the long-term efficacy of postoperative.** Therefore, it is necessary to conduct an experimental study of the clinical basis of recurrence and metastasis. Without a breakthrough in basic research, clinical efficacy is difficult to improve.

So we established the Experimental Surgery Laboratory (later established the Experimental Surgery Research Institute of Hubei College of Traditional Chinese Medicine in 1991, the research direction is to conquer cancer).

We have carried out research from the following two aspects: one is animal experimental research: one is clinical research. Based on the success of animal experiments, it is applied clinically for clinical validation. After 30 years of hard work, a series of experimental research and clinical verification work were carried out, and a series of scientific and technological innovations were obtained.

New discovery

(1) From the results of follow-up, it was found that:

1. The postoperative recurrence and metastasis are the key factors affecting the long-term efficacy of surgery.
2. The clinicians must pay attention to and study the prevention and treatment measures for the postoperative recurrence and metastasis.

(2) From the experimental tumor research it was found:

1. Excision of the thymus (Thymus, TH) can be used to create a cancer-bearing animal model. Injection of immunosuppressive agents can also contribute to the establishment of a cancer-bearing animal model. **The conclusion of the study clearly proves that the occurrence and development of cancer has a clear positive relationship with the immune organs TH of the host and the tissue function of the immune organs. It is difficult to manufacture animal models without removing the TH.** Repeated experiments repeatedly confirmed the experimental results.

2. **Whether it is immune first and then easy to get cancer or cancer first and then low immunity, our experimental results are: first, there is low immunity and then easy to have cancer, the development, if no immune function decline, it is not easy to vaccinate successfully. The results of this study suggest that improving and maintaining good immune function and protecting the thymus of the immune organs is one of the important measures to prevent cancer.**

3. The animal model of liver metastasis was established in our laboratory to study the relationship between metastasis and immunity in cancer. Group A and B were divided into groups. Group A used immunosuppressants, and group B was different. The result was that the number of intrahepatic metastases in group A was significantly higher than that in group B. **The results of this experiment suggest that metastasis is associated with immunity, low immune function or the use of immunosuppressive agents may promote tumor metastasis.**

4. Our laboratory conducted an experiment to investigate the effects of tumors on the immune organs of the body. It was found that the thymus was progressively atrophied as the cancer progressed. Immediately after inoculation of cancer cells, the thymus of the host showed acute progressive atrophy, cell proliferation was blocked, and the volume was significantly reduced. **The results of this experiment suggest that the tumor will inhibit the thymus and cause the immune organs to shrink.**

5. Through experiments we also found that some experimental mice were not vaccinated, or the tumor grew very small, the thymus did not significantly shrink. In order to understand the relationship between tumor and thymus atrophy, we experimented in a group of experimental mice transplanted solid tumors. When the tumor grew to the size of the thumb, it was removed. After 1 month, the thymus was found to have no progressive atrophy. **Therefore, we speculate that a solid tumor may produce a factor that is not known to inhibit the thymus, which needs further study.**

6. **The results of the above experiments prove that the progression of the tumor causes the thymus to progressively shrink. Then, can we use some methods to prevent the host thymus from shrinking? Therefore, we further designed and wanted to use this immune organ cell transplantation to restore the experimental function of the immune organ.** Our laboratory is investigating the atrophy of the thymus gland during suppressing tumor progression, looking for ways to restore the function of the thymus and reconstituting the immune system. The experimental study of the reconstruction of its immune

function was performed by fetal liver, fetal spleen, and fetal thymus cell transplantation in mice. The results showed that: S, T, L three groups of cells combined transplantation, the recent complete tumor regression rate was 40%, the long-term tumor complete regression rate was 46.67%, and the tumor disappeared long-term survival.

7. When we explored the effect of tumor on the spleen of the immune organs of the body, we found that the spleen has an inhibitory effect on tumor growth in the early stage of the tumor, and in the late stage of the tumor, the spleen also shows progressive atrophy. The results of this study suggest that the spleen has a bidirectional effect on tumor growth, which has a certain inhibitory effect in the early stage and loses its inhibitory effect in the late stage. Spleen cell transplantation can enhance the inhibition of tumors. This is a new discovery in experimental research and is a very important finding that should be further studied.

In summary, from the above series of experimental studies, it is found that thymus atrophy, immune dysfunction may be one of the causes and pathogenesis of cancer, and should further do research from the function and tissue structure of the thymus, immune function is low and how to promote immunity, and how immune function can be reconstructed? how to protect Thymus and increase immune function. The following part is to review the structure of the thymus and the function of the thymus, and find new ways and means of cancer treatment.

The experimental research parts:

2). Experimental observation of the influence of tumor on the thymus of immune organs

It is generally believed that the immune function of the body affects the occurrence and development and prognosis of the tumor, and the tumor also has an inhibitory effect on the immune state of the body. The two are causal and intricate. In the animal experiment of the effect of spleen on tumor growth, the author observed that many changes occurred in the thymus and spleen of the immune organs in the tumor-bearing mice. It seems that there is a certain regularity. In order to further explore the relationship between tumor and spleen and thymus and its regularity, the following experiments were designed to dynamically observe the changes of thymus, spleen and lymphocyte transformation rate at different stages in tumor-bearing mice and to explore the regularity between them.

【Materials and Methods】

(1).Experimental animals and grouping

40 Kunming mice were randomly divided into 4 groups, aged 40~50d, weighing 15~18g. Male or female.

Group I: healthy control group, healthy mice that were not inoculated with cancer cells, and the thymus, spleen and peripheral blood were taken for observation after sacrifice.

Group II: 0.1×107 Ehrlich ascites tumor cells were inoculated intraperitoneally, and sacrificed after 3 days.

Group III: Inoculated tumor cells (the same as above), and sacrificed on the 7th day.

Group IV: Observation on the 14th day of inoculation of tumor cells.

Take the experiment results of autopsy after 100 natural deaths in tumor-bearing mice in the previous experiment (the experimental study on the effect of spleen on tumor growth) as a result of changes in thymus and spleen of advanced tumor. The average diameter thymus in late stage tumor-bearing mice is (1.2 ± 0.3) mm, the average weight is (20 ± 5) mg, and the texture is hard. The spleen is extremely atrophied, with an average weight of (60 ± 12) mg. The texture is hard, the color is gray, the growth center is significantly reduced, and fibrosis occurs.

(2) Experimental method

Each group of mice was sacrificed by excretion of the eyeball at the scheduled time. Each mouse was given 1 ml of whole blood (heparin anticoagulation) for lymphocyte transformation test, and then the mice were immediately dissected to observe the tumor. Infiltration range, ascites volume and the involvement of various organs, and the anatomy of the thymus, spleen and lymph nodes were observed with the naked eye. The thymus and spleen were completely removed, and the volume was measured with a vernier caliper.

[Experimental results]

(1) The weight of thymus at different stages after inoculation of tumor cells in mice is shown in Table as the following:

Perform variance analysis on Table 1, see Table 2. The results of Tables 1 and 2 are shown by curves, and the thymus weight change curve (Fig. 1) is plotted. The weight of the thymus on the 25th and 30th days in the figure is from the experimental results in the previous.

Table 1 Comparison of thymus weights of mice in groups (mg)

Group	Group I Control	Group II on the 3rd after inoculated	Group III on the 7rd after inoculated	Group IV on the 14rd after inoculated	Group On the 25th after inoculated	Group On the 30th after inoculated
Xij	72.8 50.0 56.4 96.4 77.4 100.7 87.5 76.8 112.7 51.0	78.2 83.4 89 68 74.8 95.4 115.0 56.4 43.0	90.0 66.0 85.4 106.5 51.7 77.8 73.0 60.0 49.4	40.0 32.2 39.8 23.5 38.0 36.0 46.0 20.0 55 20	25.13 29.46 28.90 26.77 27.00 28.00 26.78 27.69 31.37 28.90	16.90 17.00 19.05 18.16 16.98 20.01 19.23 18.98 18.54 15.15
ΣX N XI ΣX^2	781.07 10 78.17 66261.79	703.2 9 78.13 58566.66	736.3 10 73.63 57033.75	350.5 10 35.05 18467.25	280 10 28.00 7867.44	180 10 18.00 6518.612

Table 2 Analysis of variance of table 1

Resources of variation	SS	V	MS	F	P
Between groups within groups	12967.10 11777.12	3 35	4322.36 336.48	12.85	<0.01
Total	24744.22				

It can be seen from Table 1, Table 2, and Figure 1 that the thymus of the tumor-bearing mice showed a regular change. Within 7 days after inoculation, there was no significant change in the thymus macroscopic view, but the weight had begun to decrease after 7 day, it is acute progressive atrophy. The diameter of each leaf of the late thymus is reduced from the normal 5~8mm to about 1mm, the weight is reduced from 76.1mg to 20mg, the texture becomes hard, and the function is also reduced or even lost. It shows that the cellular immune function of the body is increasingly manipulated and inhibited as the tumor progresses, causing the immune function to be low and the tumor to grow faster and faster.

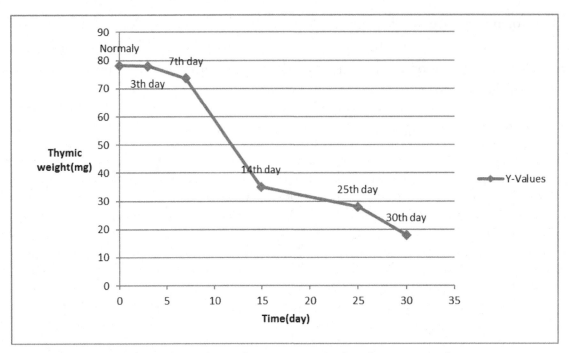

Figure 1 the curve of variation on the thymic weights

(2) Pathological changes in the thymus

Thymus: progressive atrophy throughout the course of the disease. On the third day after inoculation of the tumor cells, the thymus was slightly shrunk and the color was slightly gray. On the 7th day after inoculation, the thymus volume was significantly atrophied, cell proliferation was blocked, and mature cells were reduced. By the end of the tumor, the thymus is extremely atrophied, the volume is about the size of sesame seeds, the diameter is 1mm, and the texture becomes hard.

(3) About the effect of tumor on the thymus

The experimental results show that after inoculation of the tumor cells, the thymus is immediately suppressed, and the whole process is progressively atrophied, so the thymus quickly loses the anti-tumor immune effect. It was observed in the experiment that the thymus gland changed its morphological structure shortly after inoculation of the tumor cells, and the whole course of disease showed progressive atrophy. By the end of the tumor, the weight of the thymus was reduced from 78.13±13.2 mg to 20±5 mg, and the volume was reduced from 5 to 8 mm in diameter to 1 mm. Cell proliferation was significantly blocked.

Due to progressive atrophy of the thymus, cell proliferation is blocked, mature cells are reduced or depleted, the index is decreased, metabolism is weakened, cell viability is decreased, and thymus hormone secretion is also reduced. The cellular immune function of the body is inevitably damaged, and the defense ability of the mouse is low. The transplanted cancer cells grow and multiply. Zhang Tongwen and other similar reports have found that the thymus atrophy of tumor-bearing mice is accompanied by **the inhibition of bone marrow** cell proliferation and the decrease of nucleated cell viability, and it is considered that there is a close relationship between the two. It can be seen that the inhibition or damage effect of the tumor on the host immune function is multifaceted, affecting the entire immune system of the body. The lymphocyte transformation rate test of this group showed that the lymphocyte transformation rate decreased progressively after inoculation of cancer cells, and decreased to more than 50% in the late stage, which also indicated that the cellular immune effect was inhibited. As for why the thymus of tumor-bearing mice is inhibited and atrophied, further experimental research and observation are needed.

The thymus also produces a variety of thymus hormones that promote the differentiation and maturation of immune lymphocyte stem cells. Although the thymus is a lymphoid organ, due to the presence of the blood thymus barrier, the thymus does not directly interact with the antigenic substance to exert an effect. Thus, it is not proliferated by the stimulation of tumor-specific antigens. The tumor produces secretory immunosuppressive factors that act on the thymus, causing progressive atrophy and functional damage.

Immunotherapy for malignant tumors: many doctors are committed to the development of this field with great interest.

Since the 1980s, due to the rapid development of immunology and biotechnology, it has provided an opportunity for immunotherapy for cancer patients. The theory of biological response regulation has been proposed and a fourth therapeutic program other than surgery, radiotherapy, and chemotherapy has been established. That is tumor biotherapy (BRM). The use of biological modulators to treat tumors may be promising for the development of new therapies for effective immunotherapy for tumors.

In short, the host and the tumor are a contradiction, and have existed throughout the process of tumor development and development. In the case of a healthy function of the body's immune system, the body can restrict and destroy tumors through its cellular and humoral immune responses. On the other hand, the growing tumor has a lot of effects on the body's immune system, inhibiting the body's immune function and promoting the development of the tumor.

3). The Morphology and location of the thymus

The thymus (thymus) is a cone-shaped shape, which can be divided into left and right symmetrical leaves. The texture is soft and long and flat, and the two leaves are connected by connective tissue (Fig. as the following). The size of the thymus varies greatly from age to age. In the late embryonic development and neonates, the growth rate of the thymus is very fast. From birth to 2 years old, it is the best period for thymus development, weighing 15-20g. With the increase of age, the thymus continues to grow, but it is relatively slower than the post-natal period, reaching 25~40g in puberty. After puberty, the thymus begins to shrink and degenerate. The adult thymus still retains its original shape, but its structure changes greatly, lymphocytes are greatly reduced, and thymus tissue is often replaced by adipose tissue.

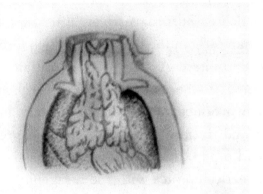

Figure 1. Morphological location of the thymus in children

The adult thymus is in the anterior portion of the mediastinum behind the sternum. The posterior is adjacent to the innominate vein and the aortic arch, and the sides are adjacent to the mediastinal pleura and lung. Thymial enlargement and thymoma can compress the above organs and have corresponding clinical symptoms.

The thymus of the child is large in volume, the upper end can extend to the base of the neck, some can reach the lower edge of the thyroid, and the lower end can extend into the anterior mediastinum to reach the front of the pericardium.

4). The structure of the thymus

(1) Capsule: The thymus surface is covered with a connective tissue film, and the film is composed of a dense collagen fiber bundle, an elastic fiber, and a matrix. The connective tissue fiber bundle in the capsule protrudes into the thymus parenchyma and divides the thymus into many leaflets. The periphery of the lobules is the cortex, and the deep side is the medulla. There is a scaffold composed of reticular epithelial cells (Fig. as the following).

(2) Cortex: The cortex of the thymus is located in the periphery of the leaflet and consists of dense lymphocytes and epithelial reticular cells. Lymphocytes in the superficial cortex are larger and belong to the original lymphocyte type. The

middle layer of lymphocytes is medium in size, and the inner layer is mostly small linba cells. There are scattered macrophages in the cortex. From shallow to deep is the process by which hematopoietic stem cells proliferate and differentiate into T lymphocytes.

(3) Medulla: The medulla of the thymus is located deep in the leaflet and consists of epithelial reticular cells and a small number of lymphocytes. There are scattered thymus bodies in the medulla. The body is round or oval, consisting of several layers of epithelium(Fig. as the following)

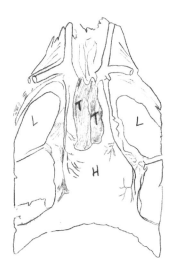

Figure 2. Upper mediastinal organ and pericardium and thymus in adult
T: thymus; L: lung; H: heart

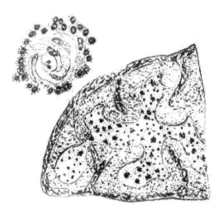

Figure 3 Structure of the thymus in children
1, small leaf interval; 2, thymus lobules; 3, thymus on the mass;
4, thymus small body; 5, the capsule; 6, medulla; 7, keratinized
epithelial cells and debris; 8, epithelial cells; 9, thymocytes

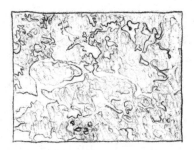

Figure 4. Thymic medulla
The scattered thymus bodies (arrows) distributed in the medulla

5). Thymus function

The function of the thymus is complex, the thymus is a lymphoid organ, and has the function of an endocrine gland. Some authors have included it in the endocrine system. **Its main function is to cultivate and manufacture T lymphocytes and secrete thymus hormone.** The cultivation of T cells in the thymus requires a suitable internal environment. The epithelial network of the thymus can secrete a variety of hormones: thymosin, thymopoietin, thymulin, thymic humoral factor (THF), and ubiguitin. These hormones together with macrophages and staggered cells in the thymus form a microenvironment for culturing T cells. Thymosin and thymosin can promote the differentiation of lymphocyte stem cells into T-cells, stimulate T cell proliferation, and stimulate the hypothalamic secretion of ACTH and LH; Thymogenin induces T cell differentiation; other hormones promote synergistic effects on early division of T cells and promotion of T cell maturation.

Primitive lymphatic stem cells have no immunity and are further developed into T cells with immune function. Then through the blood circulation to the surrounding lymphoid organs, such as lymphoid tissue, lymph nodes, spleen, etc., after antigen activation and proliferation, participate in the immune response. Although the adult thymus is atrophied and degraded, it still has the ability to secrete thymus hormone. When the lymphoid tissue of the body is destroyed, the T cells are greatly reduced, and the lymphatic stem cells that enter the thymus with blood circulation can still be converted into T cells under the action of thymus hormone.

T lymphocyte
Differentiation and development of lymphocytes in the thymus
Phenotypic changes during T cell differentiation and development
It is currently known that the main factors inducing differentiation and maturation of T cells in the thymus include: 1 Thymic stromal cells (TSC) interact directly with thymocytes via adhesion molecules on the cell surface; 2 Thymic stromal cells secrete a variety of cytokines (such as IL-1, IL-6, IL-7) and thymus hormone to induce

thymocyte differentiation; 3 Thymocytes secrete a variety of cytokines (such as IL-2, IL-4) also play an important role in the differentiation and maturation of thymocytes themselves. In addition, thymic epithelial cells, macrophages, and dendritic cells play a decisive role in self-tolerance, MHC restriction, and formation of T cell function subpopulations during thymocyte differentiation.

A T cell, or T lymphocyte, is called T cells because they mature in Thymus from thymocytes (although some also mature in the tonsils) and All T cells originate from haematopoietic stem cells in the bone marrow. In the bone marrow haematopoietic stem cells become haematopoietic progenitors; on the way to thymus haematopoietic progenitors are expanded by·cell division to generate a large population of immature thymocytes; is a type of lymphocyte (a subtype of white blood cell) that plays a central role in cell-mediated immunity. T cells can be distinguished from other lymphocytes by the presence of a T-cell receptor on the cell surface. There are several subsets of T cells, each of which has a distinct function such as Cytotoxic (Killer) or CD8+T cells, helper T cells or CD4+ T cells, Natural killer T cells, etc. Two distinct types of thymocytes are produced in the thymus: CD4/CD8. in the thymus the earlist thymocytes are double- negative (CD4-CD8-) cells, later become double-positive thymocytes (CD4+CD8+); finally mature to single-positive (CD4+CD8- or CD4-CD8+) thymocytes. About 98% of thymocytes die during the development processes in the thymus by failing either positive selection or negative selection, whereas 2% matured naïve T cells leave the thymus and begin to spread throughout the body, including the lymph nodes. As the thymus shrinks by about 3% a year throughout middle age, there is a corresponding fall in the thymic production of naive T cells, leaving peripheral T cell expansion to play a greater role in protecting older subjects.

6). Immune function of the body

In particular, the function of cellular immunity and T lymphocytes gradually decreases with age, and the thymus gradually degenerates in structure and function after adulthood. The thymus is the central organ of immune function and is the base for differentiation and maturation of T lymphocytes. Thymus epithelial cells produce and release thymosin, which plays an important role in the differentiation of precursor T lymphocytes into mature immune active T cells. The thymus is also the earliest organ of body degradation. It begins to shrink after sexual maturity, and its ability to produce and secrete thymosin gradually decreases with age.

The study of the thymus began in the early 1960s when it was found to be closely related to immune function. Miller et al. (1960) found that the immune function of the thymocytes (neonatal mice) was insufficiency and the number of circulating T cells was significantly reduced. For 50 years, the thymus has been recognized as the central organ of the animal's immune system. It is the earliest organ of the body's development. When it matures, the structure and function of the thymus reach its peak, and then gradually shrinks and degenerates with age. Immune function is gradually replaced by spleen and other lymphatic tissue in adult animals. The thymus is the core tissue of T lymphocyte development, and is the base for producing various immune factors (lymphokines, cytokines). Thymosin is the main secretory immune regulator. Now there are various thymosin (peptide). The product is used for clinical and experimental research. There are special journals abroad called "thymus", which regularly publish reports on thymus research and clinical treatment.

7). Thymic immune regulation

In the early days, it was considered to be a single self-regulating system independent of other physiological systems. It has been developed so far that It is believed that the thymus and neuroendocrine systems are interconnected and functional network systems. In the late 1970s, Besedovsky (1977) proposed the theory of neuroendocrine immune network (NIM), which has been recognized as the core idea of guiding thymus and immune function.

The thymus forms a three-point line with the central nervous system and peripheral immune response system. The central cerebral cortex, hypothalamus, and pituitary gland are superior regulatory centers; Peripheral lymphoid organs and tissues, lymphocytes and cytokines are the regulatory and executive units of the lower immune network; The intermediate hub is the thymus, which can be called the middle line of NIM. The NIM pathway can be divided into three sections:

1. Down line, that is, from the center down to the middle line and the lower line units;
2. Up line, feedback information from the cytokines of the lower line to the central part;
3. .The middle line pathway, with the thymus as the main axis, is accompanied by the spleen and other lymphoid tissues and bone marrow progenitor cells. Recent studies have shown that the thymus plays an important role in NIM activities. For example, Fabres (1983) proposed the concept of "thymus-neuroendocrine network", and Goldstein AL (1983) proposed the idea of "neuroendocrine-thymus axis", which can express the special significance of thymus in NIM network.

The thymus begins to degenerate after sexual maturity, and the secreted thymosin and other hormones are also reduced, which hinders the differentiation of T lymphocytes and reduces the immune function of the body. The main cause of aging in humans and mammals is closely related to thymic atrophy and degeneration.

As the age increases, the thymus naturally shrinks and life gradually ages. The thymus is an important factor affecting the body's immune level. Experiments have shown that removal of the thymus from adult rats (2 months old) can accelerate their autoimmune dysfunction and aging. At 6 months after the thymus surgery in rats, the immune activity of spleen lymphocytes decreased significantly, which was only 51.6% of the same age without thymus.

8). Thymus exocrine

Thymic hormone vitality can be detected by available bioassay method. The experiment proved the vitality of the thymus hormone decline with increasing age. With thymic atrophy it decreases. In the animals with removal of the thymus serum cannot be measured. Thymus is the main source of thymic hormone. Thymus hormones are substance secreted by thymocytes regulating immune function.

The thymus is the important organization of body's immune function, secrete and generate thymulin etc, and secrete IL-1 and IL-2 and other interleukins to adjust thymus intrinsic function and viability ingredient; at the same time regulated by the pituitary secretion of prolactin. Now the research about thymus immunomodulator primarily provides evidence indicating that exogenous hormone (such as prolactin, growth hormone, thyroxine, etc.) can rejuvenate the thymus recession and maintain immunomodulatory force. **Thymic involution can be reversed which is common developmental prospects of modern immunology and endocrinology.**

9). The Effect of chemical drugs on immune function

<u>**Cyclophosphamide (Cy) or hydrocortisone (HC)**</u> **is** a commonly used drug in clinical practice, which can cause a decline in immune function. Long-term injection can cause atrophy of thymus, spleen and lymph nodes, and significantly reduce immune function.

In short, Cy and HC have certain inhibitory effects on immune function, such as Cy for 3w, the thymus has shrunk, the spleen begins to shrink after 6w, and the proliferative power of peripheral blood T lymphocytes decreases significantly at 6~12w.

10). The naming and function of thymus hormone

Since the early 1960s, the well-known scientists Good and Miller first reported that the function of the thymus is the "central" organ of the systemic immune system, and cellular immunology has developed rapidly. In the early 1970s, a hypothesis about thymus secreting hormones was proposed. Several "presumptive" but not yet confirmed thymosin or hormone-like components were successively introduced. They are peptide components extracted from the whole thymus. Recent studies have shown that thymic epidermal cells (TEC) are cells that produce thymus hormone components and can be divided into two major categories: interleukins (Ils) and thymosin.

Foreign studies have shown that there are four thymus hormones: (1) thymosin-α; (2) thymulin; (3) thymopoietin; (4) thymichumoral factor (THF). Thymulin is a 9-peptide binding component that requires zinc binding to be biologically active. The thymus component is extracted from the bovine thymus in foreign countries.

11). Immunomodulation: immune promoter

In the current situation, immune promoters can be divided into several categories depending on the source.

The first class of immunostimulants is first derived **from microbial components.**

The fungal glucan containing β-1,3-glucosamine chains has been shown to have a good clinical effect. They promote MΦ killing of bacteria and tumor cells and induce the release of cellular mono-kinks such as interleukin-1 (IL-1), tumor necrosis factor (TNF), colony stimulating factor (CSF), and the like.

The second major class of immune boosters is **the thymus extract.**

Peptide components are extracted from animal thymus. Various products have been produced in various countries (including China), and all have immunological pharmacological activities, also known as thymus hormones. Zinc thymulin complex is an active component secreted by thymic epithelial cells. Other kinds of thymus crude extracts have clinical effects. Their main function is to enhance the activity of T cells in vivo, but it has no effect on producing new T cells. In other words, activation of T cells can enhance the body against microbial pathogens, anti-tumor activity and delay the decline of immune function in aging animals. Clinically used for the treatment of chronic infectious diseases and tumors.

The third major class of immunostimulating agents was **the recombination cytokine that was developed in the 1980s.**

These bioactive factors have achieved significant benefits in clinical treatment, the most prominent of which are rIFN-r, rIFN-α, IL-2 (IL-1 to IL-2), TNF, rCSF (such as GM-CSF). This can be said to be a major innovation or breakthrough in immunopharmacology. Recently, monoclonal antibodies (Mabs) and human gene antibodies (H-Ab) have emerged. These new components can be summarized as recombinant peptide immunological substances.

The purification of various immunostimulating substances has made significant progress, and a variety of effective products have been available, and there are not many chemical substances that have been proven to have clinical therapeutic effects.

12). The Research progress of Chinese medication polysaccharide anti-cancer immunopharmacology

Antitumor Research of Wolfberry Polysaccharides(Lycium barbarum polysaccharide, **LBP)**, Polyporus umbellatus Polysaccharides(PUPs), Poria Polysaccharides, Lentinan (Mushrooms Polysaccharide), **Versicolor(**Yunzhi), Ganoderma lucidum Polysaccharides and Tremella Polysaccharides **(White fungus Polysaccharide)**

Mechanism and prospect of anti-tumor effect of polysaccharide drugs

a).Progress and Advances in anti-cancer immunity of traditional Chinese medicine polysaccharides

Polysaccharides can improve the body's immune surveillance system including natural killer cells (NK), macrophages (MΦ), killer T cells (CTL), T cells, LAK cells, tumor infiltrating lymphocytes (TIL)), the activity of interleukin (IL) and other cytokines to achieve the purpose of killing tumor cells. Although many polysaccharides have a certain anti-tumor effect, the two immunopotentiators, including the two polysaccharides, have higher therapeutic effects, and the polysaccharide can be further improved by the same treatment with chemotherapy or radiotherapy.

b).Research overview and progress

Thomas and Burnet's immunosurveillance theory suggests that the in vivo **immune system has the effect of eliminating tumor cells produced by cell mutations in order to maintain a single cell type of each cell**. The body's immune surveillance system for tumors includes cellular and humoral immune functure, and cellular immunity is particularly important for tumor rejection. Immune cells that perform cellular immune functions include natural killer cells (NK) and macrophages (MΦ). Recently, LAK cells and tumor infiltrating lymphocytes (TIL) have been proposed. The anti-tumor effect of the latter is 50-100 stronger than that of LAK cells. The anti-tumor effect of the latter is 50 to 100 times stronger than that of LAK cells, and exerts a stronger effect. If these effector cells are inhibited, it is difficult to function as an immunosurveillance system. Elston reported that only 19 patients with choriocarcinoma with cellular immune response died, while 13 patients with no immune response or significantly reduced immune response had 13 deaths, indicating that the level of immune function plays an important role in tumor therapy. **Prevention and treatment of tumors by enhancing the body's immune function is undoubtedly a research field with bright prospects.**

According to the research progress of polysaccharides at home and abroad and related information, polysaccharides including LBP can play the role of antibacterial, antiviral, antitumor, anti-aging, anti-chemotherapy side effects and anti-autoimmune diseases on the one hand; There may also be various physiological activities such as lowering blood pressure, lowering blood fat, anti-vomiting, and lowering blood stasis. These aspects will also be an important direction for LBP's in-depth research and application development.

Compared with other polysaccharides, LBP is a glycopeptide with strong action, small dosage, good water solubility, stability and easy absorption by oral administration. It can be considered as a highly effective immune T cell adjuvant. However, LBP is still a crude extract. It is still to be cooperated with phytochemical experts to purify and modify LBP including degradation of oligosaccharides and oligosaccharides with different molecular weights and sulfated polysaccharides. It is expected to further enhance the immunological activity of LBP in order to find a newer, immunologically active drug.

Immunization is closely related to aging. Many scholars have further discovered that the main cause of the deterioration of cellular immune function during aging **is that the thymus shrinks with age**. It is suggested that the thymus is the **biological clock** that controls immune function during aging. LBP is the main link in aging immunity - the thymus. **The main experiments are as follows**: 1 LBP mainly chooses to act on thymic T cells; 2 Ding Yan and other reports pointed out that LBP can promote the increase of the number of thymic mature T cells, and enhance the "empty" function, so that thymocytes metastasize to the periphery to play a role in the regulation of thymus immune center and to enhance the role of resisting disease and delaying aging; 3 Our experiments have shown that aged mice drink LBP aqueous solution daily. After half a year, the thymus gland in the control group is atrophied. The thymus atrophy in the LBP group is recovered and the weight is increased, but it has not reached the normal level of adulthood. This fact suggests that LBP can reverse the retrograde thymic degeneration. Based on the above, it is clear that the thymus is related to aging.

13). Characteristics of Traditional Chinese Medicine Immunopharmacology

Compared with Western medicine immunopharmacology, traditional Chinese medicine immunopharmacology has its own characteristics or advantages, and each has its own shortcomings. The advantages of traditional Chinese medicine immunology are as follows:

First of all, long-term clinical managers have accumulated a large number of prescriptions to regulate the body's immune function, especially the beneficial Chinese medicines generally have the effect of regulating immune activity.

Traditional Chinese medicine is rich in sources. In recent years, research has increasingly proved that traditional Chinese medicine is an effective medicine for long-term clinical treatment. After extraction, it can obtain obvious pharmacological effects (including immunomodulatory effects), and the research process saves people time and has high efficiency.

Secondly, traditional Chinese medicines, whether single-agent or prescription, contain multiple active ingredients, unlike Western medicines (synthetic drugs) which are single-structured substances. The role of traditional Chinese medicine is multifaceted. In addition to regulating immune function, it has a certain effect on the whole functional system and organs. And these roles are connected and combined.

The role of traditional Chinese medicine in regulating immune function is generally beneficial, that is, within the normal adjustment range, two-way regulation is the main feature. The tonic drug can be called immunomodulatory drugs, causing a non-specific immune response.

Chinese medicines for tonics have the function of regulating the immune function of the body. Under the general experimental conditions, the correlation between dose and benefit is presented, especially in normal healthy animal experiments. When the animal is at a low level of immune activity (such as dethymus, aging animals or chemotherapy drugs cyclophosphamide inhibition and tumor animals), the tonic drugs improve the body's immunity is more significant.

Immunopharmacology is an interdisciplinary subject formed by the combination of immunology and pharmacology. Traditional Chinese medicine immunopharmacology plays a special important role in immunopharmacology in China. Traditional Chinese medicine immunopharmacology can be understood as a new discipline in the grafting of traditional Chinese medicine and modern immunopharmacology.

As early as the 1970s, **Professor Zhou Jin had been calling for the establishment of pharmacology in the integration of Chinese and Western medicine in China,** and clearly proposed to study and clarify the pharmacological effects of traditional Chinese medicine from the theory of traditional Chinese medicine.

TCM theory has its obvious overall view, emphasizing the balance of the body and maintaining balance when the internal and external environment changes. Losing balance and coordination, the body will have a medical certificate.

Modern medicine also emphasizes the stability of the internal environment. The regulatory factors for the stability of the internal environment are the three systems of nerve, endocrine and immunity. These are self-contained systems that independently exert their respective regulatory roles, while at the same time interacting with each other and interacting with each other to achieve the goal of maintaining a relatively stable internal environment. "Nerve, endocrine, immune, regulatory networks" (NIM network) is currently a research hotspot in immunopharmacology. Professor Zhou Jin developed the NIM idea through a lot of research work, and believed that the "NIM" concept has broad practical significance, is in line with the laws of life science, and coincides with the overall ideology of traditional Chinese medicine. Extensive and in-depth study of the role of traditional Chinese medicine in the NIM network can greatly develop the basic theories of Chinese medicine, so that Chinese medicine can go global faster.

14). New discoveries from cancer research experiments:

(1) Removal of the thymus (Thymus, TH) can be manufactured bearing animal model for sure;

(2) These results suggest that: the metastasis is related to immune function; immune deficiency may promote tumor metastasis;

(3) It was found that: the host thymus was acute atrophy after inoculation of cancer cells which cell proliferation is blocked and volume was significantly reduced;

(4) It was found that: When solid tumors grow to large thumb, they were removed. A week later there was no further thymus atrophy;

(5) In our laboratory we were looking for immune reconstitution methods by using mice fetal liver, fetal thymus, fetal spleen cell transplantation to reconstitute while exploring to stop thymus atrophy. The results showed that in S, T, L three groups of cell transplantation, recently complete tumor regression was 40%, long-term tumor regression rate was 46.67%.

From the above experimental findings, thymus atrophy and immune dysfunction may be one factor in cancer incidence and pathogenesis, we should start from the body's immune function, especially cellular immunity, T lymphocyte function and immune function of the thymus to explore and seek immune regulation approach in the molecule levels.

In view of the development of Chinese medicine immunity pharmacology, traditional Chinese medicine theory has its obvious overall concept, emphasizing the balance of the body and maintain balance when changes in internal and external environment, loss of balance, the body appeared syndromes.

Modern medicine also places great emphasis on a stable internal environment. Internal environment stable adjustment factors are three systems: nervous, endocrine and immune systems. "Nervous, endocrine, immune regulatory network" (NIM Network) is the research focus immune pharmacology.

There are a lot of traditional Chinese medications regulating the body's immune function, especially having generally dynamic regulation of the immune benefits. During 28 years we have conducted a series of experimental research to find new drugs from natural medications to find new anti-cancer drugs and anti-cancer metastasis, to prevent thymus atrophy and to increase immune anti-cancer medication; looking only inhibit cancer cells without inhibiting normal drugs; from traditional Chinese medication to look for preventing atrophy of the thymus and adjusting the relationship between the host and tumors, preventing recurrence and metastasis drugs.

Existing anti-cancer drugs inhibit the patient's immune function, suppress bone marrow and thymus and immune surveillance was lost so that cancer further develops. Therefore, we must strengthen the research, all the anti-cancer drug used must be able to increase immune function and protect the immune organ, and should not be immune suppression drugs.

15). the research of the action mechanism of XZ-C immunomodulatory anti-cancer medications

Looking for the new drugs of the anti-cancer, anti-metastasis in natural medicine (TCM) in the experimental work within our laboratory over a long period, a batch of 200 kinds of traditional considered to be "anti-cancer medicine," were screened in the experiments of tumor inhibition in tumor-bearing animal models, the results found that only 48 kinds do have some even better inhibition of tumor proliferation of cancer cells. Optimized combination, and then in vivo anti-tumor experiments in tumor-bearing animal models such as liver cancer, lung cancer, stomach cancer and others to consist of $Z-C_{1\sim10}$ particles, $Z-C_1$ can inhibit cancer cells, but not normal cells, $Z-C_4$ can protect thymus and improve immune function, $Z-C_8$ can protect marrow liters of blood, ZC immune regulation medicine can improve the quality of life of patients with advanced cancer, increase immunity, enhance physical fitness, improve appetite, prolong survival.

With more and deeper researches on traditional Chinese medicine, it has been proved that many kinds of traditional Chinese medicine can regulate and control the production and biological activity of cytokine and other immune molecules, which is meaningful to explain the immunological mechanism of XZ-C traditional Chinese anti-carcinoma medicine for immunologic regulation and control from the level of molecule.

I. Protecting Immune Organs and Increasing the Weight of Thymus and Spleen

That XZ-C traditional Chinese medicine can protect immune organs resulting from the following active principles.

1. XZ-C-T (EBM): Using its 15g/kg and 30g/kg extracting solution (equivalent to 1g original medicine) along with 12.5mg/kg, 25mg/kg ferulic acid suspension to feed the mice for seven days in a raw can increase the weight of thymus and spleen obviously, especially the effects of the group with high dose are more apparent. Intraperitoneal injection of EBM polysaccharide can also alleviate thymus and spleen atrophy obviously caused by perdnisolone.

2. XZ-C-O (PMT) :Extract PM-2, feed the mice with 6g/(kg·d) PMT decoction for successive seven days which can increase the weight of thymus and celiac lymph nodes and antagonize the reduction in the weight of immune organs caused by perdnisolone. Drenching the mouse of 15 months old with 6g/kg decoction (with the concentration of 0.5g/ml) for 14 days can increase the weight and volume of thymus, thicken the cortex and raise cellular density apparently. The combined use of PM and astragalus root can promote non-lymphocyte hyperplasia and benefit the micro environment of thymus.

3. XZ-C-W (SCB):SCB polysaccharide can gain weight of thymus and spleen of a normal mouse. Lavage with it enables cyclophosphane to control the gain in the weight of thymus and spleen.

4. XZ-C-M (LLA):Drench a mouse with LLA decoction for seven days resulting in increasing the weight of thymus and spleen.

5. XZ-C-L:For a 15-month old mouse, its thymus degenerates obviously. Astragalus injectio can enlarge the thymus significantly. The cortex under microscope is thickened and the cellular density increase obviously.

II. Effects on Proliferation, Differentiation and Hematopiesis of Marrow Cells

The following active principles of XZ-C traditional Chinese medicine have effects on hematopiesis of marrow cells.

1. XZ-C-Q (LBP) extracts (PM-2):

(1)Effects on the proliferation of hematopoietic stem cell (CFU-S) of a normal mouse: inject PM-2 with the dose of 500mg/(kg·d)×3d or 10mg/(kg·d)×3d LBP into the experimental mice respectively by venoclysis and kill them in the ninth day. It can be found that the number of spleen CFU-S in the group with administration increases obviously. The number of CFU-S in group PM-2 is 21% higher than that of the control group and it is 36% in the group with LBP.

(2)Effects on colony forming unit of granulocytes and macrophages (CFU-GM): the experimental results indicate that LBP with the dose of 5~30mg/(kg·d)×3d can increase the number of CFU-GM and PM-2 can also strengthen the effect of CFU-GM with the effective dose of 12.5~50mg/(kg·d)×3d. In the early stage of cultivation, most CFU-GMs are units of granulocytes and then units of macrophages increase gradually. In the anaphase units of macrophages take over the dominance.

From the above experiment, it can be found that PM-2 and LBP can promote hematopiesis of normal mice obviously. The experiment proves that during the process of restoring hematopiesis damaged by cyclophosphamide, PM-2 and LBP stimulate the proliferation of granulocytes at first, and then marrow karyocytes multiply; at last these two promote the restoration of peripheral granulocytes.

2. XZ-C-D (TSPG):

Ginsenoside, which is the active principle of ginseng to promote hematopiesis, can bring the recovery of erythrocyte in peripheral blood, haemoglobin and myeloid cell of thighbone in the mice of marrow-inhibited type, increase the index of myeloid cellular division and stimulate the proliferation of myeloid hematopoietic cell in vitro so as to make it into cell cycle with active proliferation ($S+G_2/M$ stage). TSPG can promote the proliferation and differentiation of polyenergetic hematopoietic cells and induce the formation of hemopoietic growth factor (HGF).

3. XZ-C-H (RCL):

Steamed Chinese Foxglove can promote the recovery of erythrocyte and haemoglobin for animals with blood deficiency and accelerate the proliferation and differentiation of myeloid hematopoietic cell (CFU-S) with the effect of predominance and hematosis significantly. Peritoneal injection of rehmannia polysaccharides for successive six days can promote the proliferation and differentiation of myeloid hematopoietic cells and progenitor cells as well as increasing the number of leucocytes in peripheral blood.

4. XZ-C-J (ASD):

ASD polysaccharide has no effects on erythrocytes and leucocytes of normal mice, but for those damaged by radiation, injection of ASD polysaccharide can influence the proliferation and differentiation of both polyenergetic hematopoietic stem cells (CPU-S) and hemopoietic progenitor cells. But its decoction has no obvious effects.

5. XZ-C-E (PEW):

Poria cocos (micromolecule chemical compound extracted from Tuckahoe polysaccharide) is the active principle that can strengthen the production of colony stimulating factor (CSF) and improve the level of leucocytes in peripheral blood inside the mouse's body. It can also prevent the decline in leucocytes caused by cyclophosphamide and accelerate the recovery with the effects better than sodium ferulic which is used to increase leucocytes.

6. XZ-C-Y (PAR):

Its polysaccharide can obviously resist the decline in leucocytes caused by cyclophosphamide and increase the number of myeloid cells to promote the proliferation of myeloid induced by CSF as well as the recovery and reconstitution of hematopiesis for the mice irradiated by X ray. It can also increase the number of hematopoietic stem cells and myeloid cells along with leucocytes.

III. Enhancing Immunologic Function of T Cells

The active principles of XZ-C traditional Chinese medicine and their effects are following.

1. XZ-C-L (AMB):It can raise the percentage of lymphocytes in peripheral blood obviously. The LBP in small dose (5~10mg/kg) can cause the proliferation of lymphocytes, indicating that LBP can promote the proliferation of T cells apparently. 50mg/(kg·d)×7d is the best dose in that it will have no effects if lower than the level and it will bring the effects down if higher than the level.

Oral administration of LBP can raise the conversion rate of lymphocytes for the sufferers who are weak and with fewer leucocytes.

2. XZ-C$_4$: It can regulate immune system and active T cells of aggregated lymphatic follicles, as well as stimulate the secretion of hemopoietic growth factor in T cells. Among the crude drugs of XZ-C$_4$, the extract from the hot water of atractylodes lancea rhizome can obviously stimulate the cells of aggregated lymphatic follicles, which is regarded as the base of XZ-C$_4$ immunoloregulation.

IV. Activating and Enhancing NK Cell Activity

Natural killer cell, NK cell is another kind of killer cell in lymphocytes for human beings and mice, which needs neither antigenic stimulation, nor the participation of antibodies to kill some cells. It plays an important role in immunity, especially in the function of immune surveillance as NK cell is the first line of defense against tumors and has broad spectrum anti-tumor effects.

NK cell is broad-spectrum and able to kill sygeneous, homogenous and heterogenous tumor cells with special effects on lymjphoma and leucocytes.

NK cell is an important kind of cells for immunoloregulation, which can regulate T cells, B cells and stem cells, etc. It can also regulate immunity by releasing cytokines like IFN-α, IFN-γ, IL-2, TNF, etc.

The active principles in XZ-C traditional Chinese medicine and their effects are following.

1. XZ-C-X (SDS)

Divaricate Saposhniovia Root can strengthen the activity of NK cells of experimental mice. When combined with IL-2, it can make the activity of NK cell higher, indicating that its polysaccharide can give a hand to IL-2 to activate NK cells and improve the activity.

LBP can strengthen T cell mediated immune reaction and the activity of NK cells for normal mice and those dealt by cyclophosphamide. Peritoneal injection of LBP can improve the proliferation of spleen T lymphocytes and strengthen the lethality of CTL increasing the specific lethal rate from 33% to 67%.

2. XZ-C-G (GUF)

Glycyrrhizin can induce the production of IFN in the blood of animals and human beings and strengthen NK cell activity at the same time. Clinical tests made by Abe show that after intravenous injection of 80mg GL, the raise of NK cell activity reaches 75% among 21 sufferers. Peritoneal injection of 0.5mg/kg GL on mice can strengthen the activity of NK cells in liver.

3. XZ-C-L (AMB)

Its bath fluid can promote NK cell activity of mice both in vivo and in vitro, and can also induce IFN-γ to deal with effector cells under the certain concentration of 0.1mg/ml. Cordyceps sinensis extract can strengthen NK cells activity of the mouse both in vivo and in vitro. Fluids with the concentrations of 0.5g/kg, 1g/kg and 5g/kg can strengthen NK cell activity of mice.

(5) Effects on Iterleukin-2 (IL-2)

The active principles in XZ-C anti-carcinoma traditional Chinese medicine and their effects are following.

1. XZ-C-T

EBM polysaccharide can enhance obviously the production of IL-2 for human beings when the concentration is 100ug/ml. At higher concentration (2500ug/ml and 5000ug/ml), it will lead to inhibition. Hypodermic injection of barrenwort polysaccharide for seven days in a row can significantly improve the ability of thymus and spleen of the mouse induced by ConA to produce IL-2.

2. XZ-C-Y

PAR polysaccharide has strong immune activity and is able to promote the production of IL-2. For the mouse bearing S-180 tumor, it can raise the ability of spleen cells to produce IL-2 obviously。

3. XZ-C-D

Ginseng polysaccharide has great promotion on IL-2 induced by peripheral monocytes for both healthy people and sufferers with kidney troubles. The effects are relevant to the dose positively.

IFN are broad-spectrum in resisting tumors and can regulate immunity. It can also inhibit the proliferation of tumor cells and activate NK cells and CTL to kill tumor cells. Meanwhile, IFN can cooperate with TNF, IL-1 and IL-2 to enforce anti-tumorous ability.

The active principles in XZ-C anti-carcinoma traditional Chinese medicine and their effects are following.

1. XZ-C-Z

250mg/kg or 500mg/kg CVQ polysaccharide can improve significantly the level of IFN-γ produced by mouse spleen cells.

2. XZ-C-D

Ginsenoside (GS) and panaxitriol ginsenoside (PTGS) can induce whole blood cells and monocytes of human beings to produce IFN-αand IFN-γ. It can also recover the low level of IFN-γand IL-2 to the normal.

The IFN potency of ASH polysaccharide on S-180 cell line of acute lymphoblastic leukemia and S_{7811} cell line of acute myelomonocytic leukemia produced after acanthopanax polysaccharide stimulation is 5~10 times more than that of normal control group.

3. XZ-C-E

Hydroxymethyl Poria cocos mushroom polysaccharide has many kinds of physical activity like immunoloregulation, promoting to induce IPN, resisting virus indirectly and alleviating adverse reaction resulting from radiation. Do IFN inducement dynamic experiment on S-180leukaemia cell line by using 50mg/ml Hydroxymethyl Poria cocos mushroom polysaccharide. The results indicate that its potency to induce interferon at all stages is better than that of normal inducement.

4. XZ-C-G (GL)

It can induce IFN activity. Make peritoneal injection of 330mg/kg GL on mice. IFN activity reaches the peak after 20 hours.

16). The research of cytokines which are induced by XZ-C4 anticancer Chinese medications

(1) Z-C4 anticancer medications can induce endogenous cytokines

① The experimental study: Z-C4 has a variety of immune-enhancing effect and there are closely relation with induced endogenous cytokine.

② Z-C4 can inhibit the reduction of leukocyte and neutrophils and thrombocyte.

③ Through the interleukin -1β (IL-1β) Z-C4 not only has a direct effect on the production of GM-CSF, but also can enhance the tumor necrosis factor (TNF), interferon (IFN) and other cytokines, which may be an indirect mechanism.

④ In the cancer patients Th1 cytokine which regulates the cellular immune function decreases ; however Z-C4 can raise Th1 cytokines so that it has effects on anemia and leukopenia after chemotherapy.

⑤ Z-C4 can not only protect the bone marrow, but also play a direct role in the cell differentiation through the cytokines.

In short, Z-C4 induces tumor cell differentiation and natural death due to autocrine which produce the different kind of cytokines. Autocrine is called as that the substance which is secreted by itself reversely acts on it own. Looking to the future, Z-C4 may become inducing therapy for cancer cell differentiation.

(2) Z-C4 can inhibit cancer progression and metastasis

Cancer cells obtains Invasion and metastasis of malignant nature in the proliferation process, this phenomenon is called malignant progression. To research cancer progress requires the good reproducibility animal model. Thus, the regression type of cancer cell QR-32 isolated from mouse fibrosarcoma was made into this good reproducibility animal model. Even though QR-32 was implanted subcutaneously in the mice, it was nor hyperplasia and will be completely self-limiting; it does not appear the metastatic nodules in the lung while it was injected through the vien. However, if the gelatin sponge as the foreign substances together with QR-32 was transplanted into mice subcutaneously, QR-32 becomes the proliferative cancer cell QRSP in vivo.

(3) Z-C1 + Z-C4 immune regulation and control anti-cancer medication

Z-C1 + Z-C4 immunomodulatory anticancer medication has the following characteristics:
① Overall improvement in the quality of life of patients with advanced cancer.
② Protect the thymus enhance immunity, protect the bone marrow and enhance hematopoietic function, improve immune and regulatory capacity.
③ Enhance physical fitness, reduce pain, improve appetite.
④ Enhance the therapeutic effect and reduce the side effects of chemotherapy.

17). The experiment and clinical efficacy of XZ-C immunomodulation anticancer Chinese medication

A. Summary:

(1) a. Antitumor effect of XZ-C$_1$ and XZ-C$_4$ anticancer Chinese medications on liver cancer in H$_{22}$ tumor-bearing mice

It was found that after administrating the medications for 2 weeks, 4 weeks, and 6 weeks in the H_{22} tumor-bearing mice, the tumor inhibition rate was increased with the prolonged medication administration time. The tumor inhibition rate of $Z\text{-}C_4$ at the 6th week was as high as 70%. After repeated tests twice, the results were stable, indicating that the anti-tumor effect of Chinese medicine is slow and gradually increased. That is, the anti-tumor effect is positively correlated with the cumulative dose of traditional Chinese medicine.

b. The effect of $Z\text{-}C_1$ and $Z\text{-}C_4$ anticancer Chinese medicine on the survival of H22 tumor-bearing mice:

The experimental results show that Z-C1, Z-C4 anti-cancer traditional Chinese medicine can significantly prolong the survival of tumor-bearing mice, especially Z-C4, significantly prolonging its survival time by more than 200%. Not only that, Z-C4 can significantly improve the body Immune function, protect immune organs, protect bone marrow, reduce the side effects of chemotherapy and radiotherapy drugs, and it has not seen any side effects after being fed for 12 months. The above experimental research provides a useful basis for clinical application.

(2) Clinical efficacy

On the basis of experimental research, since 1994, it has been applied to clinical cancers, mostly patients with stage III or IV. That is:

1).The advanced cancer that cannot be removed by exploration; 2).The advanced cancer has lost the indication for surgery;3)recent or long-term metastasis or recurrence after various cancer operations;

4)liver metastasis, lung metastasis, brain metastasis or cancerous pleural effusion or cancerous ascites in various advanced cancers;5)Various cancer with estimated resection, gastrointestinal anastomosis or colostomy can only be done but cannot be removed during the exploration;6)Patients who are not suitable for surgery, radiotherapy or chemotherapy.

XZ-Cl, XZ-C4 anti-cancer Chinese medicine has been clinically applied for 20 years, systematically observed, and achieved obvious curative effect. There are no side effects for long-term use. Clinical observations have shown that XZ-Cl andX Z-C4 anti-cancer traditional Chinese medications can comprehensively improve the quality of life of patients with advanced cancer, improve overall immunity, control cancer cell proliferation, and consolidate and enhance long-term efficacy. The internal and external application of XZ-C drug has a good effect on softening and reducing the surface metastasis of the tumor. Combined with intervention or intubation pump treatment, it can protect the liver, kidney, bone marrow hematopoietic system and immune organs and improve immunity.

(3) The analgesic effect of XZ-C anti-cancer is good

Pain in advanced cancer patients is more obvious and painful symptoms; the general pain medication does not have much effect for cancer pain and the narcotic analgesics are addiction and dependence; XZ-C anticancer analgesic cream has strong analgesic effect and last longer. In 298 cases it was clinically proved to have significantly effective rate 78.0%, the total efficiency of 95.3%, can be re-used with no significant side effects, non-addictive. Analgesic effect is stable and relieves pain for cancer patients to improve the quality of life.

Through experimental research and clinical validation, our experience is:

Traditional Chinese medicine with Chinese characteristics has its unique advantages in cancer treatment such as: Strong overall concept, the regulation effect is outstanding, mild side effects, alleviating the pain, relieving symptoms, significantly improving the quality of life of patients, and it can regulate the immune function of the body and the overall disease resistance and improving the treatment effect.

B. The experimental result

1. Antitumor effect of XZ-C Chinese medications on liver cancer H_{22} mice:

① The tumor inhibition rate was 40% in the second week of XZ-C1, 45% in the fourth week, and 58% in the sixth week. In the second week of XZ-C4, the tumor inhibition rate was 55%, the tumor inhibition rate was 68% in the fourth week, and the tumor inhibition rate was 70% in the sixth week (P<0.01). The tumor inhibition rate was 45% in the second week of CTX administration. The tumor inhibition rate was 45% at the 4th week and 49% at the 6th week (Fig.1, Fig. 2).The experiment results.

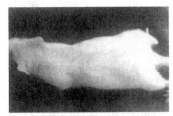 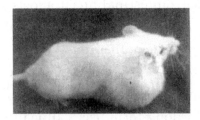

Figure 1 XZ-C1, XZ-C4 treatment group 30d after inoculation of hepatoma H_{22}

Figure 2 Control group 30d after inoculation of hepatoma H_{22}

② Effect of 2Z-C Chinese medicine on the survival of liver cancer H22 mice

The average survival days of XZ-C1, XZ-C4 and CTX groups were higher than those of normal saline control group (P<0.01). XZ-C Chinese medicines significantly prolonged survival. Compared with the control group, the life extension rate of the XZ-C1 group was 85%, the life extension rate of the XZ-C4 group was 200%, and the life extension rate of the CTX group was 9.8%. In Group B, Z-C1 and CTX groups had died within 75 days. Six cancer-bearing mice in the XZ-C4 group survived after 7 months. The effect of XZ-C medicine on the survival time of the rats bearing hepatic carcinoma H_{22}: the average survival time of XZ-C_1, $_X$Z-C_4 and CTX was longer than the one of the normal saline control group (P<0.01); XZ-C medicine played a role in obviously prolonging the survival time. Through comparison with the control group, the life elongation rate of XZ-C_1 group was 85%, the one of XZ-C_4 group was 200% and the one of CTX group was 9.8%. The rats in XZ-C_1 and CTX in Group B met with death in 75d. 6 rats bearing carcinoma in Z-C_4 survived after seven months.

(3) Both XZ-C_1 and XZ-C_4 medicine improved the immunologic function and Z-C_4 obviously improved the immunologic function, increased the white blood cells and red blood cells, **without any effect on the hepatic function and kidney function and without damage to the hepatic and kidney section. CTX decreased the white blood cells and reduced the immunologic function with the renal damage to the kidney section.** The thymus in the control group was obviously atrophic (Fig. 1-4) while the one of XZ-C_1 and XZ-C_2 therapy group was not atrophic but a little hypertrophic (Fig.1-3).

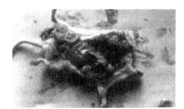 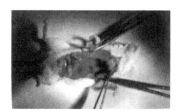

Fig XZ-C4 treatment group
30d after inoculation of hepatoma H22
Thymus hypertrophy

Figure 4 Control group
30d after inoculation of liver cancer H22
marked atrophy of thymus

Pathological section of thymus in the control group:

the cortex of the thymus was atrophic, the cells were discrete and the blood vessel met with sludge (Fig. 1-5). The pathological section of the thymus in Z-C_4 therapy group displayed that the cortical area of the thymus built up, the lymphocyte was dense, the epithelium reticulocyte increased and the thymus corpuscles increased (Fig. 1-6).

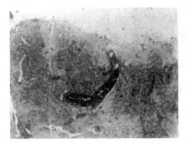 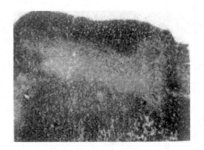

Figure 5 thymic tumor-bearing control group, HE × 100 lymphocytes decreased cortical atrophy, Cortex form a lymphocyte empty band degree

Figure 6 X Z-C4 treated thymus HE × 100 thymic cortex and medulla thickening, lymphocyte high, intravascular congestion

C. Clinical Application

1. Clinical information

(1) Hubei Branch of China Anti-cancer Research Cooperation of Chinese Traditional Medicine and Western Medicine, Anti Carcinoma Metastasis and Recurrence Research Office and Shuguang Tumor Specialized Outpatient Department had treated 4, 698 carcinoma patients in Stage III and IV or in metastasis and recurrence with Z-C medicine combined with western medicine from 1994 to Nov. 2002, among which there were 3, 051 men patients and 1,647 women patients. The youngest one was 11 years old and the oldest one was 86 years old, the high invasion age was 40~69 years. All groups of the patients were entirely subject to the diagnosis of pathological histology or definitive diagnosis with ultrasonic B, CT and MRI iconography. According to the staging standard of UICC, all the cases were entirely the patients in medium and advanced stage over Stage III. In this group, there were 1,021 hepatic carcinoma patients, among which there were 694 primary lesion hepatic carcinoma patients and 327 metastatic hepatic carcinoma patients; there were 752 patients suffering from carcinoma of lung, among which there were 699 patients suffering from the primary carcinoma of lung and 53 patients suffering from the metastatic carcinoma of lung; there were 668 gastric carcinoma patients, 624 patients suffering from esophagus cardia carcinoma, 328 patients suffering from rectum carcinoma of anal canal, 442 patients suffering from carcinoma of colon, 368 patients suffering from breast carcinoma, 74 patients suffering from adenocarcinoma of pancreas, 30 patients suffering from carcinoma of bile duct, 43 patients suffering from retroperitoneal tumor, 38 patients suffering from oophoroma, 9 patients suffering from cervical carcinoma, 11 patients suffering from cerebroma, 34 patients suffering from thyroid carcinoma, 38 patients suffering from nasopharyngeal carcinoma, 9 patients suffering from melanoma, 27 patients suffering from kidney carcinoma, 48 patients suffering from carcinoma of urinary bladder, 13 patients suffering from leukemia, 47 patients suffering from metastasis

of supraclavicular lymph nodes, 35 patients suffering various fleshy tumors and 39 patients suffering from other malignancies.

(2) Medications and the methods of drug administration : the treatment aims to support healthy energy to eliminate evils, soften and resolve the hard mass and supplement qi and blood. $Z-C_1$ is the compound, 150ml to be taken on the daily basis, $Z-C_4$ is powder, 10g to be taken on the daily basis. According to the analysis and differentiation of the diseases, anti-cancer powder shall be taken orally and the anti-cancer apocatastasis paste shall be applied externally for the solid tumor or the metastatic tumor. In case of being in pain, anti-cancer aponic paste shall be applied externally. Icterus removal soup or dropsy removal soup shall be taken orally for the patients suffering from icterrus and the ascites.

(3) Therapeutic evaluation: it pays attention to the short-term curative effect and iconography indexes as well as the survival time of long-term curative effect, quality of life and immunologic indexes. Attention shall be paid to the changes in subjective signs in administration of drugs. It will be effective when the subjective signs are improved and last over one month; otherwise, it will be ineffective. As to the quality of life (Karnofsky Performance Status), it will be effective when it is improved and lasts over one month, otherwise, it will be ineffective. As to the evaluation standard of the curative effect of solid tumor, it can be divided into four levels according to the changes in size of tumor: Level I: disappearance of tumor; Level II: tumor reduces 1/2; Level III: softening of tumor; Level IV: no change or enlargement of level tumor.

The effect of treatment

(1) The symptom was improved, the quality of life was improved, the survival time was prolonged: among the 4,277 carcinoma patients in medium and advanced stage who took Z-C medicine with the return visit over 3 months. It improved the quality of life of the patients in an all-round way, see Table 1.

Table 1 Observation of curative effect on 4 277 patients: fully improving the quality of life of the carcinoma patients in medium and advanced stage

Improvement	Vigor	Appetite	Reinforcement of physical force	Improvement in generalized case	Increase of body weight	Improvement of sleep	The restriction of improvement activity and capability released activity	self servicing normal walking	Resumption of work Engaged in light work
No. of cases (%)	4071	3986	2450	479	2938	1005	1038	3220	479
	95.2	93.2	57.3	11.2	68.7	23.5	24.3	75.3	11.2

All the patients in the group were in the middle and advanced stage. After taking the medicine, they all had different degrees of symptom improvement, and the effective rate was 93.2%. In terms of improving the quality of life (according to the Kasper's scoring standard), the average score was 50 points before medication, and after treatment, the average score was 80 points. The patients in this group had metastasis and dysfunction of different tissues and organs in stage III or above. It was reported that the median survival time is about 6 months. The longest period of this group has reached 21 years, and the average survival time of the remaining cases is more than 1 year. 1 case of primary hepatic lobe of the left hepatic lobe, recurrence of right liver after resection, treatment with XZ-C for 21 years; another case of liver cancer with XZ-C for 20 and a half years; 2 cases of liver cancer with multiple intracranial cancer, taking XZ-C Six months later, after 2 CT scans, the cancer lesion completely subsided and it has been stable for half a year. One case of double renal cell carcinoma, extensively transferred to the abdominal cavity after one side resection, was completely restored to work after taking XZ-C medicine. Three cases of lung cancer were not detected by thoracotomy. The XZ-C drug has been taken for 3 and a half years. Two cases of residual gastric cancer were treated with XZ-C for 8 years. Three cases of rectal cancer had been treated with XZ-C for 3 years. 1 case of breast cancer metastasis of liver and ribs has been taken for 8 years. One case of recurrent bladder cancer after renal cell carcinoma disappeared for 9 and a half years after taking XZ-C. All of the above cases were inoperable, and could not be used in the middle and late stage of radiotherapy and chemotherapy. They were given Z-C medicine alone and were not treated with other drugs. So far, I have come to the clinic every month to review and take medicine. After long-term medication, the condition is controlled in a stable state, so that the body and the tumor remain in a balanced state for a long time, and a better tumor-bearing survival is obtained, the patient's symptoms are improved, the quality of life is improved, and the survival period is prolonged.

(2) As to 84 patients suffering from solid tumor and 56 patients suffering from enlargement of upper lymph node of metastatic compact bone, after taking XZ-C series medicines orally and applying XZ-C3 anti-cancer paste, they met with good curative effects, see table2.

Table 2 Changes of 84 patients suffering from solid tumor and 56 patients suffering from metastatic mode after applying Z-C paste externally

Table 2 84 cases of physical mass and 56 Lymph nodes on the neck tumor after applying Z-C paste externally.

	Solid tumor				Enlargement of upper lymph node of metastatic compact bone			
	Disappearance	Shrinkage 1/2	Softening	No change	Disappearance	Shrinkage 1/2	Softening	No change
No. of cases (%)	12 14.2	28 33.3	32 38.0	12 14.2	12 21.4	22 39.2	14 25.0	8 14.2
Total effective rate (%)	85.7				85.7			

(3) 298 patients suffering from carcinoma pain obtained the obvious pain alleviation effects after taking XZ-C medicine orally and applying XZ-C anti-cancer paste externally, see Table3.

Table 3 The situation of 298 patients cases of after taking Z-C medicine orally and applying Z-C anti-cancer apocatastasis paste externally

Clinical Symptoms	Pain			
	Light alleviation	Obvious alleviation	Disappearance	Avoidance
No of cases (%)	52 17.3	139 46.8	93 31.2	14 4.7
Total effective rate (%)		95.3		

18). XZ-C immunomodulation anti-cancer traditional Chinese medications are the result of traditional Chinese medication modernization

XZ-C immunomodulation anticancer Chinese medicine,

Nor is it an old Chinese medicine formula,

XZ-C immunomodulatory anti-cancer medications are not the empirical formula, nor is the medical formula of the famous old Chinese doctor, but the combination of Chinese and Western medicine and traditional Chinese medicine with modern scientific research, are to combine modern medical methods, experimental methods in experimental tumors, and modern pharmacology and medicine efficient methods. After seven years of more than 4000 cancer-bearing animal models, the so-called 200 kinds of commonly used anti-cancer herbs are screened in batches in tumor-bearing animals, then screened out of 48 kinds of anti-cancer effect of good medicine.

Then this 48 kinds of natural medicine are composed of XZ-Cl ~ 10 number which according to the respiratory, digestive, urinary, gynecological, endocrine system are built into animal model of liver cancer, stomach cancer, colon cancer, breast cancer, Kennedy bladder cancer, lung cancer, then tested and selected XZ-Cl, XZ-C2, XZ-C3, XZ-C4, XZ-C5, XZ-C6, XZ-C7, XZ-C8, etc. series of immune regulation anti-cancer medicine for in vivo efficacy in tumor-bearing animal experiments and toxicological experiment.

The material basis of the traditional recipe playing its unique clinical efficacy is one of the chemical composition. The changes of quality and quantity of the chemical composition directly affect the clinical efficacy of prescriptions. So only study of the changes of quality and volume of chemical composition of prescription, to find out the main active ingredient preparation, molecular immunology to explore the mysteries of its unique effect can make research tradition reach a new level of prescription.

The formulation of XZ-C immune regulation medicine is Chinese medicine innovation and reform which is not mixed boiling liquid compound, but particles per herb concentrates or powders, which every membrane in every flavor raw pharmaceutical drug retains its original composition, pharmacological effect, molecular weight, constant structure and is made by using modern scientific methods, not the compound to keep the original flavor of each ingredient and function in order to evaluate and affirm the the efficacy and action of the tasting drugs.

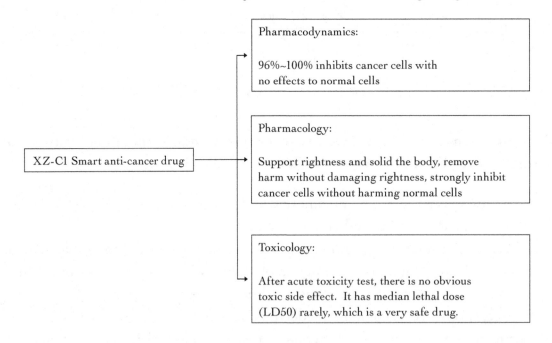

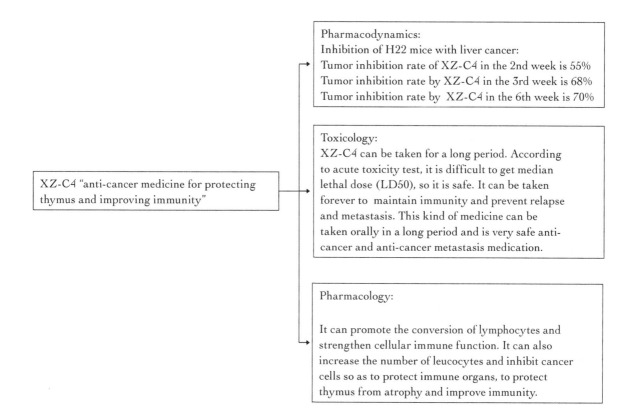

Pharmacodynamics:
Inhibition of H22 mice with liver cancer:
Tumor inhibition rate of XZ-C4 in the 2nd week is 55%
Tumor inhibition rate by XZ-C4 in the 3rd week is 68%
Tumor inhibition rate by XZ-C4 in the 6th week is 70%

Toxicology:
XZ-C4 can be taken for a long period. According to acute toxicity test, it is difficult to get median lethal dose (LD50), so it is safe. It can be taken forever to maintain immunity and prevent relapse and metastasis. This kind of medicine can be taken orally in a long period and is very safe anti-cancer and anti-cancer metastasis medication.

XZ-C4 "anti-cancer medicine for protecting thymus and improving immunity"

Pharmacology:

It can promote the conversion of lymphocytes and strengthen cellular immune function. It can also increase the number of leucocytes and inhibit cancer cells so as to protect immune organs, to protect thymus from atrophy and improve immunity.

19).Exclusive research and development products: Z-C immune regulation anti-cancer Chinese medicine series products (introduction)

The self-developed ZC (Xu Ze China) (Xu Ze-China) immune regulation and anti-cancer series of traditional Chinese medicine preparations, from experimental research to clinical verification, applied to clinical practice on the basis of successful animal experiments, clinical practice of a large number of clinical cases over the years Verification, the effect is significant. For the independent invention results, it is independent innovation and independent intellectual property rights.

To search for and screen new anti-cancer and anti-metastatic drugs from traditional Chinese medicine:

The purpose is to screen out new anti-cancer, anti-metastatic, anti-recurrent and anti-cancer drugs that have no drug resistance, no toxic side effects, and high selectivity.

To this end, In our laboratory it was conducted the following the screening tests of the new anti-cancer and anti-metastatic drugs from traditional Chinese medications

(A) The method of cancer cells in vitro, the experimental study of Chinese herbal medicine suppressor screening rates:

a. **In vitro screening tests:** The cancer cells in vitro was observed for sore drugs directly damage cells.

b. **The screening test in tube culture of cancer cells**: in vitro tests respectively allowing raw and crude drugs of crude product (500ug / ml) to be used and to observe whether there is inhibition of cancer cells or not. 200 kinds of traditional Chinese medicine herbs having anticancer function were screened one by one in vitro screening tests. And under the same conditions with a normal fiber cell culture the toxicity of these cells was tested and compared.

(B) Built cancer-bearing animal model for the screening of anticancer Chinese herbs

In vivo screening test: in cancer-bearing animal model screening Chinese anti cancer herbs, 240 mice were divided into eight experimental groups, each group 30 mice, Group 7 was the blank control group, Group 8 with 5-Fu or CTX was the control group. The whole groups were inoculated with EAC or S180 or H22 cancer cells. 24h later each rat was orally fed by crude drug powder. These medications fed the rats for long term to observe survival time and to calculate the cancer inhibition rate.

Therefore, we conducted experimental studies for four consecutive years in more than 1000 rats each year. A total of nearly 6,000 tumor-bearing animal models were made and autopsy each mice after died to observe liver, spleen, sheets, pituitary gland, kidney and to get pathological anatomy with a total of 20,000 slices to explore to find out whether There may be slight carcinogenic pathogens and the establishment of tumor micro-vessels beds and microcirculation was observed with the microscope in 100 tumor-bearing mice.

Through experimental study we first found that Chinese medication TG had a significant effect on inhibiting tumor angiogenesis. Now it has been used as anti metastasis in more than hundreds of the patients in clinic treatment.

Experimental results: In our laboratory animal experiments after screening 200 kinds of Chinese herbal medications, 48 kinds of medications with certain and excellent inhibitory effect on cancer cells and inhibition rate of more than 75-90% were selected. 152 kinds with no significant anti-cancer effects were screened-out.

48 kinds of traditional Chinese medications with having good tumor suppression rates after screening out were optimized into the combination and repeated tumor suppression rate experiments in vivo, and finally developed XU ZE Chinal-10(XZ-Cl-10) immunomodulatory anticancer Chinese medication with Chinese characteristics.

$Z\text{-}C_1$ could inhibit cancer cells, but does not affect normal cells; $Z\text{-}C_4$ specially can increase thymus function, can promote proliferation, increased immunity; Z-C_1 can protect bone marrow function and to product more blood.

Clinical validation: Based on the success of animal experiments, clinical validation was conducted. Namely the oncology clinics and the Research Group of combined Chinese with Western medicine for anti-cancer and anti-metastasis and recurrence were established. The patient medical records were retained and the regular follow-up observation system were established to observe the long-term effects. From experimental research to clinical evidence, the new questions were discovered during the new clinical validation process, then went back to the laboratory for the basic research, then applied the results of a new experiment for clinical validation. Thus, the experiment to the clinics, the experiment again and the clinical experiment again, all experimental studies must be clinically proven in a large number of patients observed 3—5 years, or even clinical observation of 8 to 10 years. According to evidence-based medicine, the long-term follow-up assessment information had gained and they have been verified indeed to have a good long-term efficacy. The efficacy of the standard is: a good quality of life, longer survival. XZ-C sectional immune regulation anti-cancer medicine was made after a lot of applications in advanced cancer patients verification and achieved remarkable results and can improve the quality of life of patients with advanced cancer, enhance immune function, increase the body's anticancer abilities, increased appetite and significantly prolong survival.

In the chinese herbal medications many of them are the immune enhancer and the biological reaction regulator and the tonic medications; many can strengthen the body immune and have anti-cancer function. The two major global diseases that threaten human life are cancer and AIDS. The former is immunocompromised, the latter is immune deficiency. **At present, the world scientists agree that tumor formation is summarized as three processes: the first step, carcinogenic factors act on the body, interfere with cell metabolism; the second step, disrupting the genetic information within the nucleus, causing cell cancer; the third step, cancer cells escape the body Immune alert defense system; the body's immune defense capability is internal causes and the external causes have the action and the function through the internal factors. Cancer cells must be escaped from the alarm system monitoring in the body, breaking the body's immune line, to develop into a tumor. Therefore, trying to improve the body immune function is the key of the measures of the anti-cancer and the prevention of cancer. How to improve immune function? Chinese herbal medication has the extremely important advantage; there are many immune herbal preparations and there are** a lot of drug sources and it should be an important anti-cancer and prevention cancer resources and it organizes the research and performs the development.

The research of the prevention and treatment of malignant tumors in the world are carried out in each country. Each country focuses on a large number of experts and scholars with the experimental research and clinical experience to study and try to overcome cancer.

We should be in the advantage areas in our country to play the advantages of our country and to catch up with the international advanced level.

In the field of cancer research, the traditional Chinese medication is the advantage of our country. To play this advantage in the function of the field of cancer research and to explore and to develop the prevention of the cancer and anti - cancer Chinese herbal medications and to play this advantage of the study should be a strategic significance of the international significance.

On the road of human conquest cancer the research and the excavation and the development of effective and reproducible anti-cancer anti-cancer new Chinese herbal medication preparations must be promising and can be excavated into effective treasure and must be carried out the strict and objective and realistic and scientific and repetitive research with the strict scientific methods and the modern experimental surgical methods. All experimental studies must be rigorously and clinically proven in a large number of patients who demonstrate that there is a good curative effect and that the standard of efficacy is good quality of life and prolonged survival.

20).A series of products of XZ-C immunoregulation anti-cancer traditional Chinese medicine

1. **XZ-C1+4: for all kinds of cancer**
2. **XZ-C1: has the stable and significant anti-cancer effects, the inhibition rate up to 98%, no harmful to normal cells.**
3. **XZ-C4: protection of thymus and increase of immune function, promote the thymus proliferation, increase the immune function**

XZ-C8: protection of bone marrow and production of blood, increase T cells, and anti-metastasis

4. **Lung cancer: XZ-C1+XZ-C4+XZ-C7**
5. **Breast cancer: XZ-C+XZ-C+XZ-C+ mushroom**
6. **Esphogus cancer: XZ-C1+XZ-C4+XZ-C2**
7. **Stomach cancer: XZ-C1+XZ-C4 or +XZ-C5**
8. **Liver Ca: XZ-C1+XZ-C4+XZ-C5 + Mushroom+ Red ginseng**
9. **Bile cancer: XZ-C1+XZ-C4+XZ-C5 + Capillaris**

10. **Pancrease cancer : XZ-C1+XZ-C4+XZ-C5+XZ-C9**
11. **Colon and rectal cancer: XZ-C1+XZ-C4+XZ-C5**
12. **Kidney and bladder cancer: XZ-C1+XZ-C4+XZ-C6**
13. **Cervical and ovary cancer: XZ-C1+XZ-C4+XZ-C5+ Lms+ MDS**
14. **Lymphma: XZ-C1+XZ-C4+XZ-C2+ Dai Dai**
15. **Leukemia: XZ-C1+XZ-C4+XZ-C2+XZ-C8+ barge pole**
16. **Prostate cancer:XZ-C1+XZ-C4+XZ-C6**

Comments: A series of XZ-C immune regulation anti-cancer traditional medications have been verified and tested for 20 years in Shuguang tumor special out-patient center on 12,000 of middle or later stage cancer patients. On clinical application they can change the symptoms, the patients have the good spirit and appetites are good, the life quality is improved, and they significantly prolong the survival time.

21). Adaptation Scope of Clinical application observation of XZ-C immunomodulation Chinese medication XZ-C$_{1-10}$ anti-cancer metastasis and recurrence

1. a variety of distant metastatic cancer, such as liver metastases, lung metastases, bone metastases, brain metastases, abdominal lymph node metastasis, mediastinal lymph node metastasis, cancerous pleural effusion, cancerous ascites, can be applied XZ-C immunization Regulate and Control anti-metastatic treatment, according to the transfer step, intervene and block the cancer cells on the way to prolong life.
2. After all kinds of radiotherapy and chemotherapy have been completed, XZ-C1-4 should be taken to control the traditional Chinese medicine to consolidate the long-term effect and prevent recurrence.
3. in the process of radiotherapy and chemotherapy, if the reaction is serious and can not continue, you can continue to use XZ-C immunomodulation therapy to resist metastasis and recurrence.
4. in the elderly or weak patient with other diseases who cannot have radiology and chemotherapy, XZ-C immunomodulation anti-metastasis, relapse treatment.
5. surgical exploration can not be cut, can be used XZ-C immune regulation treatment.
6. after palliative surgery, XZ-C immunomodulation anti-metastatic treatment.
7. after a variety of cancer radical surgery, should continue to take XZ-C immunomodulation treatment of traditional Chinese medicine anti-recurrence, metastasis, in order to improve the long-term effect after radical surgery

2. The introduction - "finding the road"

A. Step out a new road of conquering cancer in the past 30 years

a).The Research inspiration and revelation from finding a new way —the path finding

Conquering cancer, where is the road? - Where is the road? Where to go? How to find this way?

What is our new path in cancer treatment?

We are taking a new road combining Chinese and Western medicine; it is a new way of combining Chinese and Western medicine at the molecular level; it is a new way for our laboratory to find immunomodulatory methods and drugs based on the new findings of animal experiments; after years of animal experiment screening And clinical verification, finally looking for a new way of immunomodulation of XZ-C immune regulation anti-cancer Chinese medicine series.

Why should we take a new road combining Chinese and Western medicine? Why should we take a new path of combining Western medicine at the molecular level? Why should we take a new path to find immunomodulatory drugs?

The road we are looking for is step by step. After a long process of clinical verification for more than 20 years, it is not the beginning of this understanding, but a step by step to find out gradually.

b).We are taking "Chinese-style anti-cancer" new road of the combination of Chinese and Western medicine at the molecular level

The combination of Chinese and Western medicine is the characteristics and advantages of Chinese medicine. The goal of combining Chinese and Western medicine should be to combine innovation, and the goal of innovation should be to improve the treatment effect. The efficacy criteria for cancer patients should be: long survival time, good quality of life, and few complications.

In the past 28 years, we have initially embarked on a new way to use immunomodulation of Chinese medicine, regulate immune activity, prevent thymic atrophy, promote thymic hyperplasia, protect bone marrow hematopoietic function, improve immune surveillance, and combine Western medicine at the molecular level to overcome cancer.

Our experimental surgical research institute is based on the research direction and main task of conquering cancer. It is a joint research project to tackle cancer, taking the road of combining Chinese and Western medicine, and conducting

research on the combination of Chinese and Western medicine at the molecular level. On the basis of animal experiment research, And in the clinical practice to achieve the combination of Chinese and Western medicine, and then in the anti-cancer, anti-cancer transfer theory development, innovation:

Adhering to the scientific research work of combining Chinese and Western medicine with innovation, we should persevere and persevere, adhere to the road of independent innovation with Chinese characteristics, and promote the new development of the theory of modern oncology in the 21st century.

Efforts will be made to take the road of innovation in China's distinctive anti-cancer transfer, take the road of modernization of traditional Chinese medicine, promote the integration of Chinese and Western medicine at the molecular level, and integrate with international medicine modernization. We have initially embarked on a road of XZ-C immune regulation, molecular and Chinese medicine combined with cancer— "Chinese-style anti-cancer" new road.

[Notes]:

- "Chinese-style anti-cancer" is a monograph title published by Academician Tang Yu in April 2014. The wisdom of Sun Tzu's art of war is used for anti-cancer strategy and tactical thinking.
- I think that the combination of Chinese and Western medicine is only a method and it is a means. Why should we combine Chinese and Western medicine? How to combine Chinese and Western medicine? What is the goal of the combination? Academician Wu Xianzhong proposed that the goal of combining Chinese and Western medicine should be to combine to have innovation.

So what is the goal of combining to innovation? What are the hopes of combining innovation?

- I believe that the goal of combining innovation is to improve the effectiveness of treatment and benefit patients. The efficacy of cancer patients should be: long survival time, good quality of life, and fewer complications.
- The result of combining to innovation should be innovation "Chinese medicine" innovation "Chinese-style anti-cancer".

If this sentence is analyzed in a sentence, it should be:

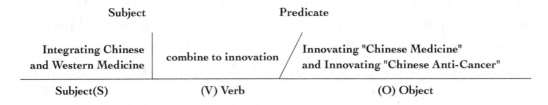

Subject	Predicate	
Integrating Chinese and Western Medicine	combine to innovation	Innovating "Chinese Medicine" and Innovating "Chinese Anti-Cancer"
Subject(S)	(V) Verb	(O) Object

This is a complete sentence, with purpose, method, and result, so I quote the word "Chinese-style anti-cancer" created by Academician Tang Yu. It is also the new way of combining the ideological understanding and research thinking of our scientific research journey that the anti-cancer and anti-metastatic research institutes have gone through in the past 28 years.

B. Pathfinding - where to find the way:

The road we have been looking for in the past 30 years has come step by step:

- **Discovery of findings through follow-up:**
(1) - Looking for ways to prevent and treat cancer recurrence and metastasis after surgery
(method, medicine, technology, basic theory)

- **Discovery through the findings of experimental research:**
(2) - Looking for ways to prevent thymus atrophy, promote thymic hyperplasia, and boost immunity
(method, medicine, technology, basic theory)
(3) - Looking for the road to immune reconstruction
(method, medicine, technology, basic theory)

- **Through our proposed anti-cancer metastasis research on the new concept of cancer metastasis, the new theory of understanding: the key to cancer treatment is anti-metastasis, how to eliminate the cancer cell group on the way to transfer.**
(4) - Looking for ways to eliminate cancer cells on the way to metastasis
(method, medicine, technology, basic theory)

- **Through the above research results: We basically found the way to take immunomodulatory therapy, and gradually established XZ-C immunomodulation therapy.**

We think this is one of the roads to overcome cancer. In order to explore the etiology, pathogenesis and pathophysiology of cancer, we conducted a series of animal experiments. From the experimental results, we obtained new findings, new enlightenment: thymus atrophy, low immune function is one of the causes and pathogenesis of cancer. Therefore, Xu Ze (Xu Ze) proposed one of the causes and pathogenesis of cancer at international conferences, which may be thymus atrophy, central immune organ damage, immune dysfunction, decreased immune surveillance, and immune escape.

Regardless of the complexity of the mechanisms behind cancer, mechanismic immunosuppression is the key to cancer progression. Removing immunosuppressive factors and restoring the recognition of cancer cells by immune system cells may effectively prevent cancer.

By activating the body's anti-tumor immune system to treat tumors, a major breakthrough in the next cancer is likely to stem from this. Immunomodulatory therapy, the prospects are gratifying.

Until 1985, I had conducted more than 5000 patient operations and in 1985 I conducted a petition with all of these patients and there were more than 3,000 patients who underwent radical surgery for various cancers to reply for my petition. It was found that most patients had recurrence and metastasis 2 to 3 years after surgery, and some even metastasized several months after surgery. This made me realize that although the operation is successful, the long-term efficacy is not satisfactory. Postoperative recurrence and metastasis are the key factors affecting the long-term efficacy of the operation. It also reminds us that prevention and treatment of postoperative recurrence and metastasis is the key to prolonging postoperative survival. Therefore, basic research must be carried out, and without breakthroughs in basic research, clinical efficacy is difficult to improve. So we established the Institute of Experimental Surgery and spent a total of 24 years conducting a series of experimental research and clinical validation work from the following three aspects.

1. First, explore the mechanism of cancer onset, invasion and recurrence and metastasis, and carry out experimental research on effective measures to regulate invasion, recurrence and metastasis.

We have been conducting laboratory research for a full four years in the laboratory. They are clinical basic research and research projects. They are all clinically raised questions to explain these clinical problems or solve these clinical problems through experimental research.

From experimental tumor research it was found:

(1) Resection of the thymus (Thymus, TH) can produce a cancer-bearing animal model;

(2) The experimental results suggest that metastasis is related to immunity, and low immune function may promote tumor metastasis;

(3) The experimental results showed that the host thymus was acutely progressively atrophied after inoculation of cancer cells, cell proliferation was blocked, and the volume was significantly reduced;

(4) The experimental results showed that when the transplanted solid tumor of the experimental mouse was long to the thumb, it was removed. After one week, the thymus was found to have no atrophy;

(5) Our laboratory is investigating the atrophy of the thymus gland in the immune system to stop the progression of the tumor, and looking for the method of immune reconstitution. The experimental study on the immune function of fetal liver, fetal thymus gland and fetal spleen cell transplantation was used to reconstruct the immune function. The results showed that the three groups of S, T, L cells were transplanted. The complete regression rate of tumors was 40%, and the complete regression rate of long-term tumors was 46.67%.

Our laboratory experimental results showed that the thymus of the cancer-bearing mice showed progressive atrophy, the volume was reduced, the cell proliferation was blocked, and the mature cells were reduced. By the end of the tumor, the thymus is extremely atrophied and the texture becomes hard.

From the above experimental studies, it is found that thymus atrophy and immune dysfunction may be one of the pathogenic factors and pathogenesis of tumors, so it is necessary to try to prevent thymus atrophy, promote thymocyte proliferation, and increase immunity. The immune function of the body, especially cellular immunity, the function of T lymphocytes, and the immune regulation function of the thymus should be explored at the molecular level, and methods for immune regulation and effective drug research should be sought.

It should further from the thymus function and tissue structure, immune function is low and how to promote immunity, immune reconstitution, how to "protect the chest lift" further research, looking for new ways and new methods of cancer treatment.

2. Second, look for new anti-cancer, anti-metastatic, anti-recurrence new drug experimental research from natural drugs.

The existing anticancer drugs kill both cancer cells and normal cells, and have large adverse reactions. We have tried new cancer drugs in cancer-bearing mice to find new drugs that inhibit cancer cells without affecting normal cells. We spent a full three years on the anti-tumor screening experiments of cancer-bearing animals in 200 kinds of Chinese herbal medicines used in traditional anti-cancer prescriptions and anti-cancer agents reported in various places. Results 48 kinds of traditional Chinese medicines with good anti-tumor effect and good effects were screened out.

To search for and screen new anti-cancer and anti-metastatic drugs from traditional Chinese medicine:

The purpose is to screen out new anti-cancer, anti-metastatic, anti-recurrent and anti-cancer drugs that have no drug resistance, no toxic side effects, and high selectivity.

To this end, our laboratory conducted the following experimental studies to screen new anticancer and anti-metastatic drugs from traditional Chinese medicine:

(1) Using the method of in vitro culture of cancer cells, screening experiments on the cancer suppression rate of Chinese herbal medicines:

In vitro screening test: The cancer cells were cultured in vitro to observe the direct damage of the drug to cancer cells.

In-vitro screening test, in the test tube for culturing cancer cells, respectively, into the crude drug product (500 ug / ml), to observe whether it has an inhibitory effect on cancer cells, we will take 200 kinds of Chinese herbal medicines that traditional Chinese medicine thinks have anti-cancer effect. Screening experiments were performed in vitro. The toxicity of the drug to the cells was tested by normal fiber cell culture under the same conditions and then compared.

(2) Making animal models of cancer-bearing animals, and conducting experimental screening of Chinese herbal medicines on cancer suppression rate in cancer-bearing animals

In vivo anti-cancer screening test, each batch of 240 mice, divided into 8 groups, 30 in each group, the seventh group was a blank control group, the eighth group with 5-FU or CTX as a control group, the whole group of mice Inoculate EAC or S180 or H22 cancer cells. After inoculation for 24 hours, each rat was orally fed with crude drug powder, and the traditional Chinese medicine was screened for a long time. The survival time, toxicity and side effects were calculated, the survival rate was calculated, and the cancer inhibition rate was calculated.

In this way, we conducted a four-year experimental study, and conducted an experimental study on the pathogenesis, metastasis, and recurrence mechanism of tumor-bearing mice for three years, and an experimental study to explore how tumors cause host death. More than 1,000 tumor-bearing animals are used each year. In the model, nearly 6000 tumor-bearing animal models were made in 4 years. After the death of each mouse, the pathological anatomy of the liver, spleen, lung, thymus and kidney was performed. More than 20,000 slices were taken to explore whether to find out whether There may be carcinogenic micro-pathogens, and microcirculation microscopy was used to observe the microvascular establishment and microcirculation of 100 tumor-bearing mice.

Through experimental research, we have found for the first time in China that TG has a significant effect on inhibiting tumor microvessel formation. It has been used in more than 80 clinical patients for anti-metastasis treatment, and the efficacy is being observed.

Experimental results: Among the 200 kinds of Chinese herbal medicines screened by animal experiments in our laboratory, 48 strains were selected to have certain or even excellent inhibitory effects on cancer cell proliferation, and the tumor inhibition rate was above 75-90%. However, there are also some commonly used traditional Chinese medicines that are generally considered to have anti-cancer effects. After screening for animal tumors in vitro and in vivo, there is no anti-cancer effect, or the effect is very small. In this group, 152 kinds of anti-cancer effects were eliminated by animal experiments.

The 48 kinds of traditional Chinese medicines with good cancer suppression rate were selected by this experiment, and then the optimized combination was repeated to carry out the experiment of cancer suppression rate in cancer. Finally, the immune-regulating anti-cancer Chinese medicine XU ZE Chinal- with its own characteristics was developed. 10 preparation (XZ-C1-10).

XZ-C1 can significantly inhibit cancer cells, but does not affect normal cells; XZ-C4 can promote thymic hyperplasia and increase immunity; XZ-C8 can protect the marrow from hematopoiesis and protect bone marrow hematopoietic function.

3. Third, how should we find new ways to regulate immune therapy?

In order to try to prevent thymus atrophy, promote thymocyte proliferation, increase immunity, we look for both Chinese medicine and western medicine. The existing medicines of western medicine can improve immunity and promote the proliferation of thymus. So we changed to look for Chinese herbal medicine.

(1) Why do you look for drugs that promote thymic hyperplasia, prevent thymus atrophy, and boost immunity? Because Chinese medicine's tonic drugs generally contain the role of regulating immunity.

1. Chinese medicine, polysaccharide Chinese medicine, tonic medicine, many have the role of regulating immunity.

The role of traditional Chinese medicine in regulating immune function is generally replenishing, and traditional Chinese medicine for tonic has the effect of regulating immune activity. Replenishing drugs can be called immunomodulatory drugs, causing non-specific immune responses.

Chinese medicines for tonics have the function of regulating the immune function of the body. Under the general experimental conditions, the correlation between dose and benefit is presented, especially in normal healthy animal experiments. When the animal is at a low level of immune activity (such as dethymus, aging animals or chemotherapy drugs cyclophosphamide inhibition and tumor animals), the tonic drugs improve the body's immunity is more significant.

2. Research on anti-cancer immunity of Chinese medicine polysaccharides is progressing rapidly. A large number of immunopharmacological studies have been carried out at the molecular level. Polysaccharides can improve the body's immune surveillance system, including natural killer cells (NK), macrophages (MΦ), and killer T cells. (CTL), T cells, LAK cells, tumor infiltrating lymphocytes (TIL), interleukin (IL) and other cytokines are active to kill tumor cells. Although many polysaccharides have a certain anti-tumor effect, the two immunopotentiators, including the two polysaccharides, have a higher therapeutic effect.

Traditional Chinese medicine and western medicine have their own strengths, each with its own shortness. Compared with Western medicine immunopharmacology, traditional Chinese medicine immunopharmacology has its own characteristics or advantages, and each has its own shortcomings. The advantages of traditional Chinese medicine immunology are as follows:

A large number of Chinese medicines have the effect of regulating the body's immune function, especially the beneficial Chinese medicines generally have the effect of regulating immune activity.

Chinese medicine is rich in source and is an effective medicine for long-term clinical treatment. After extraction, it can obtain active ingredients and have obvious pharmacological effects (including immunomodulatory effects). The research process saves people time and has high efficiency.

(2) Why look for immunomodulatory drugs from traditional Chinese medicine because of the progress in the study of traditional Chinese medicine immunopharmacology.

In view of the development of traditional Chinese medicine immunopharmacology, TCM theory has its obvious overall view, emphasizing the balance of the body, maintaining balance when the internal and external environment changes, losing balance, and the body has symptoms.

Modern medicine also emphasizes the stability of the internal environment and the regulation of the stable environment in the body. The factors are the three systems of nerve, endocrine and immunity. "Nerve, endocrine, and immunoregulatory networks" (NIM network) is currently a research hotspot in immunopharmacology.

Traditional Chinese medicine has a large number of prescriptions to regulate the body's immune function, especially the beneficial Chinese medicine has the effect of regulating immune activity. In the past 28 years, our laboratory has carried out a series of experimental studies to find new anticancer drugs for anticancer, anticancer metastasis, prevention of thymus atrophy, and elevated immunity from natural drugs, and to find new anticancer drugs from natural drugs. Looking for anti-metastatic, anti-relapsing drugs; looking for drugs that only inhibit cancer cells without inhibiting normal cells; looking for drugs that prevent thymic atrophy, regulate host-tumor regulation, and prevent recurrence and metastasis.

The existing chemotherapy anticancer drugs inhibit the immune function of the patient, inhibit the hematopoietic function of the bone marrow, inhibit the thymus, inhibit the bone marrow, and make it lose immune surveillance, so that the cancer can be further developed. Therefore, it is necessary to strengthen research so that all anticancer drugs used must be drugs that can boost immunity and protect immune organs, and should not be immune.

(3) Why do we look for drugs that promote thymic hyperplasia, prevent thymic atrophy, and boost immunity from traditional Chinese medications?

Because in the course of our research on anti-cancer and anti-cancer metastasis, we gradually discovered and recognized that the theory of traditional Chinese medicine is similar to our concept of anti-cancer and anti-cancer metastasis.

Chinese medicine theory	New concept of anti-cancer and anti-cancer metastasis research
1、a. TCM treatment believes that righteousness is not Fictitious or imaginary, evil spirits do not enter, governance and treatment must be righteous and firm the solid and increase tonic. b. And developed a series of prescriptions for tonic drugs. The essence is to maintain the overall functional balance and enhance disease resistance. c. In modern scientific language, the main role of supplemental drugs is to enhance the body's immune function. d. In Chinese medicine treatment it is to emphasize righting and is equivalent to the immune function of Western medicine.	1、a. Our experimental study found that: tumor model has thymus atrophy, immune function is low, it must try to prevent thymus atrophy, promote thymocyte proliferation, increase immunity, it must seek to enhance immune drugs to enhance immunity. b. Therefore, the theory of traditional Chinese medicine is in good agreement with the concept of the new concept and new method of cancer metastasis. c. We understand the supporting rightness and solidification of traditional Chinese medicine, which is equivalent to the immunity of Western medicine and enhance the body's disease resistance.
2、a. TCM treatment not only pays attention to righting up, but also pays attention to evil spirits, that is, helping the righteousness and removing evils or strengthening the righteousness can kill the evil spirits. b. The traditional Chinese medicine rightness and removing evils are based on the treatment of increasing immune function in Western medicine, thereby improving the treatment principle of immune surveillance to eliminate metastasize cancer cells. The two are in good agreement。	2、a. The traditional concept of Western medicine believes that cancer is the continuous division and proliferation of cancer cells, and the goal of treatment must be to kill cancer cells. b. The new concept and new method of cancer metastasis we studied believe that the treatment and cure of cancer should be regulated and controlled rather than killed. c. Protecting the thymus and improving immunity and improving immune surveillance and controlling the transfer of cancer cells are similar to the concept of evil spirits in the Chinese medicine practitioners.
3、a. Traditional Chinese medicine treatment of activation of blood and removing stasis are a common treatment principle, so it is commonly used to promote blood circulation and to remove blood stasis drugs. b. There are many drugs with circulating-blood and removing blood stasis in traditional Chinese medicine, the effect is exact, the effect is long-lasting, and it can be taken orally for a long time. It is suitable for anti-cancer metastasis drugs, because anti-cancer and anti-metastatic drugs must be taken orally for a long time. c. Traditional Chinese medication has many medications with blood-activating circulation and removing the blood stasis, which can be used for anti-cancer thrombosis and prevention of cancer thrombosis and anti-cancer metastasis. From the << new concept and new method of cancer metastasis treatmenth>> research it is believed that cancer cells in the blood circulation are gathered into a heap, surrounded by cellulose, platelets and a small amount of white blood cells to form tiny tumor thrombi. The tumor thrombus can be transported to other parts by blood flow, or stayed primary site after a certain period of time, it can penetrate the local upper wall, adhere to the solid organ cells and divide and proliferate around the blood vessel and forms the metastasis.	3、a. From the << new concept and new method of cancer metastasis treatmenth>> research it is believed that cancer cells in the blood circulation are gathered into a heap, surrounded by cellulose, platelets and a small amount of white blood cells to form tiny tumor thrombi. The tumor thrombus can be transported to other parts by blood flow, or stayed primary site after a certain period of time, it can penetrate the local upper wall, adhere to the solid organ cells and divide and proliferate around the blood vessel and forms the metastasis. b. In our research on anti-cancer metastasis, we realized that we must focus on the cancer cell population or cancer cell groups or micro-cancer plugs on the metastasis way and conduct the encircling, chasing, blocking, intercepting, and anti-coagulation. Anti-coagulation is the main point of anti-cancer. c. How to eliminate cancer cells and tumor thrombus on the way of metastasis?

4. Fourth, clinical verification work

(1) After 7 years of scientific experiments in the laboratory, the XZ-C immunomodulatory anti-cancer and anti-metastatic traditional Chinese medicines were screened from the Tianjiu drug, and the chest-protection, blood-protecting, blood-activating and blood-sucking were successfully performed in animal experiments. On the basis of the clinical validation work.

(2) Since 1985, one side of the tumor-bearing mice in the tumor-bearing mice has been tested in clinical practice.

However, there are few patients, and there is no medical record in the outpatient clinic (the medical records are all issued to patients), and it is impossible to accumulate scientific research materials.

(3) Establishing an anti-cancer research collaboration group, taking the road of scientific research collaboration and joint research, and setting up the Dawn Cancer Specialist Clinic.

(4) Resume the outpatient medical records, fill in the complete and detailed outpatient medical records, obtain complete information of clinical verification, facilitate analysis and statistics, and be conducive to outpatient clinical research to improve the quality of medical care.

(5) Retaining outpatient cases, regular follow-up, and a brief analysis of the experience and lessons of this case, in order to long-term observation of long-term efficacy.

(6) The oncology clinic outpatient medical records are designed in a tabular format, including all relevant medical information and relevant epidemiological data, in order to statistically analyze the possible pathogenic factors.

(7) Cases and outpatient medical records that have been reviewed for more than 1 year, all of which are written with medical records, and analyzed by large tables. The contents of the large table include the contents of the outpatient medical record form, which are both concise and detailed, and the Twilight Oncology Specialist The outpatient clinic has been verified for 20 years, and the large scale has accumulated nearly 10,000 outpatient clinical data for outpatient clinical research.

(8) From experimental research to clinical research, from clinical to experimental. The collaboration group has an experimental research base and a clinical application verification base. The former is in the medical laboratory, and the latter is in the Twilight Oncology Clinic. From the experiment to the clinical, that is, based on the success of the experimental research, it is applied to the clinical and clinical application process. New problems are discovered, and further basic experimental research is carried out, and new experimental results are applied to clinical verification. For example, outpatients have liver cancer with portal vein tumor thrombus, renal cancer patients with inferior vena cava tumor thrombus, some are CT reports, and some are surgery. The pathological section of the specimen was resected. In fact, the tumor thrombus is the cancer cell group on the way to metastasis. It is the third form of cancer in the human body. When the cancer thrombosis problem is discovered, we began the experimental study of cancer thrombus formation. Looking for new ways to fight against cancerous plugs and dissolve cancerous plugs, we found four traditional Chinese medicines that help to dissolve cancerous plugs and found out their active ingredients.

Such experiments → clinical → re-experiment → re-clinical, continuous cyclical rise, after 12 years of clinical practice experience, understanding is also constantly rising, summed up practice, analysis, reflection, evaluation has risen to theory, propose new understanding, new thinking, new Treatment ideas.

(9) Clinical efficacy observation: On the basis of experimental research, it has been applied to clinical cancers since 1994, mostly patients with stage III or IV, ie advanced cancer that cannot be removed by exploration; recent cancer surgery Or long-term metastasis or recurrence; liver metastasis, lung metastasis, brain metastasis, bone metastasis or cancerous pleural effusion, cancerous ascites in various advanced cancers; palliative resection of various cancers, exploration can only do stomach Thoracic anastomosis or colostomy can not be removed; patients who are not suitable for surgery, radiotherapy or chemotherapy. XZ-C immunomodulation anticancer Chinese medicine has been clinically applied for 20 years, and systematic observation has achieved obvious curative effect. No adverse reactions were observed after long-term use. Clinical observations have shown that XZ-C immunomodulatory Chinese medicine can comprehensively improve the quality of life of patients with advanced cancer, improve immunity, control cancer cell proliferation, and consolidate and enhance long-term efficacy after surgery or radiotherapy.

(10) Oral administration and external application of XZ-C medicine have good curative effect on softening and reducing surface metastasis of tumor. Combined with intervention or intubation pump treatment, it can protect liver, kidney, bone marrow hematopoietic system and immune organs and improve immunity.

In the Dawn Cancer Specialist Clinic, 4698 cases of stage III, IV or metastatic recurrent cancer were treated for long-term follow-up or follow-up.

(11) Evaluation of quality of life of patients with advanced cancer by XZ-C immunomodulation Chinese medicine: This group is middle and late stage patients, the symptom improvement rate is 93.2%, the mental improvement is 95.2%, the appetite is improved by 93%, and the physical strength is increased by 57.3. %, comprehensively improved the quality of life of patients with advanced cancer.

(12) Efficacy evaluation: not only pay attention to the short-term efficacy and imaging indicators, but also pay attention to the long-term efficacy of survival, quality of life and immune indicators, the goal is to live long patients, good quality of life. During the course of medication, it is necessary to pay attention to changes in self-conscious symptoms and improvement of self-conscious symptoms for more than one month, otherwise it is effective; it pays attention to the spirit, appetite, and quality of life (Carson's score).

From experimental research to clinical validation, new problems are discovered during the clinical validation process, and back to the laboratory for basic research, and new experimental results are applied to clinical validation. For example, experiment-clinical-re-experiment-re-clinical, all experimental research must be clinically verified. In a large number of patients, observe for 3 to 5 years, or even clinical observation for 8 to 10 years. According to evidence-based medicine, there is long-term prevention. The interview and evaluable data prove that there is a good long-term efficacy. The standard of efficacy is: good quality of life and long survival. XZ-C immunomodulation anticancer traditional Chinese medicine preparation has been proved to be effective after being applied to a large number of patients with advanced cancer. XZ-C immunomodulatory Chinese medicine can improve the quality of life of patients with advanced cancer, enhance immunity, enhance the body's ability to fight cancer, enhance appetite, and significantly prolong survival.

5, the fifth, XZ-C immune regulation of anti-cancer Chinese medicine mechanism of action

XZ-C immunomodulatory Chinese medicine can improve the quality of life of patients with advanced cancer, enhance immunity, enhance the body's ability to fight cancer, enhance appetite, and significantly prolong survival. The introduction is as follows:

With the deepening of research on traditional Chinese medicine, many traditional Chinese medicines have been known to regulate the production and biological activities of cytokines and other immune molecules. At this time, the immunological mechanism of XZ-C immunomodulation of anticancer Chinese medicines is explained at the molecular level. It is very important.

1). XZ-C anti-cancer Chinese medicine can protect immune organs and enhance the quality of thymus and spleen.
2). XZ-C anticancer Chinese medicine has obvious promoting effect on bone marrow cell proliferation and hematopoietic function.
3). XZ-C anti-cancer Chinese medicine has an enhanced effect on T cell immune function, and has obvious promoting proliferation effect on T cells.
4). XZ-C anticancer Chinese medicine has a significant enhancement effect on the production of human 1L-2.
5). XZ-C5 anti-cancer Chinese medicine has a stimulating and potentiating effect on NK cells. NK cells have a broad-spectrum anti-tumor effect and can kill xenogenic tumor cells.
6). XZ-C anticancer Chinese medicine has an enhanced effect on the activity of LAK cells. LAK cells have a broad-spectrum anti-tumor effect on solid tumor cells that are sensitive and insensitive to NK cells.
7). XZ-C anticancer Chinese medicine has the function of promoting tumor necrosis factor (TNF). TNF is a kind of cytokine which can directly cause tumor cell death. Its main biological function is to kill or inhibit tumor cells.

6. Biological response modifier (BRM) and BRM-like Chinese medicine and tumor treatment

1). Biological response modifier (BRM) has opened up a new field of tumor biotherapy. At present, BRM is widely regarded as the fourth program of cancer treatment by the medical community.

In 1982, Oldham founded the biological response modifier (BRM), or BRM theory. On this basis, in 1984, the fourth modality of cancer treatment, biotherapy, was proposed. According to the BRM theory, under normal circumstances, the dynamic balance between tumor and body defense, tumor occurrence and even invasion and metastasis are completely caused by the imbalance of this dynamic balance. If the state of the disorder has been artificially adjusted to a normal level, the growth of the tumor can be controlled and allowed to subside.

Specifically, BRM includes the following anti-tumor mechanisms:

1. to promote the enhancement of the effect of the host defense mechanism, or to reduce the immunosuppression of the tumor-bearing host, in order to achieve the immune response to cancer.
2. The natural or genetically recombinant biologically active substance is administered to enhance the defense mechanism of the host.
3. Modification of tumor cells induces a strong host response.
4. Promote the differentiation and maturation of tumor cells and normalize them.
5. to alleviate the toxic side effects of cancer chemotherapy and radiotherapy, and enhance the tolerance of the host.

2). XZ-C immunomodulation of anti-cancer Chinese medicine BRM-like effect and efficacy

XZ-C immunomodulation anti-cancer Chinese medicine after 4 years of experimental research on cancer-bearing animals and 10 years of clinical verification showed that it has BRM-like effect and efficacy, and is a drug with BRM-like effect excavated from Chinese medicine resources. XZ-C immunomodulation anticancer Chinese medicine was experimentally screened from 200 Chinese herbal medicines by Professor Xu Ze's laboratory. Firstly, the cancer cells were cultured in vitro, and 200 kinds of Chinese herbal medicines were screened in vitro to observe the direct damage of the cancer cells in the culture tube, and the tumor cells were treated with the chemotherapy drug CTX and the normal cells in the test tube. Rate comparison test. As a result, a batch of drugs that have a certain cancer suppressing rate against cancer cell proliferation were selected. Then, the tumor-bearing animal model was further made, and the experimental study on the in vivo anti-tumor rate screening of the tumor-bearing animal model was carried out on 200 kinds of Chinese herbal medicines. The scientific, objective and rigorous experimental screening, analysis and evaluation were carried out. The results showed that only 48 species had a good tumor inhibition rate, and another 152 commonly used Chinese herbal medicines were screened by the tumor inhibition rate in this group of tumor-bearing experimental tumors, which showed no anticancer effect or a small tumor inhibition rate.

The XZ-C immunomodulatory anti-cancer metastasis drug that has been screened by the above experiments has improved immunity, increased thymus weight, protected thymus tissue function, increased cellular immunity, promoted bone marrow cell proliferation, and protected bone marrow blood production. Increase the number of red blood cells and white blood cells, enhance T cell function, activate immune cytokines, and improve immune surveillance in blood flow.

The main pharmacological action of XZ-C immunomodulation anticancer Chinese medicine is anti-cancer elevation, and its anti-cancer mechanism is:

1. Activate the body's immune cell system, promote the enhancement of the host defense mechanism, and achieve the immune response to cancer.
2. Activate the immune cytokine system of the body's anti-cancer mechanism, enhance the host defense mechanism and improve the immune surveillance of the immune cells of the body's blood circulation system.
3. chest lift, protect the thymus, increase immunity, protect the marrow from blood, protect the bone marrow from blood function, stimulate bone marrow hematopoietic function, promote the recovery of bone marrow suppression, increase white blood cells, red blood cells, etc.
4. to alleviate the side effects of radiotherapy and chemotherapy, and enhance the tolerance of the host.
5. can increase the weight of the thymus, so that the thymus does not progressive atrophy, as the cancer progresses, the chest and chest progressive atrophy.

As mentioned above, the mechanism of action of XZ-C immunomodulatory anticancer Chinese medicine is basically similar to that of BRM, and the clinical use also obtains the same therapeutic effect of BRM. Therefore, XZ-C immunomodulation anticancer Chinese medicine has BRM-like effect and efficacy. Combining today's advanced molecular oncology theory with ancient Chinese herbal medicine resources at the molecular level of Western medicine, BRM theory as a bridge, and the international advanced sub-oncology advanced theory and practice.

3).XZ-C1 + XZ-C4 immune regulation anti-cancer Chinese medicine XZ-C1 + XZ-C4 immune regulation anti-cancer Chinese medicine has the following characteristics.

(1) Comprehensively improve the quality of life of patients with advanced cancer.

(2) Protect the thymus to improve immunity, protect bone marrow, enhance hematopoietic function, and improve immunity and regulation.

(3) Enhance physical fitness, reduce pain and increase appetite.

(4) Enhance the therapeutic effect and reduce the adverse reactions of chemotherapy.

7. XZ-C immunomodulation anticancer Chinese medicine is the result of modernization of traditional Chinese medicine

XZ-C immunomodulation anticancer traditional Chinese medicine is not an empirical method, nor is it an old Chinese medicine practitioner, but a scientific research achievement of the combination of Chinese and Western medicine and traditional Chinese medicine. It is a modern medical method, using experimental tumor research methods and modern pharmacology and medicine. Combining the effects of research methods, after more than 4,000 tumor-bearing animal models in 7 years, 200 commonly used anti-cancer Chinese herbal medicines were recorded in the literature, and screened in animal experiments in batches. The screening of tumor inhibition rates in vitro and in tumor-bearing animals was carried out one by one. 48 kinds of traditional Chinese medicines with good anti-cancer effects were screened out.

XZ-C immunomodulation Chinese medicine preparation is an innovation and reform of traditional Chinese medicine preparation. It is not a compound preparation for mixed decoction, but a particle concentrate or powder for each medicine. The raw material of each medicine still retains its original ingredients and pharmacology. The function, molecular weight and structural formula are unchanged, and are made by modern scientific methods, rather than compounding, keeping the original ingredients and functions of each flavor unchanged, and it is easy to evaluate and affirm the effects and effects of various medicines.

In the above series of studies, we spent 4 years exploring the mechanism and regularity of cancer metastasis, looking for an effective method for anti-cancer metastasis; and spent 3 years passing 200 scientifically controlled cancer-bearing animal models from 200 traditional anti-cancer Chinese herbal medicines. Screening of tumor inhibition rate, 48 kinds of XZ-C immunomodulatory anti-cancer and anti-metastatic traditional Chinese medicines with good tumor inhibition rate were screened out. Based on this experimental study, it has been applied to more than 10,000 patients with advanced cancer in the past 20 years, and has achieved good results. From clinical to experimental, from experimental to clinical, the implementation of basic and clinical integration, the combination of Chinese and Western medicine at the molecular level, intends to embark on a new road of anti-cancer and anti-metastasis with Chinese characteristics.

8. take XZ-C immune regulation, molecular level, Western medicine combined with the road to overcome cancer

The combination of Chinese and Western medicine is the characteristics and advantages of Chinese medicine. The goal of combining Chinese and Western medicine should be to combine innovation, and the goal of innovation should be to improve the treatment effect. The efficacy criteria for cancer patients should be: long survival time, good quality of life, and few complications.

Adhere to the direction of innovation between Chinese and Western medicine, and we should persevere.

Mr. Lu Xun once said that there is no road in the world, and many people are leaving the road. In the past 28 years, we have initially embarked on a new way to use immunomodulation of Chinese medicine, regulate immune activity, prevent thymic atrophy, promote thymic hyperplasia, protect bone marrow hematopoietic function, improve immune surveillance, and combine Western medicine at the molecular level to overcome cancer.

Achieving combined innovation and improving curative effect is the goal of combining high-level Chinese and Western medicine. It is necessary to combine the theory of traditional Chinese medicine with modern medical practice, and to use the experimental research direction to clarify the internal meaning of traditional Chinese medicine theory, modern molecular oncology Chinese medicine immunopharmacology...... the internal theory of modern oncology theory, and then in the theoretical and clinical practice to develop and innovate, thereby improving the treatment effect and benefiting patients.

Our experimental surgical research institute is based on the research direction and main task of conquering cancer. It is a joint research project to tackle cancer. It is a combination of Chinese and Western medicine. It is a combination of Chinese and Western medicine at the molecular level. On the basis of animal experiments, And in the clinical practice of clinical practice to achieve the combination of Chinese and Western medicine, and then in the anti-cancer, anti-cancer transfer theory development, innovation:

——Traditional Chinese medicine believes that righteousness is not empty, evil spirits are not allowed, and governance must be based on strengthening the foundation and attaching importance to strengthening the right. Western medicine believes that tumors are low in immune function, and must be "protected by chest" to enhance immunity.

Chinese medicine emphasizes righting up, which is equivalent to the immunity of Western medicine. The two are in good agreement.

——Traditional Chinese medicine cures not only the righteousness but also the evil spirits, that is, righting up the evil or strengthening the righteousness to eliminate evil spirits. Western medicine believes that boosting immunity and improving immune surveillance, thus eliminating cancer cells on the way of metastasis, the treatment concepts are similar or The two are very consistent.

——Traditional Chinese medicine treatment of blood stasis is a commonly used principle. In our research on anti-cancer metastasis, we realized that it is necessary to target cancer cells in the process of metastasis, and must be anti-cancer, anticoagulation, and change.

CHAPTER 7

Our cancer prevention and treatment research has reached the world frontier

- **Science is no end or endless the frontier**

TABLE OF CONTENTS

1. Introduction or Preface

1. **Carry out the "Conquer Cancer and Launch the total Attack to cancer - Prevention, Control, and Treatment at the same attention and heavy and level"**

   - Reform the current mode of hospitalization
   - Reform the current treatment model focusing on the middle and late stages of treatment
   - Change only treatment without into prevention, control, and treatment at the same lever
   - It is necessary to establish a hospital for prevention, control and treatment according to the whole process of cancer occurrence and development.
   - The way out for cancer treatment is "three early", and early cancer treatment is effective and can be cured.

2. **Walked out of a new way of cancer treatment with XZ-C immune regulation and control combined with Chinese and Western medications**

   - navigate the path
   - Pathfinding and footprinting (scientific footprints)
   - Walked out of a new way of cancer treatment with XZ-C immune regulation and control combined with Chinese and Western medications at the molecular level
   - a series of products of XZ-C immune regulation and control anti-cancer Chinese medications
   - The theoretical system of XZ-C immunomodulation and cancer treatment has been formed and are the experimental basis for the theoretical basis of cancer treatment

3. **Initiative to create the "Innovative Environmental Protection and Cancer Research Institute" and carry out anti-cancer system engineering**

   - XZ-C proposes: Sun-up or Dawning A-type anti-cancer plan, Sun-up or Dawning B-type anti-cancer plan Sun-up or Dawning D-type anti-cancer plan
   - Combine with the three major challenges, ride research, anti-pollution and pollution treatment, anti-cancer, cancer control

4. "Our cancer research work has reached the world frontier"
5. "Condense wisdom and conquer cancer" - for the benefit of mankind

- Guided information
- Guidance of word
- Guidance of action
- table of Contents

Volume1: How to overcome cancer? How to prevent cancer?
Has been published in December 2017 (published)
Volume 2: How to overcome cancer? How to treat cancer?
February 2018 (published in the next volume)
Note:

1. XZ-C is XU ZE-China, **science is borderless, but scientists have nationalities and have intellectual property rights.**
2. Cancer is a disaster for all mankind. It should arouse the common struggle of people all over the world. Therefore, **seven of these monographs are in English and distributed worldwide.**

2. The list of content(30 items)

In the past 30 years, **our scientific research achievements** using Conquer Cancer as the research direction and **scientific and technological innovation series** in this "Monograph" in the following topics are **first proposed internationally; all original papers, international initiative, international leading** which have reached the world's leading position. **Its main contents are as follows:**

(1).It is Internationally proposed for the first time:
"Thymus atrophy, low immune function is one of the causes and pathogenesis of cancer"
(2). It is Internationally proposed for the first time:
the theoretical basis and experimental basis of "protection of Thymus and increase of immune function by XZ-C immunomodulation therapy
(3) The first international initiative: **"Cancer treatment should change the concept and establish a comprehensive treatment concept"**

(4) The first international initiative: "**A new model for the combination of multidisciplinary treatment of cancer**"

(5) The first international initiative: "**Analysis, evaluation and questioning of systemic intravenous chemotherapy for solid tumors and four evaluations**"

(6) The first international initiative: "**Initiative for the reform of systemic venous chemotherapy for abdominal solid tumors as a reform initiative for traditional chemotherapy into target organ intravascular chemotherapy**"

(7) The first international initiative, "**There are three main forms of cancer in the human body**"

(8) The first international initiative, the **"two points and one line" theory during the whole process of cancer development**

(9) The first international initiative, the **"Three Steps of Anticancer Metastasis Treatment**"

(10) The first international initiative: "**Developing the third field of cancer metastasis treatment**"

How to overcome cancer? XZ-C proposes to overcome cancer and launch the general attack to cancer, this is unprecedented work.

(11) The first international initiative, the **"XZ-C Scientific Research Plan for Overcoming cancer and launching the General Attack of Cancer"**

(12 The first international initiative, the **"Necessity and Feasibility of Overcoming cancer and launching the General Attack to Cancer"**

(13) The first international initiative, **"Setting up the establishment of a full-scale hospital for cancer prevention and development"**

(14) The first international initiative, **the "to set up General Plan for Overcoming Cancer and the Basic Design of Science City"**

(15) The first international initiative, "**To conquer cancer and launch the general attack to cancer—prevention and control and treatment at the same attention and level and time**"

——Change the hospital mode of attention of treatment and light prevention

(16) The first international initiative, "**Proposing to build a scientific research basis science city to overcome cancer**" —— establish an overall framework for conquering cancer

(17) The first international initiative:<<Walking out of a new path of conquering cancer>> **to prevent postoperative recurrence and metastasis**

(18) **Independently developed a series products of XZ-C immunomodulation anticancer traditional Chinese medications**

(19) **The first international initiative: how to overcome cancer? XZ-C proposed " Dawning C-type plan No. 1-6"**

(20) The first international initiative: **how to overcome cancer? XZ-C proposes that cancer is a disaster for all mankind and it must be strived together by the people of the world and China and USA joint research.**

"Cancer moon shot" (US) and "Dawning C-type plan" (middle)— Moving forward together, heading for the science hall to overcome cancer

Why do you want to move forward together? What are you together? China and the United States each have their own advantages analysis and complementary advantages.

(21) Over the past 100 years, the history records of who has been proposed "conquer cancer"

a. Two US presidents have successively proposed a national plan to "conquer cancer"

b. A Chinese physician XZ-C proposed the general design, plan, specific plan, blueprint for conquering cancer, and published seven monographs (English version, global release)

(22)It is first proposed internationally : How to overcome cancer? XZ-C proposes two wheels, A wheel, B wheel

(23)It is first proposed internationally : How to overcome cancer? XZ-C proposes need A wheel, A runway and B wheel, B runway

(24) For the first time in the world it is proposed **that how to conquer cancer? XZ-C proposes to need three targets for A, B and C.**

(25) XZ-C proposes **that several treatments rules of traditional Chinese medication can be applied to the treatment of tumors.**

(26)It is the first proposal internationally : **XZ-C proposes: in order to conquer cancer, it is necessary to create an environmental protection and cancer prevention research institute and carry out anti-cancer system engineering, which is the first time in the world.**

1. Conduct anti-cancer research, find cancer-causing factors, detect the source of carcinogens or carcinogenic factors, and try to stop the damage caused by these carcinogenic factors.

2. The Cancer Research Institute should conduct anti-cancer research: the relationship between air pollution and cancer; water pollution and cancer; soil pollution and cancer; chemical, physical, biological factors and cancer; diet, lifestyle, clothing, food, housing, transportation, housing Renovate with cancer, study these sources of pollution and try to stop at the source.

(27) XZ-C proposes that research ethics should be advocated, medicine is benevolence, and ethics is the first

Research ethics: products should have ethical standards

Standard: it should be based on the standard of not damaging human health

Basic ethics: All products should be harmless to people and do not harm people's health, especially for children, not allowed to contain carcinogens.

(28) The postscript of Guidance reading includes **the general design and plan and program and blueprint for How to implement, how to achieve "conquer cancer"**

(29**) How to carry out "to overcome cancer and launch the general attack of cancer" in Hubei and Wuhan**

(30) **Internationally proposed for the first time: XZ-C proposed Dawning anti-cancer program A, B, D for anti-pollution and protecting pollution control and cancer prevention and anti-cancer**

As explained above, our research work is already in the forefront of the world, and it is already a first-class discipline. Under the guidance of Xi Jinping's new era of socialism with Chinese characteristics, we should make great strides forward, new era, new journey, new weather, new actions, and became a courageous person or struggler in the new era.

In short, if the above items can be implemented and realized, they should be able to overcome cancer.

(1) The goal of conquering cancer:

Reduce the incidence of cancer, improve the cure rate of cancer, reduce the cancer mortality, significantly prolong the survival of patients and improve the quality of life.

(2) reach:

1/3 can be prevented, 1/3 can be cured, and 1/3 can prolong life through treatment

I hope some universities can create this first-class discipline or subject using or considering "**overcome cancer**" as the research direction.

Suggestions:

The research of Huazhong University of Science and Technology, Wuhan University, Hubei University of Traditional Chinese Medicine and other alma mater [Note] should be pushed to the forefront of the world, and the first batch of first-class disciplines or subjects using "Conquer cancer" as the research direction in China and the world, in the new era of Xi Jinping Guided by the socialist ideology with Chinese characteristics, we will strive to follow the road of innovation in anti-cancer transfer with Chinese characteristics, adhere to the road of independent innovation with Chinese characteristics, adhere to the combination of Chinese and Western medicine, and the road of independent innovation of "Chinese-style anti-cancer", hoping to be in Hubei and Wuhan in the country and in Globe, the first batch of first-class disciplines or subject "to overcome cancer" as the research direction can be built, then to make new achievements in conquering cancer, and the achievement is in the modern age, benefits in the ages.

[Note]: I was admitted to the Central South Tongji Medical College in 1951. The hospital was formed by the merger of Shanghai Tongji Medical College and the National Wuhan University School of Medicine. After graduation, I was assigned to the Affiliated Hospital of Hubei College of Traditional Chinese Medicine. All of them are the alma mater for my study, work, and growth.

3. The crux of the international initiatives and innovation (30 items)

In the past 30 years, our scientific research achievements and scientific and technological innovation series of conquering cancer as the research direction are the first in the world. They are all original papers, international firsts, international leaders, and have reached the world's leading position. Its main contents are as follows:

(I). Internationally proposed for the first time: "Thymus atrophy, low immune function is one of the causes and pathogenesis of cancer":

1. New findings on experimental research on the etiology and pathogenesis of cancer
2. This is the result of international leading intellectual property rights. After the investigation, this is the first time in the world.
3. See the monograph "New Concepts and New Methods of Cancer Treatment" P.13

(2) Internationally proposed for the first time, 'the theoretical basis and experimental basis of protecting Thymus and increasing Immune function of "XZ-C immune regulation and control treatment"

1. Proposed the theoretical basis and experimental basis of cancer immune regulation and control therapy
2. Because of the new findings of the above experimental research, the treatment principle must be to prevent progressive atrophy of the thymus, promote thymic hyperplasia, protect bone marrow hematopoietic function, improve immune surveillance, and control immune escape of malignant cells.
3. See the monograph "New Concepts and New Methods of Cancer Treatment" P.17

(3) The first international initiative: "Cancer treatment should change the concept and establish a comprehensive treatment concept"

1. propose a new concept of cancer treatment principles
2. The target or goal o f cancer treatment must establish a comprehensive treatment concept for both tumor and host
3. it should overcome the one-sided treatment concept of simply killing cancer cells
4. See the monograph "New Concepts and New Methods for Cancer Treatment" P.28

(4) The first international initiative: "A new model for the combination of multidisciplinary treatment of cancer"

1. Initiative: A new concept of multidisciplinary combination model for cancer treatment
2. The new model of multidisciplinary treatment is:
Long-term treatment mainly: surgery + biological treatment + immunotherapy + Chinese medicine, Chinese and Western combined treatment; Short-course treatment is supplemented: radiotherapy, chemotherapy, not long-range, not excessive
3. See the monograph "New Concepts and New Methods for Cancer Treatment" P33

(5)) The first international initiative, "the analysis, evaluation and questioning of systemic intravenous chemotherapy for solid tumors and four evaluations"

1. Analysis of the problems and drawbacks of systemic intravenous chemotherapy for solid cancer
2. Question and evaluation of systemic intravenous chemotherapy for solid tumors, calculation of drug volume, evaluation of efficacy
3. See the monograph "New Concepts and New Methods of Cancer Treatment" P.57

(6)) The first international initiative, the "Initiative for intravenous chemotherapy of abdominal solid tumors should be reformed as intra-target chemotherapy for target organs, and reform initiatives for traditional chemotherapy for cancer"

1. Because systemic intravenous chemotherapy cytotoxic drugs cannot directly reach the portal system by the superior vena cava administration, the vena cava system and the portal system are generally incompatible, and it is difficult to reach the portal vein by the superior vena cava.
2. What are the cancer cells of abdominal solid tumors (stomach, colorectal, liver, gallbladder, pancreas, spleen, abdominal cavity, etc.)? Mainly in the portal system, postoperative adjuvant chemotherapy from the venous vein to the vena cava is unreasonable, does not meet the anatomy, physiology and pathology, because it can not directly enter the portal system
3. Therefore, the route of administration should be changed to the endovascular treatment of target organs
4. See the monograph "New Concepts and New Methods of Cancer Treatment" P.63

(7) The first international initiative, there are three main manifestations of cancer in the human body.

1. Proposed theoretical innovation of new concept of cancer metastasis treatment
2. This third manifestation is proposed to be a group of cancer cells on the way to metastasis. The treatment target of cancer should be directed to the above three forms of existence, especially for cancer cells on the way to metastasis.
3. See the monograph "New Concepts and New Methods for Cancer Treatment" P.38

(8) The first international initiative, the "two points and one line" theory of the whole process of cancer development

1. Proposed theoretical innovation of cancer metastasis treatment
2. One of the purposes of cancer treatment is to prevent metastasis and **the whole process of cancer metastasis development can be summarized as "two points and one line"**
3. Traditional cancer treatment only pays attention to "two points" and ignores "first line"; the new concept believes that both "two points" should be emphasized, and that "one line" should be cut off.
4. See the monograph "New Concepts and New Methods for Cancer Treatment" P.43

(9) For the first time in the world proposed : the "Three Steps of Anticancer Metastasis Treatment"

1. Proposed theoretical innovation of cancer metastasis treatment
2. Incorporate the "eight steps" of cancer cell transfer into "three stages" and try to break each transfer step.
3. See the monograph "New Concepts and New Methods for Cancer Treatment" P.47

(10) For the first time in the world proposed : "Developing the third field of anti-cancer transfer"

1. Proposed the theoretical innovation of the new concept of cancer metastasis treatment and found and proposed the third field of human anti-cancer metastasis
2. The circulatory system has a large number of immune surveillance cells and the "main battlefield" to annihilate the cancer cells on the way is in the blood circulation.

(11) For the first time in the world it is proposed : the "XZ-C Scientific Research Plan for Overcoming conquer and attacking the General Attack"

1. The overall strategic reform and development of cancer treatment in China
2. Avoid talk, should work hard, start to walk
3. No matter how far the road to cancer is, it should always start to go.
4. Proposed to overcome cancer and launch the general attack to cancerr, this is unprecedented work

(12) For the first time in the world proposed: the "Necessity and Feasibility Report on conquering cancer and vercoming the General Attack"

1. The overall strategic reform of cancer treatment in China should be changed from focusing on treatment into prevention and treatment.
2. XZ-C proposes the general idea and design of conquering cancer
3. What is the total attack on cancer and the goal of the total attack?
4. XU ZE proposes ideas, strategies, plans, blueprints of overcoming cancer and launching a general attack

(13) For the first time in the world proposed : "To construct the hospital with cancer prevention and treatment during cancer occurrence and development of the whole process " (Global demonstration cancer prevention and treatment hospital)

1. The existing problems in the current building hospital model
2. The road of how to overcome cancer is to study the establishment of prevention and treatment hospitals during the whole process of cancer occurrence and development, and reform the current mode of hospitalization for the attention to treatment with light preventon.
3. XU ZE's strategic thinking, planning sketch for the prevention and treatment of cancer during cancer occurrence and development

(14) For the first time in the world proposed : 'the "General Plan of conquering cancer and the Basic Design of building the Science City"

1. Equivalent to designing an overall framework for the design with Chinese characteristics of conquering cancer
2. How to set up the basic idea and design to overcome cancer and launch the general attack to cancer
3. How to overcome cancer? The Cancer Animal Experimental Center must be established and Innovative Molecular Oncology Medical College and Cancer Multidisciplinary Research Institute
4. How to overcome cancer? It is necessary to "prepare a medical, teaching, research, and science base to overcome cancer and launch the general attack of cancer - Science City"

(15) It is the first proposed internationally "To overcome cancer and to launch a general attack - to prevent, control, and treat at the same attention and level and the same time"

A. The key points are as the following:

1. Changed the mode of running a hospital and changed the current mode of running a hospital
2. Changed the treatment mode and changed the current treatment mode focusing on the middle and late stages of treatment
3. Change from only treatment without prevention into prevention, control, and treatment at the same level and attention
4. Proposed the design, blueprint and implementation rules and plans for launching the general attack.
5. It is necessary to establish a hospital for prevention, control and treatment according to the whole process of cancer occurrence and development.
6. Walking out of Cancer treatment is in the "three early", early cancer treatment is good and can be cured completely (See separate information for details)

B. Why do you need to conquer cancer and launch a general attack and why does it need to launch the total attack?

1. Because the goal of conquering cancer should be:
(1) reduce the incidence of cancer, Improve cancer cure rate, prolong patient survival and improve quality of life
(2) reach:
1/3 can be prevented
1/3 can be cured
1/3 can be prolonged life through treatment
2. then, how can we reduce the incidence of cancer? It should be prevention-oriented, control-oriented, and the cancer prevention-oriented should be the most important part. But for decades, the road we have traveled is to the attention of treatment with light prevent or only treatment without prevent.

I have been working in clinical oncology surgery for 62 years. Looking back on the lessons of failure for decades is only treatment with little prevention or no prevent so the incidence of cancer is increasing, and the more patients are treated and the more patients ocurr.

How to do? It should be prevention-oriented and control-oriented, and implement the prevention-oriented health work policy. Only by paying attention to cancer prevention can we reduce the incidence of cancer. Cancer prevention and cancer control and how to prevent cancer should be the top priority.

How can we implement and carry out health work guidelines or policies which are cancer prevention and cancer control that put main attention on prevention-oriented, how can we reform and correct the current hospitality model and the hospital policy of attention of treatment with light defense, or treatment without prevention? It must challenge the hospital policy of cancer treatment and it must reform and then develop.

Professor Xu Ze proposed to launch the general attack. In fact, it is the prevention, control, and treatment at the same time and attention and the same lever and put cancer prevention and control cancer into the important parts. The essence is to carry out and implement the health work **policy of "cancer prevention and anti-cancer", mainly "prevention-oriented".** Our medical predecessors, the world's medical sages put forward "cancer prevention and anti-cancer", mainly "prevention-oriented", this policy is very correct, but unfortunately, our medical juniors have not paid attention to it.

In particular, our cancer researchers and health workers have not realized this. Over the past century, prevention has been neglected, prevention has not been taken seriously, and cancer prevention has been neglected, leading to such a high incidence of cancer today. There are 8,550 new cancers in China every day, and 6 people are diagnosed with cancer every minute. Such amazing data should be a national event.

The task of health work should be "prevention and treatment of disease" and "prevention first". Health is to protect life and defend health. Launching the general attack, its essence is to put cancer prevention work at an important position, which are the most important of the cancer prevention and cancer anti-cancer and try to reduce the incidence of cancer.

(16) First proposed internationally:

"Building a Science City of Conquering Cancer" is to establish an overall framework for the fight against cancer, which is the only way to overcome cancer and to propose the overall design, blueprint and implementation rules and plans of Science City

(See separate information for details)

(17) First proposed internationally

"Walking out of a new road to overcome cancer" is the experimental research, the anti-cancer research with Chinese medicine immunopharmacology and the combination with Chinese and Western medicine at the molecular level, namely:

1. walk out of a new way of conquering cancer with XZ-C immune regulation and control combining Chinese with Western medicine at the molecular level to overcome cancer

2. Walk out of a new way of conquering cancer using Chinese medicine immune regulation and control, regulating immune activity, preventing thymus atrophy, promoting thymic hyperplasia, protecting bone marrow hematopoietic function, improving immune surveillance, and combining with Western medicine and Chinese medicine at the molecular leve.

3. We have embarked on the road of conquering cancer – the new path of "Chinese-style anti-cancer of XZ-C immune regulation and control, and the combination of Chinese and Western medicine at the molecular level". (See separate information for details)

(18). A series products Exclusive research and development of XZ-C immune regulation and control anti-cancer Chinese medications

1. Experimental research + clinical application + the typical cases + the case list

2. XZ-C (XU ZE-China), an independent research and development of immune regulation and control anti-cancer series of traditional Chinese medicaton preparations, from experimental research to clinical verification, applied to clinical practice on the basis of successful animal experiments. Over the years, more than 12,000 cases of clinical validation, significant efficacy, independent innovation, independent intellectual property rights.

3. XZ-C immunomodulatory anti-cancer Chinese medicine was 48 kinds of Chinese herbal medicines with good tumor inhibition rate screened from the more than 200 traditional Chinese herbal medicines in China through anti-tumor experiments in cancer-bearing mice. After compounding, they were tested through the Inhibition of tumor experiments in the tumor-bearing mice in vivo, the compound inhibition rate is far greater than the single-drug inhibition rate, in which XZ-C1 100% inhibits cancer cells, 100% does not kill normal cells, has the effect of strengthening the body and improving the immune function of the human body.

From our experiments on XZ-C pharmacodynamics studies, it has a good tumor inhibition rate for Ehrlich ascites carcinoma, S_{180}, H_{22} hepatocellular carcinoma.

Acute toxicity test in mice showed no obvious side effects. In the clinical long-term oral administration for several years (2-6 years), no obvious side effects were observed.

Middle and advanced cancer patients, mostly weak and fatigue, lack of appetite, XZ-C immunomodulation anti-cancer Chinese medicine 4-8-12 weeks later, can significantly improve appetite, sleep, relieve pain, and gradually restore physical strength.

(19) For the first time in the world proposed: how to conquer cancer? XZ-C proposed "Dawning C-type plan No.1-6

A. Why is "Dawning " used?

The dawn is the morning light, it is the dawn, it is the morning sun.
Vigorous, vigorous, original innovation, independent innovation
C=China
Type C = Chinese mode
About 8550 people in China are diagnosed with cancer every day, and 6 people are diagnosed with cancer every minute. Therefore, the research work to overcome the general attack of cancer, can not walk slowly, should run forward, save the wounded.
Time is money, time is money = one inch of time, one inch of gold
Time is life, time is life
Time flies, time flies
Empty talk about mistakes, hard work
Avoid empty talk, Attention to work hard, start to walk
No matter how far the road to cancer is, you should always start.
This research plan is the original innovation, it is time to declare war on cancer, and the general attack should be launched.
Our dreams are to conquer cancer and to build a well-off society and everyone is healthy and be away from cancer

B. The brief introduction of Dawning C Plan:

Dawning C plan
Formulated in July 2015

1. Dawning C-type plan No. 1: "Conquer cancer and launch the general attack"

1). Proposed the overall strategic reform and development of cancer treatment in China

2) Proposed the general idea, plan, design, blueprint and rules for conquering cancer

3).Avoid empty talk, attention to work hard, start to walk

4).No matter how far the road of conquering conquer cancer is, you should always start to walk.

(see separate article)

2.Dawning C-type plan No. 2: "Preparing or building the hospitals with the whole process of cancer prevention and treatment" (Global Demonstration Prevention and Treatment Hospital)

1) proposed Strategic reform,2) change the mode of running a hospital,3) Reforming treatment mode

(see separate article)

3.Dawnign C-type plan No. 3: "Building a science city to overcome cancer"

a. XZ-C proposed the overall design, planning and blueprint of Science City of conquering cancer and launching the general attack of cancer

b. This is the only way to overcome cancer

c. This is the "high-speed rail" and "high-speed" channel for cancer.

(see separate article)

4.Dawning C-type plan No. 4 "Building a multidisciplinary and cancer research group"

1. for the cause, pathogenesis, pathophysiology, metastasis, recurrence mechanism of cancer...

Study anti-cancer, anti-recurrence, anti-metastatic measures to improve the overall level of medical care to benefit patients

2. The standard of efficacy evaluation is: patients have long survival time, good quality of life, and no or little complications. Each school group is a provincial key laboratory. (see separate article)

5. Dawning C-type plan No. 5 "vaccine is the hope of human beings Immunological prevention"

a. Today's immunology prevention and treatment has become an extremely important field in clinical medicine and preventive medicine

b. △△study group+△△study group+△△study group→Scientific Alliance, Joint Group

(see separate article)

(6) Dawning C-type plan No. 6: A "The prospect of immunomodulatory drugs is gratifying"

a. Regardless of the complexity of the mechanisms behind cancer, immune suppression is the essential of the progression of cancer

b. Our laboratory analyzes the experimental results, obtains new discoveries, and has new inspirations:

Thymus atrophy, immune dysfunction, decreased immune surveillance and immune escape are one of the causes and pathogenesis of cancer, so the principle of treatment should be to prevent the thymus atrophy, promote thymic hyperplasia, and improve immune surveillance.

c. XZ-C immunomodulatory Chinese medications are 48 kinds of Chinese herbal medicines with good cancer suppression rate, 26 of which are better. The role of immune regulation selected from more than 200 kinds of the traditional Chinese herbal medicines through the anti-tumor experiment of the cancer-bearing mouse animal model, (see separate article)

Dawning C-type plan No. 6: B "the research group an laboratory of XZ-C immunomodulation anti-cancer Chinese medication active ingredient and the molecular level analysis"

a. Further research and development of XZ-C immunomodulatory anti-cancer Chinese medicine active ingredients, molecular weight, structural formula, molecular level analysis

b. Methods and steps: animal experiments, molecular level experiments; gene level experiments, first separating the active ingredients, making the precious heritage of traditional Chinese medicine modern and scientific. (see separate article)

C. The Aim and the Origination of Dawn C-type plan: Dawning C-type plan(China)

a. The Aim of this Dawning C type plan:

Hope: Apply to incorporate the "Dawning C-type plan" into the National Cancer Program

To report to:

the Party Central Committee and the State Council

Hubei Provincial Party Committee and Provincial Government
Wuhan Municipal Party Committee and Municipal Government
Goal: Conquer cancer
Mission: Prepare a science city to overcome the general attack on cancer
President of Science City, General Director, President of the General Academic
Committee: **Professor Xu Ze**(Previous Director of Institute of Experimental
Surgery, Hubei College of Traditional Chinese Medicine)
Science City Innovative Oncology Medical College
Innovative Cancer Research Institute Chief Dean:
Innovative Tumor Hospital Integrated Traditional Chinese and Western Medicine
Hospital Leadership Team:
General Secretary of Science City:
Dean of the Graduate School of Science City:

The chief scientist team of Wuhan Anticancer Research Association is **Professor Dr. Xu Ze**:
1).The chief designer of "To conquer cancer and launch the general attack on cancer and to create a science city to overcome cancer"
2).Project Leader of "Overcome cancer and launch the General Attack of Cancer"

"Conquer Cancer Science City" to establish the following genetic testing research groups:
(1) Establish genetic testing and cancer research groups and laboratories
(2) Establish HPV anti-cancer research group and laboratory
(3) Establish genetic testing and immunology and cancer research groups and laboratories
(4) Establish genetic testing and endocrine hormone and cancer research groups and laboratories
(5) Establish genetic testing and pathological sections, and related studies on immunohistochemistry
(6) Establish correlation analysis and research on gene detection and tumor markers
(7) Establish HPV treatment, exploration research groups and laboratories

The Expected results:

Using modern science and technology and analytical testing methods, the research on traditional Chinese medication, the material basis of the efficacy of traditional Chinese medication in clinical practice is the chemical composition contained therein. To study the anticancer effect and mechanism of traditional Chinese medicine, it is necessary to conduct in-depth research and analysis. **The active ingredients in it make the precious heritage of traditional Chinese medicine more modern and scientific.**

After 28 years of experimental research, basic research and clinical verification, a series of "protection of Thymus and Enhancement of immune function" immunomodulatory anticancer Chinese medication XZ-C1-10 has been screened. After 30 years of clinical observation, more than 12,000 cases have been verified, and the outpatient medical records have been saved and made a list of disease analysis, they can prolong life, improve symptoms, improve the quality of life, how to know and how to evaluate that they can extend the survival period? Some surgical explorations can not be cut down (all pathological sections confirmed diagnosis), or have been widely transferred, it is estimated that only 3-6 months, or 6-12 months of cases, after the treatment of **XZ-C immune regulation and control anti-cancer, anti-metastasis and recurrence medications, some patients can still survive for 4 years - 5 years - 8 years - 10 years - 15 years, with original data and complete data as well as follow-up data.**

b. The origination or innovation of Dawning C-type Plan

After a rehabilitation teacher, after a heart attack, calm down, hide in a small building, self-reliance, hard work, adhere to animal experiment basic research and outpatient clinical validation research with anti-cancer, anti-cancer metastasis and recurrence, from the year of the flower (60 years old)→to the age of the ancients (70s)→To the age of (80s), still perseverance, persevere in scientific research of overcoming cancer, because he has retired, failed to apply for projects and programs, so there is no research Funding, and working alone and fighting alone, being self-reliant, working hard, and no one cares, and no one knows, and there is nowhere to report, and there is no support and **it has been hard work for more than 20 years, has achieved a series of scientific and technological innovations, scientific research results; due to retirement In the past 20 years, no one cares, no one supports; as a retired professor, I don't know where to manage, where to support, so where the scientific research results are reported, I have to make a "monograph" for the benefit of mankind, but published a series of monographs, and** then Report to the Provincial Department of Science and Technology and the Provincial Department of Education:

1. I hope to open an international high-end academic forum;
2. report to the government to apply for cancer, launch a general attack;

3. report to the province and the government.

Hope:

Apply to establish the "National Science City to overcome cancer and launch the general attack of cancer" in Hubei and Wuhan, which is the "World's first science city to overcome the general attack of cancer."

How to implement this unprecedented event in human history?

(1) Reporting, requesting and instructions to the government,

(2) Reporting, request and instructions to the province and city,

(3) Make recommendations to the city to build: "The first national conquering cancer science city"; "The world's first Science City to overcome Cancer " in Wuhan.

(20) How to overcome cancer? XZ-C proposes that cancer is a disaster for all mankind and must be fought together by the people of the world.

"Cancer moon shot" (US) and "Dawning C-type plan" (China)

a. Moving forward together, heading for the science hall of overcoming cancer

b. Why do you want to move forward together? What are the common together?

1) Introduction to "Cancer Moon Shot"

On January 12, 2016, US President Barack Obama announced in his last State of the Union address during his term of office a national plan to overcome cancer, the "Cancer Moon Shot", which will be under the responsibility of Biden.

Biden will visit the Abramson Cancer Center at the University of Pennsylvania School of Medicine next week to discuss the plan. He said that the "new moon landing plan" is a commitment to overcome cancer in the world and will inspire a new generation of scientists to explore the scientific world.

Obama did not mention the specific plan of the plan in his speech, but he mentioned that the expenditure and tax bill passed by Congress in December 2015 has raised the financial budget of the National Institutes of Health (NIH).

The United States has just recently established a national immunotherapy alliance consisting of pharmaceutical companies, biotechnology companies and academic medical organizations. The alliance is trying to develop a vaccine immunotherapy by 2020 to overcome cancer and complete "Cancer Moon Shot".

The American Society of Clinical Oncology (ASCO) issued a statement on its website to welcome Obama's "New Moon Plan" and support Biden's leadership, arguing that the "New Moon Plan" will reduce the pain and reduce the risk of cancer for humans and the death caused by cancer. The statement mentions that "all effective treatments should be transformed from the laboratory to the clinic"; the application of "big data" technology, such as ASCO's "CancerLinQ" rapid learning system, can accelerate the pace of conquering cancer and enable physicians to better develop individualized treatment options for each patient and understand which areas are urgently needed to invest more research (Liu Quan).

(January 21, 2016, China Medical Tribune)

2) Introduction to the Dawning C plan

1). **Before** January 12, 2016, **it was proposed that the progress of the scientific research plan "to overcome cancer and launch the general attack on cancer"**

2). **Before** January 12, 2016, we have carried out scientific research and scientific innovation series as the research direction of conquering cancer.

3).The Dawning C plan

3). The plan construction of Canccer moon shot and Dawning C-type plan:

A. New moon landing plan (Cancer moon shot)
The United States
Plan Name: "New Moon Plan"
Objective: To overcome cancer
Nature: National Plan to Conquer Cancer
Announcement: Announced in the State of the Union Address
Announcer: President Obama
Announced: January 12, 2016
The person in charge of the plan: Vice President Biden
The specific plan of the plan: unknown
National Institutes of Health: increased financial budget
(NIH),

Recently formed:
pharmaceutical company
Biotechnology company   } **the national immunotherapy alliance**
Academic medical organization

The alliance is trying to develop a vaccine therapy by 2020 to overcome cancer and complete a new cancer landing program.

B. The Dawn of the C-type plan

China
Project name: "the dawn of the C-type plan"
Objective: To overcome cancer
Nature:
Advocates and the total designer : **Professor Xu Ze**
In 2011 Dr. Xu Ze proposed "to overcome the cancer and to launch the total attack" and in 2013 put forward " the total design of building the science city of conquering cancer and launching the total attack" and in 2013 put forward " the scientific and research plan of conquering cancer and launching the total attack; In July 2015 put forward the "dawn of the C-type plan" ; in July 2015 put forward the application report of four major items of the feasibility of conquering cancer and launching cancer; in August 2015 set up the Preliminary Design and Design of the establishment in Hubei, Wuhan of the Experimental Area of Cancer Working Group which will be used to apply for the government.

C. Racing with Cancer moon shot

Before the January 12, 2016, it was put forward that **the "to capture of cancer and to launch a total attack" has been carried out the research work. To put forward "conquering cancer and launch the total attack is the unprecedented work. XZ-C** (Xu Ze-China) has been running in front of 3-4 years.

4). Annex 2 :A brief description of the research environment and recent international research situation:

A."**New Moon Plan" (Cancer Moon Shot) (US)** (Introduction)

On January 12, 2016, US President Barack Obama announced a national plan to overcome cancer in his annual State of the Union speech. The plan is under the responsibility of Vice President Biden.
The name of the program: "New Moon Plan"
Goal: Conquer cancer
Nature: National plan to overcome cancer
Announced: Announced in the State of the Union Address
Announced: January 12, 2016
The person in charge of the plan: Vice President Biden
The specific plan of the plan: unknown

National Institutes of Health: increased financial budget
(NIH), **Recently formed:**

pharmaceutical company
Biotechnology company   } **the national immunotherapy alliance**
Academic medical organization

The alliance is trying to develop a vaccine therapy by 2020 to overcome cancer and complete a new cancer landing program.

1. On January 12, 2016, President Obama announced in the State of the Union address a national plan to overcome cancer, which was under the responsibility of Vice President Biden.

The name of the program: "New Moon Plan"

Goal: Conquer cancer

Nature: National plan to overcome cancer

2. In the second week of the program's announcement, Vice President Biden visited the Abramson Cancer Center at the University of Pennsylvania School of Medicine and discussed the plan. He said that the "new moon landing plan" is a commitment to overcome cancer in the world and will inspire a new generation of scientists to explore the scientific world.

3. On February 4, 2016, the American Society of Clinical Oncology (ASCO) announced the "2016 Annual Report: ASCO Clinical Oncology Progress" on Capitol Hill, Washington, and reviewed the 2015 progress, "Tumor Immunology Treatment". ASCO Chairman Julie M. Vose believes that the most important development in 2015 is the discovery of immunotherapy. She said in the foreword: "We no longer decide treatment based on tumor type and stage as in the past. In the era of precision medicine, we select or exclude treatment based on each patient and tumor genetic data. No other major advances can be translated into clinical practice like immunology, so the biggest advance in 2015 is immunotherapy." Immunotherapy opens tumor treatment New Era.

4. On April 28, 2016, a policy luncheon was held at the US Capitol to discuss "Precision Oncology in the Era of Health Care Reform: Improving Outcomes, Sustaining Innovations and Increasing Value" by Senator Tom Coburn. The third author of my fourth book <<On Inovation of Treatment of Cancer>> and translator Dr. Bin Wu was invited to the meeting.

(Note: Xu Ze's fourth monograph: "On Inmovation of Treatment of Cancer" - published on December 25, 2015 in Washington, English, globally distributed, and electronically distributed Introducing a new book.)

The introduction to the new books was the followings : The Experimental study and Chinese medicine immunopharmacology research and molecular level of combined with Chinese and Western medicine anti-cancer research have formed the theoretical system of cancer treatment with XZ-C immune regulation and control.

Walking Out of the new way of a traditional Chinese medicine with immune regulation and control and regulation of immune activity and preventing thymus atrophy, promoting thymic hyperplasia, protecting bone marrow hematopoietic function, improving immune surveillance at the molecular level combination of Chinese and Western medication to overcome cancer.

(5) In June 3, 2016 the American Society of Clinical Oncology Conference is held in Chicago which is the world's highest level of clinical oncology academic conference. The theme of the meeting focused on "focus on wisdom, to overcome cancer"; presidential presided over the meeting at the General Assembly reported the US anti-cancer "moon moon (moon Shot) division, the world a total of 50,000 participants, unprecedented, world attention.

(6) On May 25the 2016 Vice President Joe Biden visited Hopkins University and Cancer Research magazine, reported "New Moon Sword," said the future is mainly immunotherapy to conquer cancer, immunotherapy to control cancer, immunotherapy Is a new discovery by this, vigorously supporting immunotherapy, and knot Hopkins University 1-. $ 2 million in research funding. The magazine cover the photo of Vice President Joe Biden.

(7)On June 29, 2016 US Vice President Biden convenes a summit: broadcast from the National Palace from 9 am to 6 pm to the United States. National Children's Ten Cancer Centers and Societies organize physicians, nurses, scientists, volunteers, patients, families, cancer survivors, and those who have survived ... to participate in this missionary cancer leopard mission to encourage scientists to focus on cancer.

The American Cancer Society Cancer Action Network and the American Cancer Society [ACS] Chief Executive Officer and Chief Medical Officer and President attended the historic summit.

The white house called on the Americans to join them to host community activities.

Immunotherapy opens a new era of cancer treatment and it should be one billion dollars per year Yao Yu to overcome cancer research.

B."Dawn of the C-type plan" (China) (Introduction)

Project name: "dawn of the C-type plan"
Objective: To overcome cancer
Nature:
Advocate and Chief Designer:

(1). In October 2011 Xu Ze published, "the new concept of cancer treatment and new methods" monograph of Chapter 38 with a chapter of the length of "**to overcome the strategic thinking and suggestions of cancer**"

(2) In June 2013 Xu Ze also proposed "to overcome the cancer to start the general idea and design" in the international meeting, which attempted to reduce the incidence of cancer, reduce cancer mortality, improve the cure rate, prolong survival, the total attack is anti- Cancer, three carriages go hand in hand

(3) In August 2013 Xu Ze for the first time in the international community: " the XZ-C research program to overcome the cancer and launch a total attack " - the overall strategy and development of cancer treatment in China

(4) In July 2015 Professor Xu Ze proposed "the report of four of the feasibility of conquering cancer and launching the total attack to cancer" and " the research program which XZ-C proposed to conquer cancer and launch the total attack to concer "———The Overall Strategy Reform and Development of Cancer Treatment in China

① in the international first proposed:

"The report of the necessity and the feasibility of conquering cancer and launch the total attack to cancer"

② in the international community for the first time proposed :

"To build the hospital with the cancer prevention and treatment during the whole process of cancer occurrence and development " (Global Demonstration Prevention and Treatment Hospital)

"The design and vision and feasibility report of building cancer prevention and treatment hospital "—— Describe the necessity and feasibility of establishing a complete prevention and cure hospital

③ in the international first proposed:

"The general idea and the basic vision and feasibility of building the science city of conquering cancer " —— is equivalent to the design of a Chinese framework for cancer design

④ in the international first proposed:

"The report of which in building a moderately society at the same time, the proposed" ride research "- for the medical science of cancer prevention and cancer control and the necessity and feasibility of cancer prevention and control " - adhere to the Chinese characteristics of anti-cancer"

⑤ before January 12, 2016, it was put forward the research work "conquer cancer and launch a total attack" and it has been carried out 3-4 years. It was unprecedented for proposing the research work "conquer cancer and launch the total attack to cancer".

Before January 12ᵗʰ, 2016, we put conquering cancer as the research direction and have carried out the series of the scientific research achievements of scientific and technological innovation

(1) The new discovery of the experimental study:

In January 2001 Xu Ze published in its monograph "new understanding of cancer treatment and new touch type" published from the laboratory experimental tumor research new discovery:

1. Resecting Thymus can be used to make the animal model of the cancer-bearing mice and the injection of immunosuppressive agents can help the establishment of the animal model.
2. the host of the thymus inoculated with cancer cells was an acute progress and the inhibition of proliferation and the volume decrease and in the experimental observation in 6000 cancer-bearing mice model within seven years it was found that while cancer pregresses, the thymus continues having atrophy.

(2) in October 2011 Xu Ze published "the new concept and new methods of cancer treatment " in which <u>in Chapter 2 discussed the new discovery of the</u>

experimental study of cancer etiology and pathogenesis and pathophysiology: << one of the reasons of the cancar is thymus atropy and immune function reduction >>, in the chapter 3 it was put forward the revelation from the animal experiments which **the rules of treatment are to protect, regulate, and activate the anti- Cancer immune function; also also put forward << the therapy and experimental basis of XZ-C immune regulation and control with protection of Thymus and increase of immune function>>.**

(3). Exchange the cancer research results at the American Society for International Oncology Cancer Research Paper:

① received the American Cancer Research Society AACR in September 2013 in Washington, the United States International Cancer Society "XZ-C immunoregulation anti-cancer therapy", has great widespread attention in the international tumor medical community.

② In October 27-30, 2013 in Washington to participate in the American Society for Cancer Research (AACR) academic conference, the 12th International Cancer Research Conference, it was reported: "one of the reasons of cancer is thymus atrophy and reduce of immune functions", and the theory basis of the treatment rules of protection of thymus and increase immune function (protecting thymus and increasing immune function and the protection of bone marrow and increase immune system "(prevention of the stem cells in bone marrow).

(4) published monographs

Experimental research on the research direction of cancer above
Basic research, clinical validation,
In the above experimental research and basic research and clinical validation on the direction of conquering cancer research, we have gone through 28 years and have obtained a series of scientific research achievements and scientific and technological innovation series for anti-cancer, anti-cancer metastasis and recurrence research. These hundreds of original research papers on original innovation or independent innovation are published in my series of monographs.

1. in January 2000 the first book o<<new recognition and new model of cancer treatment>> was published by Hubei Science and Technology Press, the author is Prof. Xu Ze.

2. in January 2006 the second monograph "new concepts and new methods of cancer metastasis therapy" was published by Beijing People's Medical Publishing House, the author was Xu Ze, in April 2007 the People's Republic of China issued the certificate of the original book publication of "Three of one hundred"

3. In October 2011 the third monograph "new concepts and new methods of cancer treatment" was published in Chinese version by Beijing People's Military Publishing House and Xu Ze, Xu Jie are the authors.

4. In March 2013 the fourth monograph <<New concepts and new ways of cancer treatment>> was published in the English version

5. In 2015, the fifth monograph "On Innovation Of Treatment Of Cancer" was published in English version (Cancer Treatment Innovation on the first volume) by Washington, the United States, the global distribution, and the issue of electronic Edition

6. In 2016 the sixth monograph "the road to overcome cancer " was published.

7. In 2017 the seventh monograph "condense wisdom and conquer cancer for the benefit of mankind — —how to conquer cancer? how to prevent cancer?" was published in English version in the United States, the global distribution, and the issue of electronic Edition.

8. In 2018 the eighth monograph" condense wisdom and conquer cancer for the benefit of mankind——how to conquer cancer? How to treat cancer? Was published in English version in the Unite States, the global distribution, and the issue of electronic Edition.

9. In 2018 the ninth monograph" New progress of cancer treatment" was published in English version in the Unite States, the global distribution, and the issue of electronic Edition.

(5)innovation —— after 30 years of anti-cancer, anti-cancer metastasis of the basic and clinical research it has been walked out the new way of cancer treatment with Chinese-style of anti-cancer and immune regulation and control of the combination of western and Chinese medication; we have 30 years of the experience in more than 12000 cases of the application: it can be introduced or pushed to the country and to go on the world and it can connect the generation and the way and make Chinese medications to walk into all of the world and it is "Chinese Style anti-cancer of the combination of Chinese medications and West Medications with immune regulation and control not only develop and enrich the content of the treatment of cancer, but also it makes the modernization of Chinese medications merge with the international so that it walks to the forefront world.

(21) In the past 100 years, the history record of the "conquering cancer" program or plan has been proposed internationally

A. There are three persons in the world who proposed "conquer cancer ".

The two presidents have successively proposed the National Plan for "Conquering Cancer" and **A Chinese doctor XZ-C proposed** a series of blueprint, designing, planning, and programs of conquering cancer, and published the monographs (a full-English version, globally distributed).

(1) In 1971 the US Congress passed a "National Cancer Regulations", which the **"anti-cancer declaration"** was issued by President Nixon, therefore it was put the considerable human and financial resources in order to conquer cancer in one fell swoop.

In December 1971, President Richard Nixon presented the anti-cancer slogan in the United Nations.

(2) On January 12th, 2016, US President Barack Obama announced a national plan to "to conquer cancer" in his annual State of the Union address, which was run by Vice President Joe Biden.

The name of the program: "Cancer moon Shot"
Objective: To overcome cancer
In June 29th, 2016 Vice President Biden convened a summit in the White House from 9 am to 6 pm to broadcast the United States "national cancer lunar landing program" lively and the dozens of cancer centers and the doctors, nurses, scientists, volunteers, patients, family members, cancer survivors, rehabilitation in the communities organizations .. ... participating in this publicity activity to prevent cancer, encouraging the scientists to focus on the wisdom of cancer.
The White House calls on Americans to join them to host the community activities.
Immunotherapy opens a new era of cancer treatment and it announced that $ 1 billion per year will be used for the cancer research.

(3) In 2011 Chinese physician Xu Ze put forward " the strategic ideas and suggestions of conquering cancer " in his published monographs; in August 2013 at the International Conference on Cancer for the first time it is put forward: " XZ-C Research plans of conquering cancer and launching a total attack ". In July 2015 it was proposed "the dawning C-type plan of conquering cancer and launching a total attack."

- **In the 38 chapters in the third monograph "new concepts and new methods of cancer treatment"** with the length of a chapter Xu Ze addressed " the strategic ideas and the suggestions of conquering cancer "

1. How to overcome the cancer by **I see one**: the road to scientific research is the experimental basic research of exploring cancer Etiology, pathogenesis, pathophysiology.
2. How to overcome the cancer by **I see two**: the road to scientific research is the scientific research of studying the prevention and treatment during the whole process of cancer occurrence and development.
3. How to overcome the cancer by **I see three**: the road to scientific research is to carry out multidisciplinary research and to set up the formation of cancer-related research group and to specialize in clinical basis and clinical scientific research in-depth.

The book was translated into English in 2013, entitled "New Concept and New Way of Treatment of Cancer". The English text was published in Washington, DC in March 2013 and is released worldwide.

- **Xu Ze's fourth monograph "On Innovation of Treatment of Cancer"**
The English edition is published in Washington, DC in December 2015 and is electronically distributed worldwide

The Introduction of this book : the experimental study and the anti-cancer research of Chinese medication immunopharmacology and of the combination of Chinese and Western medications on the molecular level; XZ-C immune regulation of anti-cancer has formed the theoretical system.

Walking out of the new path of an immune regulation of traditional Chinese medication with regulating immune activity, preventing thymic atrophy, promoting thymic hyperplasia, protecting bone marrow hematopoietic function, improving immune surveillance at the molecular level of the combination of Chinese and Western medications to overcome cancer.

- Xu Ze's fifth monograph **"The Road To Overcome Cancer"**
The English edition was published in Washington, DC, on December 6, 2016, and is available electronically and worldwide.

In this book:

Chapter 11 the initiative of conquering cancer and launching a total attack
—— The overall strategic reform of cancer treatment
Section I: the necessity to launch a total attack
Section II: the feasibility of launching the overall attack
Section III: the XZ-C plan of conquering cancer and launching the total attack

Chapter 12 to strengthen the anti - cancer prevention and treatment research, to change the status of light defense and the attention of treatment
The first section: It must be aware of the existing problems and the clear research direction
Section II: In order to overcome cancer it must pay attention to the prevention and the treatment effect is in the "three early"

Chapter 13: the suggestions on the Cultivation of Scientific and Technological Talented Personals and the Transformation of Scientific Research Achievements
The first section: In order to overcome cancer the science and technology talented persons are the key
Section II : To build a good laboratory

Chapter 14 Adhering to the new path of anti-cancer with Chinese characteristics

This book is a full English version and has been published in all of the global for more than six months. Therefore, China, Hubei, Wuhan should catch up to capture cancer research work. Because conquering cancer and launching the total attack is in China; it is put forward by Wuhan professor in China and the monographs have been published. It should be carried out in the country to catch up to conquer cancer and to launch a total attack and should be applied to the provincial and municipal.

In the contemporary era and now chinese physicians do the research work of conquering cancer the most and the earliest and published the monographs and there are the experimental research and the theory and the clinical practice.

<u>**The original hope was that our leadership can report to the United Nations about conquering cancer and launching a general attack, but the US president has announced the conquering cancer national plan, called the United States and the global scientists condense wisdom to capture cancer.**</u>

<u>**It should remember the story of smallpox and Vaccinia in the Ming Dynasty Cattle! Putting Vaccinia was invented by a Chinese physician, but after this**</u>

research result was spread to France; however it was reported by the French physician.

How to do? To apply to hold an international tumor academic conference in November 16- 18th, 2018 in Wuhan : " the peak of the academic forum to overcome the cancer and to launch a total make the international announcement of which China has made the first series of scientific research of conquering cancer and launching a total attack.

B. Why is it said as moving forward together? What is inside in common?

(1) It was put forward: "conquer cancer" in Chapter 38 in Xu Z e's third monograph "new concepts and new methods of cancer treatment" which was published in Beijing in 2011 (Chinese version), and then published in Washington, 2013 (in English)

In " the strategic thinking and suggestions of conquering cancer " it was put forward "conquering cancer"

1. How to overcome the cancer by I see one: the road to scientific research is the experimental basic research of exploring cancer Etiology, pathogenesis, pathophysiology.
2. How to overcome the cancer by I see two: the road to scientific research is the scientific research of studying the prevention and treatment during the whole process of cancer occurrence and development.
3. How to overcome the cancer by I see three: the road to scientific research is to carry out multidisciplinary research and to set up the formation of cancer-related research group and to specialize in clinical basis and clinical scientific research in-depth.

The book was published by the American medical scientist Dr. Bin Wu in English and published in Washington, DC, in June 2013, published in Europe and America.

This book focuses on: to conquer cancer and to launch a total attack

(2) Xu Ze's fourth monograph "On Innovation of Treatment of Cancer"

The English edition was published in Washington, DC in December 2015, with electronic and global distribution

This book focuses on: immune regulation of anti-cancer

The experimental study: the anti-cancer research of Chinese medication immunopharmacology and of the combination of Chinese and Western medications on the molecular level; XZ-C immune regulation of anti-cancer has formed the theoretical system.

Walking out of the new path of an immune regulation of traditional Chinese medication with regulating immune activity, preventing thymic atrophy, promoting thymic hyperplasia, protecting bone marrow hematopoietic function, improving immune surveillance at the molecular level of the combination of Chinese and Western medications to overcome cancer. The above two books:

The former focuses on: to overcome cancer
The latter focuses on: immune regulation cancer treatment

(3) In January 12, 2016 US President Barack Obama in the State of the Union address put forward the national cancer plan: to overcome cancer.

The program name is: "Cancer moon shot", by that Vice President Joe Biden is responsible for the implementation. Biden proposed the focusing on the study of immunotherapy and the immunization prevention; the immunotherapy opens a new era of cancer treatment.

On June 29th, 2016, Vice President Biden convened a summit to broadcast to the United States from 9:00 am to 6:00 pm at the White House. The National Cancer Monthing Program encourages the scientists to focus on intelligence to conquer cancer and announced $ 100 million per year for the research on cancer.

The above goal: to overcome cancer

Methods and pathways: the immune anti-cancer treatment and immune prevention

In short, in Chapter 39 of Xu Ze's third monograph it was proposed: to overcome cancer and how to overcome cancer; in the fourth book there was the whole Chapter which was discussed : the immune regulation treatment of cancer and walking out of a new way to overcome cancer.

In the United States the goal of the "new moon program (Cancer moom Shot)" is to conquer cancer and its method and way are immunotherapy.

The above two goals are to overcome cancer, its methods and pathways are the immune therapy and the immune regulation and the immune prevention; the two goals and methods are the same way.

Therefore, it is put forward to going forward together. Rush toward the science hall to overcome cancer.

22) how to overcome cancer? XZ- C proposed that it needs two wheels: A wheel and B wheel

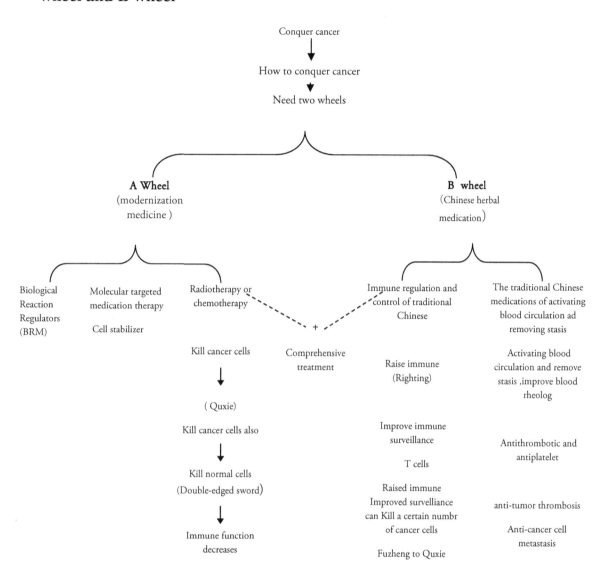

(23) how to overcome cancer? XZ-C put forward to require A wheel and A runway, and B wheel and B runway

Overcome cancer
▼
How to overcome cancer?
▼
Need two wheels and two runways

A
one wheel
A runway
(life sciences and
biomedical)

B
one wheel
A runway
(the clinical basis)
Etiology, pathogenesis, pathophysiology and
related factors

The A wheel and A runway are :

a. the DNA found
Under a variety of internal and external factors the
body occurs the mutation or error, causing DNA
structure and function changes, resulting in cancer.

b. the gene mutation
1928 it was considered that gene mutation is the
root cause of cancer and tumor occurrence and
the development is involved in genes and the
basic life activities such as the cell proliferation,
differentiation, apoptosis and other etc, therefore,
it is now recognized as a disease of the tumor.

c. the Philadelphia chromosome
opens targeted therapy
In 1960, the researchers in Philadelphia found
that there was a chromosomal abnormality in
patients with chronic myeloid leukemia (CML),
and that years later it was found to be the result of
chromosomes of chromosome 9 and chromosome 22.
The chromosome became the target of CML targeted
therapy for 40 years. In 2001 it was the first time
confirmed to the drug of being against Philadelphia
chromosome molecular defects - imatinib.

°

The B wheel and B runway are :
a. The virus
• 1951 it was found that virus can
transmit the mice leukemia.
• In 1960 the African sub-Saharan region reported
that Hodgkin's lymphoma was thought to be caused
by a virus and later confirmed as an AIDS virus.
• 1983 human papillomavirus infection is
one of the factors of cervical cancer.
• Preventive vaccines for cervical cancer in
2006 were approved by the US FDA.
b. the immune
• in 2001 in the Animal experiments it
was found that removal of thymus can
produce a mouse model of mice.
Mouse thymus had the acute progressive
atrophy after inoculated with cancer cells and
cell proliferation was blocked and the immune
function was low, the volume was significantly
reduced, thymus atrophy, immune function was
slow and it could promote cancer metastasis.
c. the hormones
• in 1916 it was found that removal of ovaries can
reduce the incidence of breast cancer, suggesting that
ovarian can promote the occurrence of breast cancer.
• in 1941 the hormone dependence of the
prostate cancer was confirmed and the injection
of androgen could promote metastasis.

d. the environmental pollution

• In 1907, the sun exposure was
associated with skin cancer
• in 1978 the nitrosamines in tobacco leaves were
confirmed to be carcinogens in cigarettes and
were found to be carcinogenic in animal models

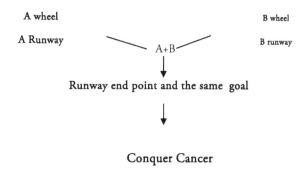

(24) It was first proposed internationally:how to overcome cancer? XZ-C proposed the need to aim for A, B, C three targets in order to conquer cancer

The treatment of the diseases must aim on the cause, pathogenesis, pathophysiology for the prevention and the treatment. The prevention of cancer and cancer treatment must also aim on the mechanism of the cause, pathogenesis, cancer metastasis for prevention and treatment. How does the tumor happen? It should carry out research and conquer by each aims or targets according to the process of tumorogenesis. Tumorogenesis is that under the influence of genetic and environmental factors, the gene occur mutation and abnormal expression or loss, resulting in a common feature of tumor cells - uncontrolled infinite reproduction.

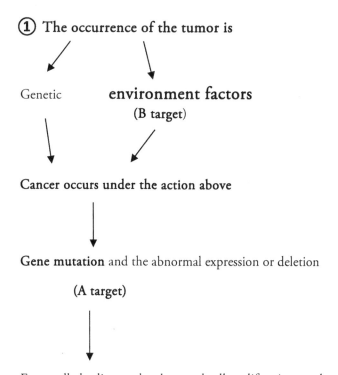

the body's normal immune system

it can identify, recognize, and remove tumor cells
(C target)
(it should adjust the immune system, thus identify and remove the tumor cells)
③

but the process of interaction between tumor cells and immune system

is regulated by a large number of immune activation / or inhibition of molecular regulation
(C target)
(C target) (in the application of up-regulated immune activating molecules; thereby inhibiting immune escape and inhibiting tumor growth)

tumor cells through either the up-regulation of immunosuppressive molecules or the down-regulation of immune activating molecules

Inhibiting the body's anti-tumor immune response

To achieve immune escape and excessive growth

According to the above brief description of the process of the occurrence of the tumor, XZ-C proposed: the goal or target to overcome the cancer should be:

A target: it should be directed against gene mutations and the abnormal expression or deletion

However: are the gene mutation and the abnormal expression or deletion the cause of cancer? Or is it the result of cancer?

Why does the mutation occur? What is the cause of its mutation? What are the consequences of the mutation?

It is the environmental factor that causes genetic mutation.

B target: it should aim on environmental factors.

B target is the goal of anti-cancer.

The environmental factors:

The external environment - air, water, soil, physical, chemical, biological factors, clothing, food, shelter and travel

The Internal environment - microscopic, ultramicro, immune, endocrine, neurohumoral

It is the environment (inside and outside) → lead to gene mutation

Therefore, we must create "anti-cancer research institute" to carry out anti-cancer system engineering.

C target: it should adjust the normal immune system, thereby remove the tumor cells.

- the Large amounts of immune activation and the up-regulation activation make the balance between the tumor and immune system interact with each other.
- the Immune activators should be up-regulated to inhibit immune escape and inhibit tumor growth.
- the Immunization and immunotherapy and vaccination are human expectations.

(25) XZ-C proposes that several treatments of traditional Chinese medicine can be applied to the treatment of tumors.

Professor Xu Ze (XZ-C) proposed several treatments for traditional Chinese medicine, which can be applied to the treatment of tumors and the combination of Chinese and Western medicine; Experimental research and clinical basic research on the combination of Chinese and Western medicine should be carried out, as well as clinical application verification observation.

A. The rule of Chinese medicine: **Fuzheng Guben(support Righting and firm Essence) matches** Western medicine treatment principles: **improve immunity, immune regulation and control and immunity reconstruction; it should carry out the research of** anticancer immunological pharmacology and the research of the mechanism of action of anticancer immune regulation and control of traditional Chinese medications; Experimental study on the combination of anticancer Chinese and Western medicine should be carried out at the molecular level.

B. TCM treatment: activate the blood circulation and remove the blood stasis **matches western** medicine treatment principles: anti-cancer metastasis, anti-cancer thrombosis, anti-micro-transfer and anti-formation of cancer plugs or thrombosis so that it must resist blood clots and improve blood circulation; activating blood circulation can remove the blood stasis and can paralyze and avoid the formation of cancerous plugs; Eliminate cancer cells on the way to metastasis must resolve cancerous plugs and micro-cancers thrombosis so as to prevent cancer cell metastasis

C. TCM treatment: removing inflammation and detoxification matches western medicine treatment principles: some cancers may be related to chronic inflammation, stubborn ulcers such as chronic atrophic gastritis, chronic pelvic inflammatory disease, cervicitis, chronic hepatitis, etc., some are cancer pre-lesion which can be treated with heat-clearing(inflammation) and detoxifying Chinese medicine to control

D. TCM treatment: soften solids and firm and dissolving the nodules **matches western medicine** treatment principle: in the current examination CT, sometimes reported that there are multiple small nodules, small, only a few millimeters in the certain organ, which can not be operated by chemotherapy and radiotherapy, can be treated by these softening Chinese medicine, and have the dynamic observation, **often have a good effect.**

(26) <u>**XZ-C proposed to attack the cancer and to launch a total attack, it must establish cancer prevention research institute and cancer prevention system engineering, which is the first international**</u>

To do the cancer prevention research, to find carcinogenic factors, and to detect the carcinogenic or carcinogenic factors and to try to prevent these carcinogenic factors on the human body damage, the cancer prevention research institute should carry out cancer prevention research and there are a lot of contents that is urgently needed to be studied and they are very rich and very broad.
<u>**Track the source of carcinogens or carcinogenic factors.**</u>
During the process of that human beings searches for cancer etiology and conditions of the process, the most prominent is that more than 90% of the cancer are caused by environmental factors.

1. **the relationship between air pollution and cancer**
Humans have developed tens of millions of tons of coal, oil and natural gas as fuel and energy **such as transports : thermal power generation, smelting steel, automobiles, aircraft, etc. and the production and life of family life fuels, day and night kept a lot of tar, bituminous coal, dust and other harmful substances being discharged into the atmosphere, causing air pollution.**

Air pollution can cause many diseases, especially respiratory diseases, the most serious is lung cancer.

2. **water pollution and cancer**

Water pollution is mainly caused by industrial and agricultural production and urban sewage. There are many types of pollutants in the water; **the farm drugs and pesticides are one of the important pollutants in water; the neutral detergent in the surfactant also is promote cancer.**

3. the soil pollution and cancer

A large number of industrial waste water and pesticide **fertilizer pour into the soil so that it deteriorates the soil quality; the poison continues the accumulation which threatens the human health and is also carcinogenic factors.**

4. chemistry and cancer
5. physical factors and cancer
6. biological factors and cancer
7. diet and cancer
8. lifestyle and cancer
9. clothing, food, live, line, house decoration and cancer

It should study the method of the effect of so many carcinogens or carcinogenic factors.

It is to study these sources of pollution and to try to stop at the source.

It is to study these carcinogenic mechanisms, its carcinogenic effects.

It is to study how to reduce or prevent the prevention of these carcinogens.

Because cancer patients cover the whole world and the industrial and agricultural waste water and the waste residue and waste gas pollution are also covered the world, therefore, it must be the whole world to attack cancer and to launch a total attack.

Professor Xu Ze suggested:

1. **various countries, provinces, all states should establish cancer prevention research institute (or institutions) and carry out cancer prevention system engineering for their own country, the province, the city to carry out anti-cancer work.**

2. **the countries to establish cancer prevention regulations and to carry out (some should be legislation)**

3. **I will recommend this project to the World Health Organization to launch cancer prevention action, the goal is to try to reduce the incidence of cancer.** To overcome cancer is the forefront of science, is a worldwide problem,

cancer is a human disaster covering the whole world, people around the world are eager to one day to overcome cancer, for the benefit of mankind.

(27) Professor Xu Ze XZ-C proposed:

Scientific ethics should be advocated, medicine is benevolence, and ethics is the first:

Research ethics: products should have ethical standards

Standard: should be based on the standard of no harm or damaging on human health

Basic ethics: All products and people are harmless and do not harm people's health, especially for children. (To become the beautiful living environment and living environment)

The health administrative department shall guard, have protection, and protect the health. It shall control, lead, support, and guide anti-cancer measures, anti-cancer projects, anti-cancer tests, and anti-cancer monitoring.

Cancer is a disaster for all mankind. It must fight globally. The people of the world must work together. Human beings should not sit still. Physicians should not do nothing. The health administrative department should not do nothing. It should guide and lead the series of anti-cancer research projects, and work together and move together with complementary, leadership and guidance to overcome cancer and launch a general attack.

(28) The review of the guideance information includes the overall design, program, plan, blueprint of conquering cancer such as how to implement and how to achieve this "Condense wisdom and conquer cancer - benefiting mankind". This is the medical monograph with the relatively complete, systematic, comprehensive design, more specific planning of how to overcome cancer. The book is divided into two parts: 1) How to overcome cancer? How can I prevent cancer? I see; 2) How to overcome cancer? how to treat cancer? I see

1.This monograph discussed the specific plans, programs, and blueprints of how to prevent cancer in four tenths of an article and proposed how to overcome cancer? How can I prevent cancer? I see. It set up the research goals or "targets" on how to reduce the incidence of cancer.

The current status quo is: the more treatment and the more cancer patients, and the incidence of cancer is continuing rising and the mortality rate is high. The road which walked through for a century is to focus on treatment and to ignore the defense or only treatment and no defense. It was done very little in the prevention work and it almost did not do. The cancer prevention did not attach importance; the prevention did not pay attention so that the incidence of cancer is rising.

How to prevent cancer? Where is the target or goal of the cancer prevention? It must have a specific prevention cancer object and a clear goal so that it can have operational.

Professor Xu Ze proposed how to prevent cancer I see (a), (b), (c), (d) proposed that it should analyze what causes or which factors lead to an increase in cancer incidence. Currently the more number of patients and the more treatment; the incidence is on the rise and 90% is related to its environment. It should study and explore for the environmental carcinogenic factors (the external environment and the internal environment).

The causes of cancer are related to the carcinogenic factors of the external and internal environment. If we have a better understanding of the causes of cancer, then in the future it will be able to put forward:

How to prevent which carcinogenic factors? how to monitor which carcinogenic factors? how to clean which carcinogenic factors? so that we can stay away from cancer and prevent cancer. Therefore, Professor Xu Ze proposed: it should prevent cancer from the big environment and the small environment and it should be from the clothing, food, live and walking to prevent cancer.

2. 60% of the length in this book is the disscussion of how to treat cancer. The study of the target or "target" is located in how to improve cancer cure rate, extends the survival of cancer patients, improve the quality of life and put forward how to cure cancer by I see.

We are taking the new road of cancer treatment in the molecular level of the combination of Western medication and Chinese medication and it is the new road of finding the immune regulation methods and drugs on the basis of new discoveries in animal experiments in our laboratory. After years of animal experiment screening and clinical validation it finally found out this new road of immune regulation of cancer with XZ-C1-10 immune regulation of anti-cancer Chinese medication series.

A. From our laboratory experiments it was found that: thymus of the host was acute progressive atrophy and the volume was significantly reduced after the host was inoculated with cancer cells.

B. From the above experimental results it was found that thymus atrophy, immune dysfunction may be one of the etiology and pathogenesis of the tumor so the principle of treatment must try to prevent thymic atrophy, promote thymocyte proliferation, increased immune function.

C. In order to prevent thymic atrophy and to promote thymocyte proliferation and to increase immune function, we look for from both the traditional Chinese medication and Western medication. Western medication which can improve immune function and promote the proliferation of thymocytes is very rare. So we changed to find from the Chinese medication because the traditional Chinese medication tonic drugs generally have immune regulation.

D. After 7 years of laboratory scientific research, we selected XZ-Cl-10 immune regulation anti-cancer, anti-transfer traditional Chinese medication with protecting thymus and increasing immune function and protecting bone marrow and hemotesise from the natural drug. on the basis of the success of the animal experiment the clinical validation work was conducted. After 20 years of more than 12,000 cases of clinical application in the cancer specialist outpatient center it achieved the good results.

E. After the experimental study, with anti-cancer research of Chinese medication immunopharmacology and the combination of Chinese and Western medication on the molecular level, it walked out of the new path of conquering cancer with XZ-C immune regulation, regulating immune activity, preventing thymus atrophy, promoting thymocyte proliferation, protecting bone marrow hematopoietic function, improve immune surveillance.

3. This medical monograph is the outline of the practical and the applied and the research and the implementation of how to overcome cancer.

The main project of this medical monograph is:

The Main Project {

1. To conquer cancer and to launch cancer the total attack: the prevention and the control and the treatment at the same level and at the same attention the same time and moving together

2. To create the cancer - related research base with a multidisciplinary -- - Science City

Two wing works:
A wing - how to prevent cancer - to reduce the incidence of cancer
B wing - how to cure cancer - to improve cancer cure rate

The goals and the aims:
A: to reduce the incidence of cancer
B: to improve cancer cure rate and to extend the survival of patients and to improve the quality of life. If it is implemented and it achieves this total design and planning blue of conquering cancer, it is possible to overcome cancer.

4. The next step is how to implement the work, how to achieve this total design and the programs and the planning and the blueprint.

It should set up the research team of conquering cancer and launching the total attack".

In order to capture cancer and to launch the total attack, the talent is the key and the first thing is to set up research team

The conditions of the research team and the academic members:

Genuine talent; in the cancer research, basic research or clinical work it has academic achievements, academic achievements, monographs, editor, special issue, international papers; has the practical clinical experience and the experimental research results, its direction of the research and academic is to capture cancer.

The leadership leaders who leads and organizes to conquer cancer should support anti-cancer research and support cancer research; the scientists and the entrepreneurs and the leaders and the volunteers of conquering cancer must have both ability and political integrity and medicine is benevolence and the legislation is for the first.

To overcome the general attack of cancer, talent is the key. First, the organization should organize a research team and issue an invitation to form:

1. The Wuhan Anti-Cancer Research Society will tackle the general attack of the cancer attack team.
2. Invite domestic colleagues to participate in the research team to overcome the general attack of cancer
3. Inviting international fellows to participate in the research team to overcome the general attack of cancer

Invitation from the chief designer of the "Science City for the General Attack on Cancer and the Establishment of a Multidisciplinary and Cancer-Related Research Base"

Invite famous experts, professors, academic leaders or leading scientists to support scientists, entrepreneurs, leaders and volunteers who have overcome the general attack on cancer.

Drafting

Within the province: Invitation to the team

Domestic: Invitation to the team

International: Invitation to the team

"Overcoming the General Attack of Cancer and Creating a Scientific Research Base for Cancer Research - Science City"--- Chief designer ⟶ Professor Xu Ze(Wuhan)

"Overcoming the General Attack of Cancer" --Project Leader

(29) How to carry out "conquer cancer and launch the general attack of cancer" in Hubei and Wuhan?

It should propose:

1. **Conducted an academic report on "Proposal to Overcome the General Attack of Cancer Attack"**
2. **set up a team to set up a "conquering cancer attack"**
3. **To formulate the tasks and achievements of each team member, not to name but to seek truth, to strive to achieve results, must be truly practical, must have both ability and political integrity, medical is benevolence, ethics first.**

The contribution of each team member, the tasks and indicators of each member, the tasks and indicators of the team, must clearly define the goals and objectives, and strive for innovation.

1. Can cancer be conquered?

It should be able to be conquered because 90% is caused by the environment.

Environmental factors lead to genetic mutations that lead to chromosomal deletions and abnormalities.

Environmental factors are possible or can be managed to find ways to solve them.

<<**Condense wisdom and conquer cancer – for benefiting the mankind**>> is a comprehensive design, specifically planning how to overcome cancer medical monographs, is the outline of how to overcome cancer, this set of scientific research plans and scientific research plans and blue maps are available everywhere to become as the Reference application.

2. Do cancers need to be overcome?

It must be and urgently overcome, because the incidence rate is rising and the mortality rate is high. The number of cancer deaths worldwide is 8.18 million. About 8550 people in China are diagnosed with cancer every day, and 6 people are confirmed to be cancer every minute. Therefore, the scientific research work of overcoming cancer and launching the total attack to cancer can not walk slowly, should run forward, save the wounded. Because people all over the world are eager to hope that one day they will be able to overcome cancer and stay away from cancer for the benefit of mankind.

3. How should I get rid of it?

(1) should conquer cancer and launch the general attack of cancer, prevention + control + treatment at the same time and at the same level and at the same attention

And (Change the current mode of hospitalization with attention to treatment and little prevention, and change the current treatment mode that focuses on the middle and late stages of treatment)

(2) It should be implemented and realized in accordance with the report on "conquer cancer and launch the general attack on cancer" and the proposal book.

The next step is how to implement, how to achieve this overall design, plan, program, blueprint for conquer cancer.

The steps, plans, programs, and general design of how to achieve the general attack on cancer have been completed, and have been published in the books and distributed worldwide.

Why publish English books worldwide? Because cancer patients cover the whole world, industrial and agricultural wastewater, waste residue, and exhaust gas pollution also cover the whole world. Therefore, it is necessary to globally start to launch conquering cancer and launching the total attack to cancer.

(3) The above-mentioned plan, planning, general design, and blueprint for conquering the general attack of cancer can be applied to a country, a province, a state, and a market reference application to conquer cancer and even conquer cancer.

4. How to implement the creation of this anti-cancer research, XZ-C proposed the general design of prevention cancer and cancer prevention system engineering

Professor Xu Ze suggested:

(1) All countries, provinces and states should establish cancer prevention research institutes (or institutions) to carry out cancer prevention system projects and carry out cancer prevention work for their own country, province, state and city. (Because there are a large number of cancer patients in various countries, provinces and cities)

(2) Each country should establish cancer prevention regulations and comprehensively carry out (some should be legislated)

(3) I will use this project to recommend the World Health Organization to hold the cancer prevention campaign with the goal of reducing the incidence of cancer.

Conquering cancer is a frontier of science and a worldwide problem. Cancer is a disaster for human beings. The whole world and the people all over the world are eager to hope that one day they can overcome cancer and benefit mankind.

(4) Scientific ethics should be advocated, medicine is benevolence, and ethics is the first

Research ethics: Products, achievements, and patents should all have ethical standards.

Standards: The bottom line should be based on standards that do not harm human health. In particular, it must not contain carcinogens.

Basic ethics: All products, achievements, patents, goods and people are harmless and do not harm people's health, especially for children. Do not contain carcinogens.

(5) XZ-C proposed scientific ethics, and **should recommend to WHO that all products, achievements, and patents should be the bottom line of moral standards that do not harm human health, especially the carcinogens**. E.g:

1. Women's cosmetics, hair dyes, children's toys... should be tested without carcinogens, without damaging human health
2. house decoration, materials ... should be tested without carcinogens
3. food additives, preservatives, food processing packaging ... should be tested without carcinogens
4. leather products, cloth dyes ... should be tested, no carcinogens
5. The feed of collectively fed pigs should not contain hormones, auxins, vegetarian meat, growth-promoting hormones... all should be tested without carcinogens.
6. group feed chicken, duck feed must not contain hormones, auxin ... should be tested without carcinogens

(6) The health administrative department shall protect life and protect health, and shall lead, fugle, support, and guide anti-cancer measures, anti-cancer projects, anti-cancer tests, and anti-cancer monitoring.

(7) XZ-C proposes to establish the "Cancer prevention Research Institute" and carry out cancer prevention system engineering:

- The way in which so many carcinogens or carcinogenic factors should be studied
- These sources of pollutants should be studied and managed to stop at the source
- These carcinogenic mechanisms should be studied, their carcinogenic effects, and environmental factors leading to genetic mutations.
- It is necessary to study the "two-type society" resource-saving and environment-friendly community to prevent cancer (to achieve a green living environment and a living environment where birds and flowers are fragrant).

(30) It internationally proposed for the first time: XZ-C proposed Dawning anti-cancer program A, B, D for anti- pollution and pollution control and anti-cancer, anti-cancer

Dawning A-type plan: goal: to prevent air pollution, to prevent respiratory diseases and lung cancer

Dawning B-type plan: goal: to prevent water pollution, to prevent liver cancer, stomach cancer, colon cancer, pancreatic cancer in the digestive tract...

Dawning D-type plan: goal: to prevent soil pollution to prevent cancer

How to overcome cancer? How to prevent cancer? I see:

Professor Xu Ze proposed that the "Innovative Environmental Protection and Cancer Research Institute" should be established and the anti-cancer system project should be carried out.

Where is the target or "target" of cancer prevention? How to prevent?

The more cancer patients are treated the more and more cancer incidence, the incidence is rising, and 90% of them are related or closely related to environmental carcinogenic factors. Therefore, the target or "target" of cancer prevention r should be researched and discussed in response to environmental carcinogenic factors (external environment, internal environment).

XZ-C proposes the general design of prevention of cancer and cancer prevention system engineering: Since the disaster of cancer covers the whole world, industrial and agricultural waste gas, waste water and waste residue also cover the whole world. **Therefore, it is necessary to establish "Innovative Environmental Protection and Cancer Research Institute" and carry out cancer prevention engineering system.**

Why must we prevent and control the three major pollutions? First, we should study the relationship between the environment and cancer.

There are many examples of **how to prove the relationship between environmental pollution and cancer.** In particular, environmental pollution such as air pollution, water pollution, and soil pollution has a serious impact on human carcinogenesis.

1. **Air pollution and cancer in environmental pollution**: Every minute of human life is inseparable from air. Air pollution can cause many respiratory diseases, the most serious of which is lung cancer.

2. **Water pollution and cancer in environmental pollution**: Human beings are inseparable from water every moment in production activities and life. Water pollution is mainly caused by industrial and agricultural production and urban sewage. In China, industrial pollution has intensified due to the rapid development of township and village enterprises. Water pollution is related to the high incidence of liver cancer, and it is related to the occurrence of gastric

cancer, intestinal cancer and esophageal cancer. Drinking water that does not meet the standard is not able to induce or promote cancer.

3. **Soil pollution and cancer in environmental pollution**: Fertilizers, pesticides and pesticides in agricultural production can cause soil water quality in farmland, soil pollution is serious, agricultural workers are exposed to a variety of pesticides, herbicides and fertilizers, and some are known. Human carcinogens.

Pollution prevention and pollution control actually are cancer prevention and cancer control. It can effectively prevent the effects of first-class anti-cancer. It must prevent and control the three major pollutions; pollution prevention and pollution treatment and overcome difficulties. It can certainly achieve the benefits of cancer prevention and cancer control to reduce the incidence of cancer.

The Cancer Research Institute will carry out anti-cancer system engineering, conduct microscopic, ultra-micro, high-tech research, monitor and analyze carcinogenic factors, and try to eliminate it. We have developed four Dawning Cancer Prevention Programs:

1 Dawning A-type plan and goal: to study the microscopic study of air pollution caused by air pollution, and try to remove it to prevent air pollution leading to lung cancer.

Why is the anti-cancer system project the first to solve air pollution? Because the current global respiratory cancer has the highest incidence rate, 1.295 million / 8.18 million, both male and female are the first, therefore, how to solve the problem of preventing lung cancer is a top priority.

Ways and methods: Through the microscopic, ultra-micro, high-tech monitoring and analysis of carcinogenic factors, try to detect, monitor, and try to remove it.

2 Dawn B type plan

Objective: To study the microscopic study of carcinogenic factors of environmental pollution caused by water pollution, and to eliminate cancers such as liver cancer, stomach cancer, and intestinal cancer caused by waterproof pollution.

Why do you currently have to pay attention to water pollution and cause cancer? Because the global mother river is polluted by industrial and agricultural sewage, urban sewage, river water pollution, carcinogens have increased significantly.

Ways and methods: "target"

Solve the pollution of industrial and agricultural sewage, the first should try to reduce fertilizer

To solve urban and rural drinking water, it must be purified

Resolve drinking water and drink standard water

3. Dawning C-type plan

Already mentioned above

4. Dawning D-type plan

Objective:

To study the microscopic study of the carcinogenic factors of soil pollution to the environment

Try to solve the problem of chemical fertilizers, pesticides, genetic modification and cancer

Try to detect the presence or absence of carcinogenic factors from clothing, food, housing, and samples, and take samples of carcinogens from microscopic monitoring.

Ways and methods:

Conduct microscopic detection and monitoring of cancer prevention, and put forward ethical standards for cancer prevention.

Through the above-mentioned Dawning A, B, and D plans, antifouling and pollution control of the atmosphere, water, and soil are actually a first-class anti-cancer, which can reduce the incidence of cancer. It can reach the green hills, the green waters, the mountains and rivers, the ecological environment of birds and flowers, and the living environment of human beings.

Professor Xu Ze proposed how to overcome cancer, how to prevent cancer
Situation analysis: (1) - how to prevent cancer, cancer incidence is rising
Situation analysis: (2) - Cancer incidence is related to the environment

1. Why does the increase in cancer incidence have a relationship with the environment?
2. The cause of cancer is related to the external environment and the carcinogenic factors of the internal environment.
3. If we have a deeper understanding of the causes of cancer, then we can come up with more valuable suggestions in the future: how to prevent cancer-causing factors, how to monitor which carcinogenic factors, and which cancer-causing factors to clear, so that we can stay away from cancer, prevent cancer.

Situation analysis: (3) - Prevention should be prevented from carcinogenic factors that improve external (external) and internal (internal) conditions.

Professor Xu Ze proposed: the establishment of an innovative anti-cancer research institute and an innovative anti-cancer system project. This is an unprecedented work and must be practiced in person to seek health and welfare for mankind.

XZ-C proposes anti-cancer general design and anti-cancer system engineering.

Situation analysis: (4) – a. The establishment of the Environmental and Cancer Research Group

b. Monitor environmental pollution-causing factors and data, develop anti-cancer, cancer control measures, and research and development interventions.

a, from clothing, food, shelter, anti-cancer

b, from the big environment of life to prevent cancer

c, from the small living environment to prevent cancer

d, from life behaviors, life hobbies, living habits to prevent cancer

Under the guidance of Xi Jinping's characteristic socialism under the new era, he will strive to open a new phase of scientific research in the new era and overcome the scientific research work of cancer. Strive to follow the path of independent innovation with Chinese characteristics and adhere to the road of independent innovation of Chinese and Western medicine combined with "Chinese-style anti-cancer".

Innovation - Our 30 years of anti-cancer, anti-cancer metastasis based on basic and clinical research has initially emerged a "Chinese-style anti-cancer", Chinese and Western medicine combined with immune regulation and treatment of cancer, we have accumulated more than 12,000 clinical cases in 20 years Application experience can be pushed to the whole country, can go to the world, can connect with the "Belt and Road", make Chinese medicine to the world, make "Chinese-style anti-cancer", Chinese and Western medicine combined with immune regulation and treatment of cancer, not only develops and enriches immunology The content of cancer has brought China's medical modernization into line with international standards and is at the forefront of the world.

4. Postscript

Where did these 8 medical monographs come from? Some of the first drafts came from the original record of "Morning in the morning" and then compiled into a manuscript. I sent it to the street to copy the typing room and put it into a book. From the years of the flower, to the age of the ancient, to the year of the shackles, sent to the street copying typing room to type hundreds of times. Sometimes my wife and I went to the typing room to print the manuscript. She was the first reader and supporter of my "Monograph".

After I retired at the age of 63, I continued to research, self-reliance, self-financing, and the journey of Science was non-stop. Still struggling, arduously climbing, four different scientific research stages of one scientific research footprint, four different levels of mountain results. A mountain is better than a mountain scientific research landscape. Perseverance, perseverance. Since 1980, I have insisted on scientific research diaries, scientific research records, the accumulation of these scientific research materials and the record of scientific thinking, and some have also been selected as the material of this series of "monographs".

I read five years of private school in my childhood (then in the early 1930s, there was only one elementary school in a county, and the villages were mostly private). I loved the ancient books and poems for Self-sufficiency. In addition to medical research, you can enjoy yourself. For example, as the following two poems:

晨起想到
二〇〇六年春

万籁无声寂
鸡鸣报晓时
曙光潜入内
轻唤已黎明
一夜酣甜睡
醒来脑清新
灵思一闪现
靶点豁然明
丑起披衣坐

自咏
二〇〇六年春

年逾古稀犹自奋
赛因征途不停蹄
躲进小楼研机理
灵思一现靶点明
老骥伏枥志未已
为控转移究歧黄
十栽卓然成夙志

5.Keeping the complete medical record of each patient as the following examples: Chinese part is the original; English part is the translation.

A. Chinese example:

B. English part example:

Liver cancer cases.

a. XZC immunomodulatory anticancer medicine treatment of liver cancer in some cases list

Liver cancer(translation)

Number	Name	Medical record	Gender	Age	Hometown	Profession	Address	Diagnosis	Test
1	Shi	6101204	Male	57	Zhaoyang	Farmer	Zhaoyang	Liver cancer	CT, MRI(06/22/1998)
2	Lan	6201222	Male	35	Dawu	Teacher	Dawu	Right lobe of huge liver cancer	CT(08/1998)
3	Lu	6201229	Male	38	Danyang	Land management personnel	Danyang	Right liver cancer	Ultrasound and CT(07/07/98)
4	Liu	6201230	Male	30	Gongen	Engineer	Gongen	Huge Liver cancer	Ultrasound and CT(07/07/98)
5	Zeng	6301242	Male	50	Zhongxiang	Farmer	Zhongxiang	Primary liver cancer	CT(08/98)
6	Ke	6301244	Male	54	Huangshi	ABC bank	Huangshi	Liver cancer	CT(08/98)
7	Song	6301257	Male	37	Yinchen	Elementary principle	Yinchen	Huge liver cancer	Ultrasound(07/01/98)
8	Yang	6401263	Male	51	Erzhong	Attending doctor	Erzhong	Liver cancer after surgery	Ultrasond(09/98)
9	Jiang	6401264	Male	57	Henan	Radio factory welders	Xiaogan	Huge liver cancer	Ultrasound(02/98)

1

Number	Hospital	Habbits Somking year	Habbits Somking amount	Habbits Drinking year	Habbits Drinking amount	Eating frenqently Pickle	Eating frenqently Pickles	Eating frenqently Bacon	Eating frenqently Salted fish	Eating frenqently Pickle
1	Zhaoyang hospital	30 years	1-2 package/day	30 years	3-4 oz/ meal		+		+	
2	Dawu County hospital and xiehe hospital			10		+	+			
3	Xiehe hospital	6-7 year	little							
4	Gongen county erzhou city	More than 10 years	1 package/day	10 year	2-3oz/ meal					
5	Zhongxiang city hospital					+	+		+	+

6	Huangshi hospital and xiehe hospital	30	1-2 package/day	More than 10 years	16oz/meal					
7	Yinchen city renmein hospital and xiehe hospital									
8	Erzhong city hospital and xiehe hospital									
9	Shanjianghangtan hospital and xiehe hospital	20year	1 package	More than 10 years	32oz/meal					
10	Railroad hospital and xiehe hospital									+

2

Number	Eat frequently Sausage	Eat frequently Fried food	Eat frequently Pepper	Eat frequently Garlic	Eat frequently Onion	Eat frequently Freshly vegatable	Eat frequently fruit	Eat frequently Mildew food	Drink frewunly Green tea	Drink oftern tea	Drink often others
1						+			+		
2			+			+			+		
3			+	+		+			+		
4			+	+		+			+		
5		+		+		+					
6			+	+		+			+		
7						+					
8						+			+		
9			+	+						+	
10		+				+	+				

3

Number	Drink water	Eat often Meat	Eat oftern Ribs soup	Eat often vegeteran	Work condition General	Work condition High pressure	Character Condition Cheerful	Character Condition Dull irriability	Exercise oftern
1	Well water	+						+	
2	Tap water					+	+	+	
3	Tap water							+	No
4	Tap water	+							
5	Pony water					+	+		

227

6	Well water	+							
7	Tap water	+				+	+	+	No
8	Well water							+	
9	Tap water	+	+	+		+	+		No
10	Tap water			+		+		+	

4

Number	Chronic medical history	Family medical history of three generation	Patch Pain medication disappear	Patch Pain medication reduction	Patch Pain medication effective	Patch removing swellen Bump size and site	Patch removing swellen Size change after using medication
1	1 years suffering from pleurisy, as puncture yellow liquid	No		+		06/22/1998 Check intrahepatic two placeholders ranging 1-3cm	
2	In junior high school suffering from jaundice, hepatitis, in 80 acute jaundice, hepatitis	Father passed away by esaphagus cancer				08/18/1998right abdminal and 12x10cm	
3	In 83 hepatitis B;96,97 Hepatitis B three positive	no					
4	Hepatitis B positivie and have nose bleeding	no				98.7 CTshow right liver lobe2.5x2.5x3 cm	
5	89 years was found to schistosome recurrent massive ascites,	Brother liver cancer				CT show right liver lober8x20cm	
6	Schistosome and lung T.B calification	No					

7	Hepatitis B half year	no				07/1998 right liver 8.7x7.5cm	
8	Hapetitis B two months ago	Father				09/1998 liver bump8.7x7.5cm	
9	67 had hepatitis B and hospitalization for three month. T.B, stamach ulcer	No				02/10/1998 ultrasound showed 15.4x12cm	
10	Debetis	no				9/29/1998CT showed that left liver 4.3x9.9cm	

5

Number	Treatment Operation way	Treatment intervention	Treatment Radiotherapy chemotherapy	Treatment When metastasis and where and size	Medication Time, kind and results	Comment
1	No	08/05/98 to 9/2015 two time of liver intervention			On July 14,1998 to 09/22 Taking XZ-C1,4,5,2 and XZ-C3 outside patch. After taking the medication, the pain in liver region reduce significantly and after intervention, the lesion decreased from 3.2x3.9cm2 to 2.2x2.4cm2	
2		08/98 to 11/98 three times of intervention			08/14/98 to 12/25/98 taking XZ-C1,4,5 AND C3 patch, the spirit well and appetite good and walking well and right sides of belly was softer than before and volume reduce from 10x10cm2 to 11x8cm2	After intervention the vessels were blocked and couldnt get up of the bed and the patients have great pain.

3					On 08/14/1998 to 12/25/1998 taking the medication XZ-C1,4,5 the patients spirit well and appetites well and looked like the normal person	
4	No	Four times of intervention			After taking the medication, the patient can walk well and pain reduced	Chemotherapy mitonisyan 5Fu Heparin, The right lung has T.B bump
5					After two month taking the medication, the patient felt much better and walked well.	The brother had liver cancer remove and after the surgery passed away and the mother have liver problems.
6	Open surgery and couldn't remove the cancer	Two times of hepatic artery of intervention		Inside metastasis in liver	The patient felt much better after taking our medication	
7	Opened surgery and couldn't remve the cancer			Lung metastasis	The patient felt much better ; however after the chemotherapy the patient condition got worse	The patient had great pain after once liver cancer bleeding.
8	Liver lobe and galdbladder removed a				The patient felt much better after taking XZ-C1,4,5 and spirit well	
9	NO			CT show galdbladder metastasis	After taking XZ-C4, the pain reduces and felt much better	The patient couldn't talk clear after four times of intervention
10	No			Lung metastasis	After taking our medications of XZ-C1,4,5 the patient didn't have any pain and no swellen	

CHAPTER 8

The Introduction of the monograph "Condense Wisdom and Conquer Cancer" - for the benefit of mankind

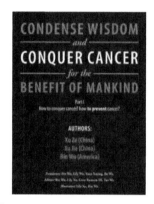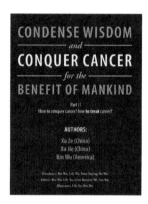

Volume I: How to overcome cancer? How to prevent cancer? Published in December 2017
Volume II: How to overcome cancer? How to treat cancer? Published in February 2018
Published in Washington, English-language, global distribution

TABLE OF CONTENTS

1. Table of Contents of the books <<Condense Wisdom and Conquer Cancer—for the benefit of mankind

Table of Contents
(Volume 1)

1. The historical records of putting forward the "to conquer cancer" program internationally within a hundred years
2. Why is it said the common progress or moving forward together?
3. To do an unprecedented event for the benefit of mankind
4. How to overcome cancer? XZ-C proposed "two wheels", "three targets"
5. Why do we put forward "the race" (the scientific and technology race)?
6. How to overcome cancer? XZ-C proposed the four major contributions
7. The exclusive scientific research products: XZ-C immunomodulation anti-cancer traditional Chinese medication series (Introduction)
8. How to conquer cancer? XZ-C put forward the scientific research achievement and the scientific and technological innovation series
9. How to conquer cancer? XZ-C proposed to conquer cancer and to launch a total attack which is unprecedented work
10. How to conquer cancer? XZ-C proposed to condense wisdom and to move forward together to conquer cancer
11. The Dawn of the C-type plan No. 1-6
12. The situation analysis
(a) Prevention of cancer and anti-cancer and walking forward together to conquer cancer
13. The situation analysis
(b) why is Chinese herbal medication the advantage of our country in cancer research?
14. The situation analysis
(c) how to overcome cancer? Can traditional therapy (surgery, chemotherapy, radiotherapy) be relied on to overcome cancer
15. The situation analysis
(d) moving forward together toward the scientific hall to conquer the cancer.

Table of Contents
(Volume II)

Table of Contents
(Volume III)

(5) The anti-cancer research work cannot walk slowly and should run forward and save the dying and help the hurting

(6) how to improve the research work of the cancer cure rate

3. How to prevent cancer I see three:

(A) why does it need to launch a total attack in order to conquer cancer?

(B) the catastrophe of cancer covers the whole world

(C) XZ-C proposed to the advice and suggestions of the establishment of the anti-cancer research institute and the anti-cancer system engineering

4. How to prevent cancer? I see four

How to prevent cancer from "two types of society"?

(A) the construction of "two-oriented society", which has the great relevance to the cancer prevention and anti-cancer

(B) the environmental pollution can increase the incidence of cancer

(C) why should we build a "two-oriented society" environment-friendly society?

(D) I think the current energy-saving and the emission reduction and the pollution prevention and the pollution treatment; to create a "two-oriented society" is I level prevention to prevent cancer and to anti-cancer. Its purpose and effect can achieve Class I prevention.

(E) So far there is no practical solution to carry out the cancer prevention and the cancer control; it can be not only from the technical and the tactical to proceed but it should focus on from the strategic; the implementation is the people-oriented and fundamentally it emphasizes the harmony between people and the environment. The scientific research must be carried out to explore the innovation.

Table of Contents
(Volume IV)

6. while building a well-off society at the same time, it is suggested "ride research" —— the necessity and feasibility of cancer prevention and cancer control of medical research and cancer prevention and treatment

7. Several suggestions of the construction of the personnel training, laboratory construction and the results transformation of the innovative countries on scientific and technological innovation

8. the strategic ideas and suggestions on the capture of cancer

Table of Contents
(Volume V)

1. It has formed the theoretical system of XZ-C immune regulation and control of cancer treatment and has walked out of the new path of conquering cancer for more than 30 years which has been experiencing the clinical application and observation and verification

1). The new discovery of anti-cancer and anti-cancer metastasis research

2). The experimental observation of tumor impact on the immune Thymus

3). The shape and location of Thymus

4). The structure and function of Thymus

5). The body's immune function

6). Thymus immune regulation function, NIM doctrine

7). Thymus exocrine function

8). The impact of chemotherapy on immune function

9). Thymic hormone name and function

10). Immune regulation and immune enhancers

11). The research progress of Chinese medication polysaccharide anticancer immune pharmacology

12). The features of the traditional chinese immune pharmacology

13). The discovery from cancer experimental research

14). The research of mechanism of XZ-C immune regulation and control anti-cancer medication

15). The research of the cytokines induced by XZ-C anti-cancer medication

16). The experimental and clinical efficacy of XZ-C immunomodulatory anticancer medication

17). XZ-C immunomodulatory anticancer medications are the achievement of the modernization of traditional Chinese medications

2. Finding the way

1), to explore the pathogenesis, invasion and recurrence and metastasis mechanism of cancer and to carry out the experimental study of the effective measures of the regulation of cancer invasion, recurrence and metastasis

2), the new drug experimental situation of finding the new anti-cancer, anti-metastasis, anti-recurrence from the natural medication

3), how to find the new ways of immunoregulatory therapy

4), the clinical validation work

5), the research of the mechanism of XZ-C immunoregulation anti-cancer traditional Chinese medication

6), XZ-C immunomodulation anti-cancer traditional Chinese medication is the achievement of the modernization of Chinese medication

7), Walked on the road of conquering cancer with XZ-C immune regulation and control in the molecular level of combining Chinese with Western medication

3. The innovation content of the research theory of the new concepts and the new methods of cancer metastasis therapy

Table of Contents
(Volume VI)

1. It has formed the theoretical system of XZ-C immune regulation and control of cancer treatment and has been experiencing the clinical application and observation and verification

(1) the concept of cancer treatment

(2) the cause and the development mechanism of cancer

(3) the theoretical basis and experimental basis of cancer treatment

(4) the principles of cancer treatment

(5) the cancer treatment model

(6) the principles of cancer metastasis therapy

(7) the new concept of cancer metastasis therapy

(8) how to do anti-cancer metastasis? the three steps of anti-cancer metastasis therapy

(9) the methods and drugs of cancer treatment

(10) the research on new concepts and new methods of cancer metastasis therapy

(11) the theoretical system of the formation of XZ-C treatment

Table of Contents
(Volume VII)

- The suggestions for improving and improving chemotherapy
7. the basic model and specific programs of anti-cancer metastasis
- The basic pattern of anti-cancer metastasis
- The specific treatment plans of anti-cancer metastasis
- Immunotherapy plays an important role in anticancer treatment
8. The new models and new methods of cancer treatment
- To strengthen immunotherapy, to improve adverse reactions to chemotherapy
- To change the intermittent treatment into the continuous treatment
  To change the damage to the host into protecting the host
- To change the potential of the tumor and the host, and strive imbalance into the balance
- To change from damaging the central immune organs into protecting the central immune organs
- To change the injury therapy into non-injury therapy
9. "three steps" of anti-cancer metastasis therapy
- The transfer step should be understood so that the goal of treatment is more specific
- Try to break each step by step
- three major anti-cancer metastasis treatment s(trilogy)
10. the review and analysis of clinical cases of cancer postoperative adjuvant chemotherapy
- The cases of which cancer postoperative adjuvant chemotherapy failed to prevent recurrence
- The cases of which cancer postoperative adjuvant chemotherapy failed to prevent metastasis
- The cases of which chemotherapy promotes immune failure
11. The review and prospect of surgical treatment of tumors
- The achievement of surgical resection of the tumor in the 20th century
- 21st century surgical goal should be prevention and treatment research for cancer recurrence and metastasis after surgery radical resection
- The design of tumor radical surgery should be further studied and perfected
- The molecular biology basic research and clinical basic research of metastasis should be strengthened after the radical resection
- To prevent cancer recurrence and metastasis should be done from the surgery

Table of Contents
(Volume VIII)

5). The cases of simply using Z-C anti-cancer traditional Chinese medicine after radical surgery without chemotherapy and radiotherapy

6). Chemotherapy plus Z-C Chinese medicine treatment of typical cases of acute lymphoblastic leukemia

17. The Immune function of Chinese herbal medications in patients with advanced cancer

18. The anticancer function of the cell immune

Table of Contents
(Volume IX)

1. List of cases of cancer treatment with XZ-C immune regulator and control chinese medications

1).List of partial typical cases of **Liver cancer** treatment with XZ-C immune regulator Chinese medications(case 1 to case 189)

2). List of partial typical cases of **Pancreas cancer** treatment with XZ-C immune regulator Chinese medications(case 190- case218)

3).List of partial typical cases of **Stomach** cancer treatment with XZ-C immune regulator Chinese medications(case219-case288)

4).List of partial typical cases of **Lung** cancer treatment with XZ-C immune regulator Chinese medications(case289-case358)

5).List of partial typical cases of **Esophagus cancer** treatment with XZ-C immune regulator Chinese medications(case359-case446)

6).List of partial typical cases of **Breast cancer** treatment with XZ-C immune regulator Chinese medications(case447-case481)

7).List of partial typical cases of **Colon, Rectal cancer** treatment with XZ-C immune regulator Chinese medications(case482-case649)

8).List of partial typical cases of **Bile duct cancer** treatment with XZ-C immune regulator Chinese medications(case650-case679)

2. The Partial typical cases of malignant cancer with XZ-C immunoruglation and control of anti-cancer Chinese medications

1). some typical cases of liver cancer treatment

2). some typical cases of Pancreatic cancer after adjuvant treatment

3). some typical cases of gastric cancer after adjuvant treatment

4) some typical cases lung cancer postoperative adjuvant treatment

5). some typical cases of esophageal cancer postoperative adjuvant treatment

6). some typical cases of breast cancer postoperative adjuvant treatment

7).some typical cases of colon and rectal cancer postoperative adjuvant treatment

8). some typical cases of gallbladder cancer after adjuvant treatment

9). some typical cases of Renal cancer and bladder cancer after adjuvant treatment

10). some typical cases of Thyroid cancer and retroperitoneal tumor and other postoperative adjuvant treatment

11). some typical cases of Non-Hodgkin's lymphoma treatment

12). some typical cases of Chemotherapy XZ-C traditional Chinese medicine treatment of acute lymphoblastic leukemia

13). some typical cases of Ovarian cancer and cervical cancer treatment of some typical cases

3. The Observation of Experimental and Clinic Curative Effect on Z-C Medicine Treating Malignancy

Table of Contents
(Volume X)

1. The new discovery of the experimental tumor research of anti-cancer and anti-metastasis and anti-recurrence

2. The Experimental Research Parts

1). The experiment research of searching etiology of cancer factor and pathogenesis and pathological physiology to seek for the effective regulation and control methods

a. The experimental research of making cancer animal models

b. The experimental research of searching the relation between tumors and immune organ to seek the methods of immune organ control

c. The experimental research of searching the methods of inhibition of thymus shrinkle during the tumor growth and reconstruction of thehost immune function

d. Searching the medicine of inhibiting the new vascular formation from nanetural drug

2). The experimental Observation of the effects of tumor on Thymus and Spleen

3).The experimental Study of the effects of the spleen on the growth of tumor

4). The experimental study of treatment of malignant tumor by adoptive immunologic reconstitution through combined transplantation of fetal cells

a. Experiment on Adoptive Immunologic Reconstitution of Fetal Liver, Spleen and Thymus Cells through Combined Transplantation

b. Progress of Study on Treatment of Tumor by Adoptive Immunity through Transplantation of Immunocyte with the Origin of Embryo

5). TG'S INHIBITION ON ANGIOGENESIS OF TRANSPLANTATION TUMOR OF MICE

a. the Experimental Study of the Observation of Angiogenesis of Transplantation Tumor at Mouse's Abdominal Muscle
b. the Experimental Study of the Effects of TG with Different Dosages on Immunologic Function of Mice
c. the Experimental Study of the Inhibition of TG of Different Dosages on Angiogenesis of Transplantation Tumor at Mouse's Abdominal Muscle
d. The Significance of Inhibition of Angiogenesis in Treatment

2. the guidance to read

1), In this medical monograph the book is divided into the next two parts, a total of 10 volumes, which wisdom are condensed to be used to conquer cancer?

Part I (Volume 1-4) condense how to conquer cancer and how to prevent cancer by my opinions

Part II (5-10 volumes) condense how to conquer cancer and how to treat cancer by my opinions?

Prevention cancer and anti-cancer, and the prevention is as the main which is a health policy, especially for the top priority, so that people can be away from cancer and reduce cancer incidence.

This is a medical monograph with the more complete and more systematic and more comprehensive design and more specific planning of how to conquer cancer which can be used for the various countries and the provinces and the states to carry out the implementation of how to overcome cancer? How to prevent cancer? How to control cancer? How to treat cancer?

2), the agglutination of the following wisdom which can be used to overcome cancer:

Part One: condense how to conquer cancer? how to prevent cancer I see.

Volume I

(A), How to overcome cancer? XZ-C proposed three targets

After analysis: XZ-C proposed that the target or the goal of conquering cancer should be:

A target: it should be directed against the gene mutations and the abnormal expression or the deletion.

B target: it should be for environmental factors:

The external environment —— air, water, soil, physical, chemical, biological factors, clothing, food, shelter.

The internal environment ——immune, endocrine, neurohumoral

It should create "the environmental protection research institute" and carry out the prevention cancer system engineering research.

C target: it should be to adjust the normal immune system and to restore the immune system to identify cancer cells, thereby remove tumor cells, and conduct the immunotherapy and the immunoprophylaxis.

(B), how to overcome cancer? XZ-C presents: two wheels

The details of the situation analysis (a), (b), (c), (d)
The basic situation is:
The United States:

life sciences, biomedicine, genetic engineering, targeted therapy, drugs, minimally invasive techniques, instruments, and precision medicine are far ahead.

China:

It has the rich resources of the immune regulation and control traditional Chinese medication and the immune regulation traditional Chinese medications, the traditional Chinese medications with activating blood and removing stasis and anti-microvascular thrombosis and anti-micrometastasis as well as the traditional Chinese medication which controls precancerous nodules by soften the firm and scatter the knot.

It should cooperate complement each other and move forward together.

(C). Why is the cooperation between China and the United States?

Because:

in 1971 the US Congress passed a "national cancer regulations", and President Nixon issued "anti-cancer declaration" in order to overcome cancer in one fell swoop.

In January 12, 2016 US President Barack Obama announced **"the national plan to conquer cancer**" and the plan is responsible by Vice President Joe Biden.

The Plan name: **"Cancer moon shot"**

The Goal: to overcome cancer

(3) In 2011 Chinese doctor Xu Ze put forward in his published monographs: " the strategic thinking and suggestions of conquering cancer."

In August 2013 at the International Cancer Conference it was put forward " the XZ-C research program of conquering cancer and launch a total attack"

In July 2015 it proposed" the dawn of the C-type plan of conquering cancer and launch a total attack"

In December 2016 in the English version of the monograph it was put forward "the initiative of conquering cancer and launch the general attack."

Therefore: China and the United States both are conducting the scientific research of conquering cancer and it should be co-operation and move forward toward the scientific hall of conquering cancer.

The second volume (Volume II)

What wisdom is condensed which can be used to overcome cancer?
Its focus is:

- How to prevent cancer I see and how to carry out conquering cancer and launching a total attack?
- How to create the scientific research bases and the Science city with a multidisciplinary and cancer research group?
- it must create an "Innovative Oncology School" and a graduate school in order to o overcome cancer.
- it must set up To overcome the cancer, it must create " the prevention and treatment hospital with innovative tumor integrated traditional Chinese and Western medications during tumor whole process and the prevention, control and treatment of cancer are at the same attention in order to conquer cancer.
- it must create an "Innovative Molecular Cancer Institute" in order to overcome cancer.
- it must create "Innovative Environmental Protection Cancer Research Institute" and prevention cancer system engineering.

Volume III

What wisdom is condensed which can be used to conquer cancer?
Its focus is:
How to prevent cancer I see: how to prevent cancer from the big environment and the small environment?

- How to prevent cancer from clothing, food, shelter, and walking?
- it should be carried out prevention cancer from improving carcinogenic factors in external causes (external environment) and internal causes (internal environment).
- Environmental and cancer research groups should be set up to study the relationship between environment and cancer.
- To study what the carcinogenic factors are in the environment and how should they be prevented?
- XZ-C proposes to create the "Innovative Environmental Protection Institute" and the prevention cancer system project
- How can we prevent cancer from "two types of society"?
- The catastrophe of cancer is the global and the people of the world must struggle with it and struggle together.

Volume IV

What wisdom is condensed which can be used to conquer cancer?
Its focus is:

- the proposals was put forward "cancer treatment reform, innovation and development"
- XZ-C proposes a plan to tackle the total attack on cancer
- it was put forward the necessity and feasibility of proposing a total attack on cancer
- it was proposed "the general design and imagine of conquer cancer and the basic design of the Science City" and the feasibility report
- it was put forward the suggestions that at the same time when a well-off society is constructed, the ride research is built and the scientific research on prevention cancer and anti-cancer is conducted.

Part II: The agglomeration of how to overcome cancer? Each opinion I see of how to treat cancer.

Volume V

What wisdom is condensed which can be used to conquer cancer?
Its focus is: "walking out of a new way to overcome cancer"

- From the experimental results it was found that: the host of the thymus inoculated cancer cells, that was acute progressive atrophy, cell proliferation was blocked, the volume was significantly reduced.
- From the above experimental study found that thymic atrophy, immune dysfunction, may be one of the etiology and pathogenesis of the tumor, it must try to prevent thymic atrophy, promote thymocyte proliferation, increased immune function.
- In order to try to prevent thymic atrophy, promote thymocyte hyperplasia, increased immunity, we from the traditional Chinese medicine, Western medicine to find both. Western medicine can improve immunity and promote the proliferation of thymocytes. So we changed from the Chinese medicine to find, because the traditional Chinese medicine tonic drugs generally have immune regulation.
- After 7 years of laboratory scientific research, we selected from the natural drug XZ-C1-10 immune regulation of anti-cancer, anti-transfer of traditional Chinese medicine, chest lifting, birth control. In the animal experiment on the basis of the success of clinical validation work, after 20 years of more than 12,000 cases of cancer specialist clinical application, and achieved good results.
- After experimental study, Chinese medicine immunopharmacology and molecular level of Chinese and Western medicine combined with anti-cancer research, out of a XZ-C immune regulation, regulate immune activity, prevent thymus atrophy, promote thymocyte proliferation, protect bone marrow hematopoietic function, improve immune surveillance, Combination of Chinese and Western medicine to overcome the new path of cancer - "Chinese - style anti - cancer" new road.

Volume VI

What wisdom is condensed which can be used to conquer cancer?
Its focus is:

- More than 20 years has been out of a new path to overcome the cancer, has initially formed XZ-C immune regulation of the theoretical system, is undergoing clinical application, observation and verification.

- The new model that considers cancer treatment is that healing should be done through immunoregulation rather than a single killer, and the last step in curing cancer is to regain the control of the host's immune regulation rather than destroy the last cancer cells.

- From the experimental results to analyze thinking, the new revelation: thymus atrophy, immune dysfunction is the cause of cancer and pathogenesis of one of the factors, so Xu Ze (XU ZE) Professor is the international academic conference on the cause of cancer, one of the pathogenesis, May be thymus atrophy, central immune organ motility damage, immune dysfunction, immune surveillance capacity decline and immune escape.

- Based on the findings of the laboratory above experimental results, so the treatment principle must be to prevent thymus atrophy, promote thymic hyperplasia, protect bone marrow hematopoietic function, improve immune surveillance, control malignant cells immune escape.

- XZ-C (XU-ZE-China) immunoregulation therapy was first presented by Professor Xu Ze in his book "New Concepts and Methods for Cancer Transfer Treatment" in 2006, and he believes that under normal circumstances, cancer and Body defense is in a dynamic balance between the occurrence of cancer is caused by dynamic imbalance. If the state has been adjusted to the normal level, you can control the growth of cancer and make it subside.

- It is well known that the occurrence, progression and prognosis of cancer is determined by a combination of two factors, namely, the biological characteristics of cancer cells and the host body itself, the ability to control cancer cells, such as the balance between the two can be controlled if the two imbalance The development of cancer.

- Cancer treatment should be changed to observe and establish a comprehensive treatment concept.

The goal of treatment only kill cancer cells, but for one aspect, compared with one-sided treatment concept, can not overcome cancer. The goal of treatment should be for the host and cancer cells in two areas, both cancer cells and protect the host, enhance immunity, chest lifting, birth control, enhance the host anti-cancer ability, this is a comprehensive treatment concept, it is possible to overcome cancer.

Therefore, the principle of cancer treatment should change the concept, the establishment of a comprehensive treatment concept.

Volume VII

What wisdom is condensed which can be used to conquer cancer?

Challenge the status quo of cancer treatment and reform can develop.
Its focus is:

- the review and the analysis and the questioning of the three major treatments for cancer
  Through the review and the analysis and the reflection it is found the traditional problems and shortcomings of traditional therapy.
- The analysis and the evaluation and the questioning of systemic intravenous chemotherapy for solid tumors:
  Whether the method and method of administration of systemic intravenous administration are scientific and reasonable analysis and questioning.
  Whether the method of calculating the dose of systemic intravenous chemotherapy is reasonable analysis and questioning.
  The analysis and query on the evaluation standard of Intravenous Chemotherapy and Curative Effect of Solid Tumor
- the century review, analysis and comment of the three major treatments for cancer

Respectively, the problems existing in the surgery and the radiotherapy and the chemotherapy are analyzed and commented:

The Surgical treatment:

Comments:

It is the future of cancer to overcome the main technology and the main treatment. The surgical treatment of cancer is the exact and effective method.

The Radiation Therapy:

Comments:

The radiotherapy is for local treatment and the transfer is the entire body and the systemic problems which is a major contradiction. The reason for its failure is not for the transfer and is not for controlling the transfer because the main problem of cancer treatment is to anti-transfer and how to play its role during anti-transfer therapy which must be carefully considered and in-depth study.

The Chemotherapy:

Comment 1:

Comment on the route of administration of systemic intravenous chemotherapy

This route of administration is not the real point of targeted administration, but through the heart pump to the blood spray to the body and has the whole body cytotoxic distribution and the whole body target so that the whole body organs obtain the cytotoxic. It is very unreasonable and is very unscientific. The result is:

① very few foci cancer, only about 0.4%, the effect is minimal (because the foci accounts for a small body surface area and is very small proportion).

② 99.6% of the cytotoxic kill to the body of normal cells, causing brain, heart, liver, lung, kidney, gastrointestinal system, hematopoietic system, the immune system, endocrine system poison reaction.

The toxic side effects of these chemotherapy is irrational route of administration, which should be avoided.

Therefore, this route of intravenous chemotherapy is unreasonable, unscientific, easily lead to iatrogenic toxic side effects.

How to do? Should be reformed, should change the route of administration, to target organ intravascular chemotherapy pathways, the drug directly to the "target" organs, so that the dose is very small, effective, no side effects, is conducive to patients.

Comment 2:

Assessment of solid body tumor intravenous chemotherapy dose calculation, is the experience and methods of leukemia treatment to solid tumor treatment, the guiding ideology is calculated by the body surface area, which is unwise, unreasonable, easy to lead Iatrogenic toxic side effects.

why?

Because solid tumors are confined to an organ, it should not be calculated with whole body surface area, which is unreasonable and unscientific.

Comment 3:

evaluation of solid tumor systemic intravenous chemotherapy efficacy evaluation criteria evaluation:

The current assessment criteria for the efficacy of solid tumors are:

a, the size of the tumor; b, remission, remission (CR, PR) - as the name suggests, ease is not cured, but a few short weeks of shortening, after this short-term improvement, will progress, increase, transfer, so ease Not the purpose of treatment, it can not be cured, can only alleviate, and only short-term relief, so the patient is not the desired purpose, should not be the goal of treatment.

Comment 4:

Why abdomen solid tumor after adjuvant chemotherapy, failed to prevent recurrence, metastasis? Abdominal solid tumor (gastric cancer, cardiac cancer, colorectal cancer, liver cancer, gallbladder cancer, pancreatic cancer, abdominal tumor), postoperative adjuvant chemotherapy are systemic intravenous chemotherapy, this way from the vena cava can not directly reach the portal vein.

Abdominal solid tumor cancer cells mainly in the portal vein system, vena cava system and portal vein system is generally not connected by the superior vena cava can not reach the portal vein, so this route of administration is unreasonable, does not meet the anatomy, not scientific.

Comment 5:

There are some important errors and shortcomings in current chemotherapy.

Chemotherapy can suppress immune function and inhibit the bone marrow hematopoietic function so that the overall immune function decreased. In cancer patients thymus is inhibited and chemotherapy can inhibit bone marrow, as "snow adds frog or worse" so that the entire central immune organs are damaged and it promotes the further decline in immune surveillance and it may cause that while chemotherapy, cancer metastasis ; the more treatment, the more chemotherapy.

Volume VIII

What wisdom is condensed which can be used to conquer cancer?
The Study on Anti - cancer Traditional Chinese Medication by XZ - C Immunomodulation
Its focus is:

(1) In our laboratory the experimental study of finding and screening anti-cancer, anti-transfer drug was conducted from the Chinese medications:

1) The in vitro culture method of cancer cells was used to study the anti-tumor rate of Chinese herbal medicine.

a, in vitro screening test: the use of cancer cells in vitro culture to observe the direct damage to cancer cells.

b, test tube screening test: in the culture of cancer cells in the tube, were placed in biological crude products (500ug / m), to observe whether the inhibition of cancer cells.

2) To make the experimental study on the tumor inhibition rate of Chinese herbal medicine in the carcasses.

Each group of mice were divided into 8 groups, each group of 30, group 7 for the blank control group, group 8 with 5-F or CTX as the control group. Whole mice were inoculated with EAC or S180 or H22 cancer cells. After 24 hours of inoculation, each mouse was orally fed with crude crude drug powder, and the selected Chinese herbal medicine was fed for a long period of time. The survival time, toxic and side effects were observed, and the survival rate was calculated and the tumor inhibition rate was calculated.

In this way, we conducted four consecutive years of experimental study, each year with more than 1,000 animals only animal model, 4 years to do a total of nearly 6000 Dutch animal model, each mouse died after the liver, spleen, kidney, lung, Thymus of the pathological sections, a total of more than 20,000 slices.

The experimental results:

In our laboratory through animal experiments screening 200 kinds of Chinese herbal medicine, screening out 48 kinds of certain, even excellent tumor inhibition rate of 75% -90% or more. During the experimental screening tests 152 kinds of Chinese herbal medication with no obvious anti-cancer effects were gotten rid of.

(2) The clinical validation:

On the basis of the success of the animal experiments clinical validation was conducted and establish cancer specialist outpatient and retain outpatient medical records and each outpatient record is recorded.

It establishes the regular follow-up observation system to observe long-term efficacy.

The standard of the Observation of the efficacy of the standard is: the survival of patients with the long and good quality of life.

After 20 years of the clinical application and verification in the cancer specialist outpatient service in more than 12000 cases of advanced patients XZ-C immunoregulation anti-cancer traditional Chinese medication preparation has achieved significant effect. XZ-C immunomodulatory medications can improve the quality of life of patients with advanced cancer and enhance immune function and increase the body's anti-cancer ability and enhance appetite and significantly extend the survival period.

Volume IX

What wisdom is condensed which can be used to conquer cancer?
The focus is:

(1) how to carry out clinical research data summary and collation and expression

① China is a large country with 1.3 billion population and thus it is a large resource for cancer cases. China has a large number of cancer cases for the clinical observation and the analysis.

In the daily clinical work clinicians conduct the subtle observation of cancer and the careful thinking and the analysis and actively explore the study. After the long-term accumulation of the practice medical experience it will also have some discovery and the development and the continuous progress; the medical research is to improve clinical diagnosis and treatment work, The medical research is to Improve the quality of medical care and medical level and thus the clinical research work is also an important part of clinical work.

② it creates a table form of scientific research materials which can be achieve that is is both concise and comprehensive and easy to read and easy to understand. Through a few decades of the bitter and meticulous clinical research work it received a lot of scientific research data and experimental data and the summary and the collation and the collection. Through the table form for the narrative expression it is concise and structured and the readers can understand their core content in ten minutes.

③ to retain the outpatient medical records and the information accumulation about the outpatient visits, treatment, rehabilitation and follow-up; to fill in a complete detailed table outpatient medical records so as to obtain clinical validation of complete information and it is easy analysis, statistics and in order to facilitate follow-up treatment of patients.

If there is no preservation of the outpatient medical records, the analysis and the statistics of the outpatient efficacy of scientific research work can not be carried out.

④ to stay outpatient medical records is to observe the long-term efficacy, is conducive to clinical research outpatient to improve the quality of medical care.

Volume X

What wisdom is condensed which can be used to conquer cancer?
Its focus is:

- How to overcome the cancer I see one: the road to scientific research is to explore the cause of cancer, pathogenesis, pathophysiology of experimental basic research.
- **the experimental surgery is extremely important in the development of medication. It is a key to open the medical closed area, many diseases prevention and control methods are after many animal experimental research, achieved a stable effect was applied to clinical and promote the development of medical career.**
- We conducted a series of animal experiments to explore the etiology, pathogenesis and pathophysiology of cancer. We have obtained new findings from the experimental results. The new findings: thymus atrophy and the immune dysfunction are one of the the cause and pathogenesis of cancer.
- As a result of our laboratory study, we found that thymus atrophy, central immune sensory dysfunction, decreased immune function, and low immune surveillance in the cancer-bearing mice. and the principle of treatment must be to prevent thymic atrophy and promote thymus Cell proliferation and protect bone marrow hematopoietic function, improve immune vision. For the immune regulation of cancer, it provides a theoretical basis and experimental basis.
- XZ-C believes that under normal circumstances cancer and body defense is in a dynamic balance. The occurrence of cancer is caused by dynamic imbalance. If the state has been adjusted to the normal level, you can control the growth of cancer and may make it subside.
- **No matter how complex the mechanism behind cancer, immunosuppression is the key to cancer progression.** Removal of immunosuppressive factors and restoring the immune system to cancer cell recognition can effectively inhibit cancer. More and more evidence shows that by regulating the body's immune system, it is possible to achieve the purpose of cancer control. Through the activation of the body's anti-tumor immune system to treat tumors is currently the majority of researchers excited areas.

3. XZ-C proposes that several treatments of traditional Chinese medicine can be applied to the treatment of tumors.

Professor Xu Ze (XZ-C) proposed several treatments for traditional Chinese medicine, which can be applied to the treatment of tumors and the combination of Chinese and Western medicine; Experimental research and clinical basic research on the combination of Chinese and Western medicine should be carried out, as well as clinical application verification observation.

A. The rule of Chinese medicine: **Fuzheng Guben(support Righting and firm Essence) matches** Western medicine treatment principles: **improve immunity, immune regulation and control and immunity reconstruction; it should carry out the research of a**nti-cancer immunological pharmacology and the research of the mechanism of action of anticancer immune regulation and control of traditional Chinese medications; Experimental study on the combination of anti-cancer Chinese and Western medicine should be carried out at the molecular level.

B. TCM treatment: activate the blood circulation and remove the blood stasis matches western medicine treatment principles: anti-cancer metastasis, anti-cancer thrombosis, anti-micro-transfer and anti-formation of cancer plugs or thrombosis so that it must resist blood clots and improve blood circulation; activating blood circulation can remove the blood stasis and can paralyze and avoid the formation of cancerous plugs; Eliminate cancer cells on the way to metastasis must resolve cancerous plugs and micro-cancers thrombosis so as to prevent cancer cell metastasis

C. TCM treatment: removing inflammation and detoxification matches western medicine treatment principles: some cancers may be related to chronic inflammation, stubborn ulcers such as chronic atrophic gastritis, chronic pelvic inflammatory disease, cervicitis, chronic hepatitis, etc., some are cancer pre-lesion which can be treated with heat-clearing(inflammation) and detoxifying Chinese medicine to control

D. TCM treatment: soften solids and firm and dissolving the nodules matches western medicine treatment principle: in the current examination CT, sometimes reported that there are multiple small nodules, small, only a few millimeters in the certain organ, which can not be operated by chemotherapy and radiotherapy, can be treated by these softening Chinese medicine, and have the dynamic observation, **often have a good effect.**

CHAPTER 9

The initiative and academic report of executing "To conquer cancer and launch the general attack to cancer"

TABLE OF CONTENTS

Preface

How to prevent cancer? What can be prevented? How should it be prevented or done?

a. Find problems and ask questions from follow-up results (Hint: To study how to prevent postoperative recurrence and metastasis is the key to improve long-term outcomes after surgery)

b. Pathfinding

(to conquer cancer, where is the road? Where can you find it?)

c. Pathfinding and footprint

(anti-cancer, anti-cancer metastasis research and scientific research results, scientific and technological innovation series)

d. Published cancer monographs (3 Chinese editions are exclusively distributed nationwide, 7 full English editions are published worldwide)

e. Participate in the International Congress of Oncology (AIACR Academic Conference, Washington)

f. Visiting the Stirling Cancer Institute in Houston, USA (2009)

g. Basic and clinical research on anti-cancer and anti-cancer metastasis in the past 30 years

h. More than 12,000 clinical application experience in 20 years

I.a). Walk Out of a new road of cancer treatment with the immune regulation and control combination of Chinese and Western medicine at the molecule level

b). Walking out of a new road to conquer cancer with "Chinese-style anti-cancer", and a new way of Chinese and Western medicine combined with immune regulation and treatment of cancer

c). Published the English monograph "The Road to Overcome Cancer on December 6, 2016 in USA, globally distributed

d). Published the English monograph "Condense Wisdom and Conquer Cancer" in December 2017 (volume 1), February 2018 (Volume 2) in USA, full English version, globally distributed.

1.How to overcome cancer? XZ-C (XU ZE-China) (Xu Ze - China) proposed: Carry out "To conquer cancer and launch the general attack of cancer"

1). Why is it proposed to overcome cancer? Please look at the current situation:

(1). The current situation of cancer incidence is: the more patients are treated and the more cancer patients occur.

The incidence of cancer in China today is 3.12 million new cases of cancer each year, with an average of 8550 new cancer patients per day, and 6 people diagnosed with cancer every minute in the country.

(2), the status quo of cancer mortality is: high, has been the first cause of death in urban and rural areas in China

Today's cancer death rate in China is 2.7 million deaths per year due to cancer, with an average of 7,500 deaths per day from cancer, and one in every seven deaths due to cancer.

Cancer is so high in China, the more patients are treated and the more cancer patients occur, the higher the mortality rate stay without decrease. It should be a major problem for the national economy and the people's livelihood. It should be a major problem for the people's health. It should be a major disaster and disaster for the people.

Human beings should not sit still, doctors should not do nothing, leaders should not do nothing, I think that we should propose "to overcome cancer", we should gather wisdom and overcome cancer.

2) Why did you propose to overcome cancer and launch a general attack? Look at the current state of cancer treatment:

1. Current status of cancer treatment:

Despite the application of traditional three major treatments for nearly a hundred years, thousands of cancer patients have been exposed to radiotherapy and chemotherapy, but what is the result? So far, cancer is still the leading cause of death. Although patients undergo regular, systematic radiotherapy or chemotherapy, or radiotherapy + chemotherapy, they have not stopped cancer metastasis and recurrence, with little success.

2. Current status of the current hospital or oncology hospital model

(1) Focusing on treatment, focusing on the treatment of cancer in the middle and late stages, it has exhausted human and financial resources, and failed to reduce mortality, prolong survival, and reduce morbidity. Cancer is still the leading cause of death in urban and rural areas.

(2) Only treatment without prevention, or attention to treatment with little prevention, the more cancer patients occur while the patient is treated.

(3) Ignore the "three early" and ignore the precancerous lesions.

(4) Neglected prevention.

The masses or people: while talking about cancer, the skin changes the color.

Patient and family: unbearable or don't know what can be done

Doctors and nurses: Inability to do anything, medical treatment stays in the three major treatments, and the efficacy is not good.

People recognize attitudes: a variety of chemical, physical, biological environmental carcinogens appear in large numbers, various carcinogens into the human body or various carcinogens affect the human body, people seem to be enveloped in the ocean of environmental carcinogens, some people talk about cancer discoloration, It seems that the grass is all soldiers, some people are insensitive, and they are doing their own thing in life. Cancer is not terrible. **What is terrible is that we do not have simple knowledge of prevention in this area. With this basic knowledge, most cancers can be avoided and prevented.**

(5) Many large hospitals and university affiliated hospitals have not established laboratories and cannot carry out basic research or clinical basic research of cancer, because without the breakthrough of basic research, clinical efficacy is difficult to improve, and "oncology" is still the most backward discipline in each subject among the current medicine. why? It is because the etiology, pathogenesis, and pathophysiology of "oncology" are not well understood. People still lack sufficient understanding of the mechanism of its pathogenesis and cancer cell metastasis. Therefore, the current cancer treatment plan is still quite blind. Therefore, it is necessary to establish a laboratory for basic research and clinical basic research.

The status quo is:

a. **In the past century the road that has passed and the mode of running the hospital are attention of treatment and little prevention, or only treatment so that the result is: the more treatment and the more cancer patient occurrence.**

b. **In the past century the road that has passed and the treatment mode are to focus on the advanced patients in the middle and late stage of invasion and metastasis, the human and financial resources are exhausted, and the result is: the mortality rate remains high.**

What should be done? It should change the current treatment mode, hospital mode, propose to overcome cancer, launch a general attack - prevention, control, and treatment at the same level and attention and the same time.

3). XZ-C proposes to plans and programs for conquering cancer and launching the general attack of cancer.

Xu Ze proposed in Chapter 38 in his third book, "New Concepts and New Methods for Cancer Treatment" (Beijing Publishing, 2011), which is the first time in the world that "to conquer cancer and launch the general attack of cancer"

(1). What is called as conquer cancer and launch the total attack on cancer?

The general attack is to carry out the three-stage work of cancer prevention, cancer control and cancer treatment in the whole process of cancer occurrence and development, and carry out the simultaneous prevention and treatment at the same lever and same attention.

What is cancer prevention, cancer control, and cancer treatment?
Namely:
Cancer prevention - before cancer formation
Cancer control - precancerous lesions with malignant tendencies
Treating cancer - has formed a cancerous foci or metastasis
Change the current hospital mode
Change current treatment mode
Namely:
change the current hospital-oriented mode
Change the current treatment mode focusing on the middle and late stages of treatment
Change only treatment without the defense into the prevention, control, and treatment at the same time and the same level
How to implement this new mode of running a hospital?
It is necessary to establish a hospital for prevention, control and treatment according to the whole process of cancer occurrence and development.

The way out for cancer treatment is "three early" (early detection, early diagnosis, early treatment)

<u>Early cancer treatment is good, can heal, especially precancerous lesions, well treated, can be cured.</u>

The goal of the total attack:

<u>reduce the incidence of cancer, reduce cancer mortality, improve cure rate, prolong survival, improve quality of life, and reduce complications.</u>

Professor Xu Ze (XU ZE) proposed the idea, strategy, and planning sketch for conquering cancer and launching the general attack as the following:

How to overcome cancer

Where is the road?

Our ideas, strategies, and plans should be divided into three parts (or three stages).

Prevention and treatment of the whole process of cancer occurrence and development

Before the formation of cancer - **for the prevention part** - anti-mutation

Precancerous lesions that may have a malignant tendency - **part of the intervention**

Therapeutic parts of anti-metastatic treatment for primary cancer that has formed a cancerous foci

Prevention of susceptibility stage precancerous lesions cancer metastasis

Early, not transferred, transferred

Prevention cancer Control Cancer Cancer treatment

(2). Why is conquering cancer proposed and is need to launch a general attack?

(1) Because the goal of conquering cancer should be:

1) reduce the incidence of cancer

Improve cancer cure rate, prolong patient survival, improve quality of life, and reduce complications.

2) reach

1/3 can prevent

1/3 can be cured

1/3 can prolong life through treatment

(2) So, how can we reduce the incidence of cancer?

It should be prevention-oriented, control-oriented, and prevention-oriented as the main part or the important part.

But for decades, the road we have traveled is to attention of treatment with little prevention or only treatment without prevention.

I have been working in clinical oncology surgery for 62 years. Looking back on the lessons of failure for decades, it was only treatment without prevention so that the incidence of cancer is increasing, and the more patients are treated and the more incidence.

What should it be done? It is necessary to implement a health work policy based **on prevention.** Only by paying attention to cancer prevention can we reduce the incidence of cancer.

How can we implement cancer prevention, cancer control, and prevention-oriented or prevention as the main part health work guidelines? How can we correct the current hospitalization model of attention to treatment with little prevention or defense, or treatment only? We must reform the current hospital treatment model for cancer treatment, only reform can have development or progress.

Professor Xu Ze proposed to launch a general attack, which is to prevent, control, and treat, and to mention cancer prevention and cancer control as the important parts. The essence is to implement the health work policy of "cancer prevention and anti-cancer" and "prevention-oriented" as the main or important parts. Our medical predecessors, the world's medical sages put forward "cancer prevention and anti-cancer" and "prevention-oriented" as the main part and the important part, this policy is very correct, but unfortunately, our medical juniors have not paid attention to it.

In particular, our cancer researchers and health workers have not realized this. Over the past century, we have neglected prevention and neglected cancer prevention, which led to such a high incidence of cancer today. There are 8,550 new cancers in China every day, and 6 people are diagnosed with cancer every minute. Such amazing data should be a national event. XZ-C is proposing to accelerate anti-cancer research to reduce the incidence of cancer.

The task of health work should be "prevention of disease and treatment of disease" and "prevention first". Health is to protect life and defend health and should execute "prevention as the main part". Launching the general attack, its essence is to put cancer prevention work at an important position, as the most part among cancer prevention and cancer treatment and to focus on reducing the incidence of cancer

2. XZ-C proposes how to overcome cancer, how to prevent cancer I see: (1 - 6)

A. The environment and cancer (the situation analysis 1-5)
a. How to overcome cancer? how to prevent cancer?

I see one:

(1) Situation analysis: How to prevent cancer? the incidence of cancer is rising

1. From what I saw in my 86-year-old society this year:

I feel deeply that the incidence of cancer, a major disease that threatens people's health, is rising.

(1) I came to Zhongnan Tongji Medical College in Wuhan in 1951. I graduated from Tongji Medical College in 1956 and was assigned to the Surgical Work of the Affiliated Hospital of Hubei College of Traditional Chinese Medicine. Successively, I was the director of surgery and the director of the Institute of Experimental Surgery of Hubei College of Traditional Chinese Medicine.

When the Central South Tongji Medical College moved from Shanghai to Wuhan in 1951, at that time, for the teaching, I was looking for a case of lung cancer to train my students and classmates. It was difficult to find one patient a week earlier while I made the phone calls to each hospital.

At that time (1950s - 1960s), all hospitals in Wuhan had no oncology department and no oncologists. Only one hospital in Wuhan had a medical doctor to see blood diseases. Tongji Hospital had a gynecologist and saw or treat gynecology tumor.

But now, (65 years later) cancer is a common disease, frequently-occurring disease, more common in hospitals, cancer patients are queued for registration, each of the top three hospitals have oncology which are busy with cancer treatment. I have done 62 years of oncology surgery. The more patients are treated, the more our doctors should think and review. **Why? Why are patients getting more and more? What causes or what causes the incidence to rise? What should I do?**

I have been engaged in medical clinical work for 62 years. I have been conducting basic research and clinical verification for cancer research for 30 years. I have deeply realized that cancer should not only pay attention to treatment, but also pay attention to prevention, so as to stop cancer at the source. Promoting the decline in the incidence of cancer, the way out for cancer treatment is "three early" (early detection, early diagnosis, early treatment), and the way to fight cancer is prevention.

b. How to overcome cancer how to prevent cancer I see two:

(2) Situation analysis: (2) - Cancer incidence is related to the environment

So how should we prevent it? What to prevent? How to prevent it? Where is the target or "target" of cancer prevention? How to control? What to control? How to control? Where is the target or "target" of cancer control?

There must be specific anti-cancer targets, clear goals, operability, and motivation and effect.

The more patients are treated and the more the incidence is rising, and 90% of

them are related to the environment. Why? Professor Xu proposed that the goal or "target" of cancer prevention should be to study and explore the carcinogenic factors (external environment and internal environment) of the environment.

1 Why does the increase in cancer incidence have a relationship with the environment?

Because cancer is a malignant abnormal cell proliferation, it is caused by external factors (external environment) or internal factors (internal environment). Cells are always in a controlled dynamic balance of proliferation, survival, and death during normal development. **However, under the influence of external factors (external environment) or internal factors (internal environment), the proliferation of a cell is abnormal, breaking through the normal restriction mechanism and rapidly proliferating, forming a tissue mass, which is formed by abnormal proliferation. The group is called a tumor.** Tumors are benign, malignant, and only proliferate without spreading, called benign tumors; but not only abnormally rapid proliferation, but cells can spread and metastasize, called malignant tumors, malignant tumors are cancer.

2. The cause of cancer is related to the carcinogenic factors of the external environment and of the internal environment.

After years of worldwide research, people have now achieved a consensus:
That is, carcinogenesis is a evolution process with multi-factor, multi-stage and multi-gene that one side is external and the one side is the body genetic (substance).
The so-called external factors refer to factors other than the cytogenetic factors themselves, including chemical factors, physical factors, biological (bacterial, viral, etc.) factors in the living environment other than the human body, as well as human lifestyles and eating habits, as well as physical Internal environment, such as hormonal status, disease infection, and mental factors.
Genetics refers to genetic material DNA or genes. There are two basic factors which can lead to cancer: one is an intrinsic genetic factor; the other is an external environmental factor. Most cancers are the result of a combination of these two factors.

3 If we have a deeper understanding of the cause of cancer, then we can come up with more valuable suggestions in the future: how to prevent cancer-causing factors, how to monitor which carcinogenic factors, and even which carcinogenic

factors are removed, so that we can stay away from cancer and prevent cancer.
For example, you should not smoke, you should not eat pickles and smoked products, you should avoid strong sun exposure, these are the important ways to reduce the incidence of cancer in the future.

Analysis from the above situation (1)

It prompts and suggests:

1. In Wuhan City in the 1950s and 1960s, there were few cancer patients; there was neither oncology nor oncologists.

But now (65 years later) cancer is a common disease, frequently-occurring disease, patients line up registration, each of the top three hospitals has oncology, is busy with cancer treatment.
It is proved that the incidence of cancer is rising.

2. The analysis : what is the cause or what causes the cancer incidence to rise? What factors lead to cancer incidence increased?

Why? What should we do? **Whether from this point to do in-depth analysis or not to find out the factors that lead to the increase in cancer incidence, and find ways to prevent cancer and control cancer?**

The Analysis from the above situation (2)

It prompts and suggests:

1. **Cancer is a malignant transformation of abnormal cells, which is caused by external factors (external environment) or internal factors (internal environment).**

The so-called external factors refer to factors other than the cytogenetic factors themselves, **including: chemical factors, physical factors, biological (bacteria, viruses) and other factors in the living environment other than the human body, as well as people's lifestyles, eating habits, and the internal environment of the body such as endocrine hormones, mental factors and so on.**

2. **To Analyze what causes or factors that lead to an increase in cancer incidence?**

Today's people's living standards continue to improve, and various high-tech products have brought us a better life, but also brought a variety of chemical, physical, biological environmental carcinogens. Various carcinogens enter the human body or various carcinogenic factors affect the human body. People seem to be shrouded in the oceans of environmentally harmful carcinogens.
From this point of view, the rise in the incidence of cancer is causey or can be

searched for the causes. The target or "target" of cancer prevention is also very clear and very specific. How should cancer be prevented? How to control? What to prevent? It is clear, specific, and operable.

It's just that while some people talk about cancer the skin changes color or they are discoloration, and they seem to be arrogant or it seems that the grass is all soldiers; others are insensitive, and they are doing their part in life

Cancer is not terrible. What is terrible is that we don't have a simple basic knowledge of cancer prevention because most cancers are preventable.

c. How to overcome cancer how to prevent cancer I see three:

(3) Situation analysis: (3) - Prevention should be carried out from the improvement of external factors (external environment) and internal factors (internal environment).

How to prevent? We should prevent carcinogenic factors from the above external factors (external environment) and internal factors (internal environment)

Professor Xu Ze proposed: the establishment of an innovative anti-cancer research institute and an innovative anti-cancer system project. This is an unprecedented work and must be practiced in person to seek health and welfare for mankind.

How to implement the creation of this cancer research institute.

Professor Xu Ze XZ-C proposed the general design of anti-cancer and proposed anti-cancer system engineering:

(1) Personal prevention: improve cancer prevention knowledge (see separate article)

(2) The government should carry out cancer prevention engineering

1.   What is cancer prevention engineering?

a.   That is, the above-mentioned each department will monitor, characterize, quantify, and set the bottom line standards for the causative cancer factors, and prevent them from even legislating and the division of labor is responsible

b.   This is the responsibility of the government to arrange the engineering details of the anti-cancer system.

c.   The division of labor is responsible for each department, and the anti-cancer research institute conducts technical monitoring.

d.   macro, micro, ultra-micro, sampling, provide effective reporting.

2. **From which departments and scope to test?**

Xu Ze proposed that there should be no carcinogenic factors from clothing, food, housing, and transportation.

a. [clothing]: - Light industry department is responsible for receiving investigations and tests: clothing, cosmetics, toys, etc., causing the detection of Ca factors, exceeding the standard to warn or stop.

b. [Food]: - The agricultural department and the food department are responsible for receiving investigation and research, water, soil, fertilizer, agricultural genetic modification, food, fish, meat, chicken, duck, packaged food, food, oil, feed... carcinogenic factors Detection.

c. **[Stay or living]**: - The building construction department is responsible for receiving investigations and tests: monitoring of carcinogenic factors such as decoration materials, supplies, and design. Those who exceed the standards will be warned and blocked.

d. **[walking or transportion]**: - The industrial department is responsible for receiving investigations, trains, cars, aircrafts, ... tail gas hazards, testing is not allowed to exceed the standard should be legislated.

e. **Environment:** The environmental protection department shall be responsible for, monitoring, investigating, monitoring, investigation, garbage disposal, air pollution, water pollution, factory chimneys, etc., from macroscopic and microscopic monitoring, qualitative and quantitative detection of carcinogen content, those who exceed the standard will be warned or prevented.

f. **Education department**: large, medium and small teachers should be teachering models

No smoking allowed(Smoking has Hundreds of damages without benefits; smoking is a non-knowledge performance, smoking harms others, harms people)

Primary, secondary and primary school students

The content of the textbook adds or plus:

1.Physical hygiene; 2.Health care, basic moral knowledge; 3.Anti-cancer, anti-cancer and other knowledge

g. **Professor Xu Ze proposed that research ethics should be advocated, medicine is benevolence, and ethics is the first**

Research ethics: products should have ethical standards

Standard: should be based on the standard of not damaging human health

Basic ethics: All products and people are harmless and do not harm people's health, especially for children.

(To become the living environment and living environment with beautiful **scenery and bird language and floral)**

h. **the health administrative department protect lives and protect health and should lead, guide, support, instruct cancer prevention measures, anti-cancer engineering, anti-cancer detection, cancer prevent monitoring, cancer is a disaster for all mankind, people all over the world are eager to one day to overcome cancer. It is urgent to hope that experts and scholars can find out cancer prevention measures to keep people away from cancer.**

Cancer is a disaster for all mankind. It must fight globally. The people of the world must work together. **Human beings should not sit still. Physicians should not do nothing. The health administrative department should not do nothing. It should lead and instruct the series of cancer protection research projects, and move forward together** and work together and have complementary, leadership and guidance to overcome cancer and launch a general attack.

Environmental pollution, air pollution, water pollution, and the incidence of cancer are rising. This is not a country or a region. It is a global problem. It is a by-product and interlude in industrial development. It should be analyzed and studied. It should be led by the World Health Organization. Research, prevent all environmental pollution carcinogenic projects, defend the beautiful living environment on which human beings depend, the harmonious and friendly environment on which human beings depend, and stay away from cancer.

d. How to overcome cancer how to prevent cancer I see four:

(IV) Situation Analysis: (4) - Formation of Environmental and Cancer Research Group
(4) How to implement the establishment of the Cancer Research Institute, the Environmental and Cancer Research Group should be established:
(1) In-depth intervention study on investigation and detection of common cancer risk factors
(2) **Monitoring pollution-causing cancer data, research and development of cancer prevention and cancer control measures**
For

a. food, food, packaging, additives
b. water pollution, beverages
c. house decoration, materials
d. air pollution, factory chimneys, car tail steam

e. soil, fertilizer, genetic modification

(3) Monitoring environmental pollution carcinogenic data and researching cancer prevention measures

Research and develop intervention measures

(4) Establishing the cancer prevention and cancer control information and communication report (publication) - "Cancer Prevention Mass Medicine"

Preventing cancer from living environment, living environment, and staying away from cancer

(5) Several tasks:

a. monitoring environmental pollution caused by cancer (data) e, science (anti-cancer) publicity and education
b. spot check the incidence of cancer in high cancer area f, "three early" popular learning
c. Establishing anti-cancer and anti-cancer information and communication report g, how to self-early discovery
d. research and development of anti-cancer technology, tools, products

(6) Several aspects:

a. from clothing, food, shelter, anti-cancer
b. from the big environment of life to prevent cancer
c. from the small living environment to prevent cancer
d. from life behaviors, life hobbies, living habits to prevent cancer

(7) Three key points in the 21st century anti-cancer:

a. smoking ban (smoking cessation) - "smoking has no harm"
b. limited alcohol - limit the amount of alcohol
c. weight loss - not suitable for obesity

(5) How to implement the establishment work of the cancer prevention system engineering for cancer prevention research project?

First of all, it must understand the history record of the relationship between environmental pollution and cancer research

Xu Ze proposed them in Chapter 38 in his third book, "New Essentials and New Methods for Cancer Treatment"

e. (5) Situation analysis: (5) - the relationship between environment and cancer

In the process of searching for the cause and condition of cancer, human beings have carried out extensive exploration and accumulated rich knowledge. More than 90% of cancers were found to be caused by environmental factors or closely related.

The environment in which human beings live includes the natural environment and the social environment. The natural environment, that is, the various natural factors surrounding people, such as everyone breathing air, drinking water and food, all of these common physical environment are called **the big environment.**

Everyone must engage in certain work and adopt a certain lifestyle, such as occupation, living habits and hobbies, to form a living environment called **a small environment**.

Whether it is a large environment or a small environment, it is the external environment on which human beings depend for survival and activity.

The physiological condition of the human body is called the internal environment.

The external environment substances have a close relationship with the internal environment through the ingestion, digestion, absorption, metabolism and excretion of the body, which has a huge impact on the human body.

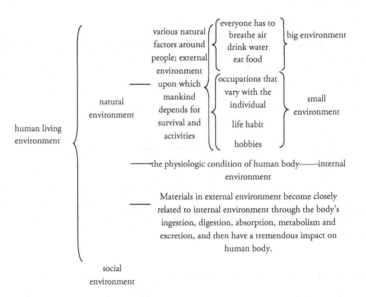

How to prove the relationship between environmental pollution and cancer? There are many examples in history:

In 1775, Dr. Pott of the United Kingdom confirmed that there were many **scrotal skin cancers among workers who cleaned the chimney, mainly due to long-term exposure to coal tar. This is the first historical example** of linking cancer to the environmental factors.

After 100 years, German doctor VolklTlaYl also realized that the high incidence of skin cancer among workers may be related to exposure to coal tar.

In 1907, some scholars discovered that <u>sun exposure was associated with skin cancer</u>, and first reported epidemiological studies of sunlight and skin cancer. It was a common phenomenon for researchers to observe early exposure of crew members to solar radiation and cause chronic skin diseases. Later, animal models confirmed that sunlight and ultraviolet rays can cause skin cancer.

In 1915, an animal model of the first chemical-induced tumor was established. Repeated tar application can cause skin cancer in rabbits. <u>This study added experimental basis for the establishment of a chemical carcinogenic theory based on scrotal cancer in 1775</u>. Later, the active ingredient, coal tar, was confirmed and isolated.

In the 20th century, it was confirmed that <u>high-initiated bladder cancer was produced among workers producing Methylnaphthylamine, Ethyl naphthylamine and Benzidine dye and almost all workers who had engaged in such occupations subsequently developed bladder cancer</u>.

In 1930, the first chemical carcinogen, benzopyrene, was separated from coal tar. The known carcinogenic environmental substances, coal tar, are separated into different components, and **the carcinogenic effects of these chemical components are clarified by animal model experiments.**

In 1938, the study found that the chemical carcinogenesis process is divided into two different stages, the excitation phase and the initiation phase. Non-specific stimuli promote tumors after low-dose carcinogens, such as tar on rabbit ears or **Papillomavirus.**

In 1940, researchers discovered that limitation of heat could reduce the occurrence of tumors for mice. **<u>It was proved that the intake of heat could encourage the occurrence of several kinds of tumors like breast carcinoma, liver cancer and skin cancer induced by benzoapyrene</u>**. Until today when obesity is popular worldwide, this project is attached with importance again by people.

In 1950, epidemiological studies found **<u>that smoking was associated with lung cancer</u>**. A retrospective analysis of lung cancer patients with smoking habits has shown that smoking is associated with lung cancer. Later, studies in male doctors have shown that smoking has a significant relationship with lung cancer mortality.

For many risk factors for cancer, it can increase the cancer mortality rate by about 30%.

In 1958, food additives banned by **<u>food additive improvement agencies were shown to induce cancer in humans or animals</u>**.

In 1964, American surgeon Luther L Terry suggested that smoking is associated with lung cancer.

Vinyl chloride is the main raw material for the plastics industry. It was not until 1974 that scientists discovered that this chemical is a potentially potent carcinogen **that can cause liver cancer.**

Epidemiological investigations in recent decades have found that many occupational workers are exposed to carcinogens in the production environment, and the incidence of cancer in certain parts is greatly increased. When these occupational exposures are eliminated or avoided, the onset of these cancers can be gradually reduced or even disappeared, indicating that environmental factors play a major role in the tumorigenesis process.

The long-term effects of various environmental factors other than the human body are the main causes of most cancers. Therefore, the effects of these environmental, life, and behavioral factors on the human body should be minimized.

Let's talk about the serious effects of environmental pollution such as air pollution, water pollution and soil pollution on human carcinogenesis.

② Air pollution in environmental pollution and cancer: **Every minute of human life is inseparable from air. Air pollution can cause many diseases, especially respiratory diseases, including the most severe lung cancer.**

At the beginning of the 20th century, lung cancer mainly occurred in a few mines, mining and smelting occupational environment. After the First World War, lung cancer mortality began to rise. In the late 1930s, with the development of modern industry, **atmospheric pollution, occupational carcinogens, tobacco and cigarette production or consumption soared, male patients in western industrialized countries experienced a rapid increase in lung cancer mortality.** In the UK, the mortality rate of lung cancer was 10/10 million in 1930, 53/100,000 in 1950, 99.7/100,000 in 1966, and 120.3/100,000 in 1975. It has grown 12 times in the 45 years from 1930 to 1975.

From 1934 to 1974, male lung cancer in the United States jumped from the fifth cause of death, and its mortality increased from 3.0/100,000 to 54.5/10, a 17-fold increase. Female lung cancer moved from the eighth to the top three. From 2/100,000 to 12.4/100,000, it also increased by 5.2 times.

By the early 1980s, lung cancer in 24 countries and regions including the United Kingdom, France, the Netherlands, Germany, and North America was listed as the leading cause of death in patients with malignant tumors. Since the middle of the 20th century, the rapid rise of lung cancer in the western industrialized countries has been formed.

In industrialized countries, harmful gases such as power generation, steelmaking, automobiles, aircraft, fuel, energy, **and large amounts of smoke are emitted into the atmosphere, polluting the air, and people are irritated by the respiratory tract, leading to an increase in the incidence and mortality of lung cancer.**

③ Water pollution of environmental pollution and cancer: Human activity in production and life depend on water at all times. Water quality pollution is mainly caused by industrial and agricultural production as well as urban pollution discharge. In China, township enterprises are having a fast development, which worsen industrial pollution.

According to the survey, many major rivers are facing a serious pollution increasingly. Fertilizers, farm chemicals and pesticides in agricultural production lead to the serious pollution of water quality.

Some rural areas of China have a habit of using pond water. **The research of Qidong County in Jiangsu Province has found that the high incidence of liver cancer in this area is related to drink pond water.** Fusui County in Guangxi Province also has the similar report. **All of these explain that water pollution is relevant to the incidence of liver cancer**. Haining County in Zhejiang Province also finds that people drinking pond water are over seven times easier to suffer from colon cancer than people drinking well water.

In recent years, **due to the advance of analysis technology of water quality, more than 100 different kinds of organic substances in water are found to have actions of carcinogenesis, cancer-promoting and mutagenesis**. Animal experiments have proved that drink water mixed with the following chemical compounds can cause liver cancer, such as benzene hexachloride, carbon tetrachloride, chloroform, trichloroethylene, perchlorethylene, and trichloroethane, etc. Furthermore, there are some limnetic algae toxins, such as **blue-green algae has an obvious action on the promotion of liver cancer**.

Mulberry fish pond area of Shunde in Guangdong Foshan is low lying and easy to generate water-logging and water accumulation, so **the water quality pollution is more serious. The incidence of liver cancer of local population is higher**.

While the neighboring Siping residents drink deep well water, the water quality is good, and the incidence of liver cancer is relatively low. According to a large number of research data from the World Health Organization and the International Association for Research on Cancer, **drinking substandard water can induce or promote cancer. Tests have shown that drinking water contains more nickel, which is more susceptible to oral cancer, throat cancer and colorectal cancer. Those with more cadmium, esophageal cancer, laryngeal cancer and lung cancer are more susceptible to gastric cancer and intestinal cancer. Ovarian cancer and**

various lymphomas; iron and zinc containing more chemical elements are prone to esophageal cancer.

④ **Environmental chemical pollution and cancer——**chemical carcinogenesis: Chemical carcinogen refers to chemical substances that can induce the generation of tumor.

In the mid-20th century, the problem of chemical carcinogenesis attracts widespread attention, mainly because modern tumor incidence rate and mortality rate continue to rise. The age of suffering from cancer has a younger tendency. Environmental chemical pollution is also found to have a close relation to the incidence rate of tumor. **World Health Organization also indicates that more than 90% of human cancers are relevant to environmental factors, which are mainly chemical factors.**

The following chemical substances have been studied and proved to have carcinogenic action.

Chloroethylene: In 1974, people began to realize that this substance is the cause of professional cancer. **Experimental study has found liver cancer, brain cancer, renal carcinoma, lung cancer and cancer of lymphatic system in experimental animals exposed to Chloroethylene.** But the related personnel cannot timely realize the hazardness of these substances from experimental results. Therefore, they fail to take measures to protect workers in time. Until recently, workers start to stop using the spraying agent of Chloroethylene; and plastic factory also change manufacturing technique to prevent workers from exposure.

Here is which it is needed to point out that Chloroethylene is an important raw material for record, packaging material, Medical test tube, household appliances, bathroom equipment and other kinds of plastic products. Plastic products themselves have no risk, but the liver cancer risk of workers in **Chloroethylene factory is 200 times higher than that of common people.**

Benzene: It is a kind of harmful chemical material, which can destroy the hematopiesis of marrow. If exposed in the environment filled with benzene, people may suffer from aplastic anemia that can change into leucocythemia after a long period. The first case of "leucucythemia led by benzene" was discovered in 1928.

Other countries have also shown that benzene is an occupational hazard. Italian scientists reported 200 years ago that **the risk of leukemia in printing and shoe factories is 20 times higher than in the general population.**

Certain activities and certain hobbies in human daily life are often closely related to environmental carcinogen polycyclic aromatic hydrocarbons. Smoking produces polycyclic aromatic hydrocarbons, which are important factors in

inducing human lung cancer. <u>In the cooking, cooking, and smoking of fats and oils, there are also carcinogenic polycyclic aromatic hydrocarbons. It is a carcinogen that poses a great threat to human health. We must pay enough attention to it</u>.

In addition, benzopyrene in asphalt and hot asphalt is associated with a high incidence of cancer among road workers and roofing workers. <u>Agricultural workers are exposed to a variety of pesticides, herbicides and fertilizers, some are known to be human carcinogens, some have been induced in experimental animals, and</u> others have been shown to be mutagens after short-term trials. Pesticides will enter the food chain and will accumulate in biological systems

⑤ **The physical factors in environmental pollution and cancer——ionizing radiation:**

With the development of technology, frequent nuclear tests, the applications of nuclear energy and radioactive nuclides are increasing, so as the radioactive substance poured in human environment. Therefore, people pay increasingly more attention to environmental pollution by ionizing radiation.

The ionizing radiation means the rays radiated by some radioactive substance in the process of transmutation. This kind of rays can give the absorbed substance adequate energy to divide ionize molecules and atoms. Some ionizing radiations are electromagnetic radiations like X-ray and γ-ray.

The sources of artificial radiation include nuclear tests which increase the radioactive environmental pollution, the exploitation, processing and retreat of nuclear fuel, for instance, in the exploitation of mineral radon gas and radioactive dust can pollute atmosphere. As the sources of energy in the world are less and less, more and more nations have been beginning to build nuclear power stations currently. This nuclear power industry can all discharge radioactive waste gas, water and residue which will pollute environment if mishandled.

Although radioactive nuclide can be applied extensively in industry, agriculture and medicine, the radioactive waste can still pollute environment.

The effects of ionizing radiation on the human body are mainly physical injuries such as chronic radiation sickness, malignant tumors, cataracts, and decreased fertility. <u>Radiation is carcinogenic, and its carcinogenic effect has a long incubation period, such as leukemia, skin cancer, lung cancer, and bone cancer. Genetic damage causes hereditary diseases in the offspring.</u>

⑥ <u>**Carcinogens that enter food from environmental pollution**</u>: With the development of science and technology, the food processing process is increasingly industrialized, and the external environment or the process of manufacturing food itself may cause various foreign substances, **including chemical and biological carcinogens, possibly Contaminated food.**

<u>In the processing of food raw materials, artificial additives are added, and smoking, frying, baking, etc. are used, and as a result, carcinogenic hybrids may occur in the food.</u>

Food products often have to be transported and shipped to reach consumers, thus providing an additional source of carcinogen-contaminated food.

<u>To study the sources of carcinogens on human food and how to eliminate such pollution is a very important issue.</u>

<u>B. How to prevent?</u> <u>The important link of cancer prevention : Carcinogenic factors(the situation analysis 6)</u>

As early as the 1980s, many experts and scholars at home and abroad believed that more than 90% of cancers were caused by environmental factors. Protecting and restoring a good environment is an important part of preventing cancer.

How to prevent cancer? How to prevent it? It must first understand what the carcinogenic factors are and its carcinogenic process, then it can propose preventive measures.

<u>(6) Situation analysis (6) – What are the carcinogenic factors in environmental factors? How to prevent it?</u>

1. Chemical factors are the main cause of human cancer, and 90% of human cancers are caused by environmental factors. More than 75% of them are chemical factors.

The earliest observations of chemical factors and human cancers date back to the 1870s. **Percivall Port** found that men who had been chimney sweepers in childhood had an increased rate of scrotal cancer. Although the nature of carcinogens was not known at the time, this finding by Port suggests a link between occupational exposure and tumor onset. Since then, many examples have clarified the relationship between various chemical carcinogens and human tumors, providing a series of experimental evidence for scientists to study and understand chemical carcinogenesis.

2. What is a chemical carcinogen? It refers to a chemical substance that has the ability to induce cancer formation.

The chemical carcinogenic problem in the middle of the 20th century has caused widespread concern, and it has been found that environmental chemical pollution is closely related to the incidence of cancer. **The World Health Organization has**

also pointed out that 90% of human cancers are related to environmental factors, mainly chemical factors.

The treatment of the diseases first should understand the cause of the disease in order to cure the disease; and prevention cancer is also appropriate to understand what the carcinogenic factors in the environment are and how to avoid it?

Common chemical carcinogens mainly involve the following types of chemicals:

The types of chemical carcinogens are:

Species Examples of

1. alkylating agent mustard gas, chloromethyl ether,
   formaldehyde, ethylene oxide,
   diethyl sulfate, ethylene,
   benzene, butadiene,
   carcinogenic alkylating agent
2. polycyclic aromatic hydrocarbons such as benzopyrene, dimethyl benzene anthracene, diphenyl anthracene, 3-methylcholanthracene and coal tar pitch
3. aromatic amine benzidine, ethyl naphthylamine, nitrobenzene
4. metal and metal arsenic, nickel, chromium, beryllium, cadmium, selenium
5. mold and phytotoxin aflatoxin, microcystin and so on
6. nitrosamines and nitrosamides
7. asbestos and silica
8. hobby cigarettes, tobacco, betel nut, excessive alcohol and beverages
9. the thermal cracking products of food
10. the drug includes certain hormones
11. cancer products have some chemicals only promote cancer, should be classified here, such as croton oil and its purified phorbol ester. Some promote cancer also has a starting effect

3. **There are many kinds of chemical carcinogens**. It is necessary to systematically and deeply study chemical carcinogens. It is necessary to classify them. There are three main classification methods, namely, according to the action mode of chemical carcinogens, according to relationships between chemical carcinogens and human tumors and classification by chemical nature.

(1) Classification according to the action mode of chemical carcinogens

According to the action mode of chemical carcinogens, they can be divided into three categories: direct carcinogens, indirect carcinogens and carcinogens.

1. <u>**Direct carcinogen**</u> refers to a chemical carcinogen that can directly affect the cells of the body after it enters the body and can directly induce cancer in the body without metabolism. These chemical carcinogens have strong carcinogenicity and rapid oncogenic effects, and are often used for malignant transformation studies of cells in vitro such as **various carcinogenic alkylating agents, nitrosamide carcinogens and the like.**
2. **Indirect carcinogens** are chemical carcinogens that are activated by the in vivo microsomal mixed function oxidase and become chemically active forms of carcinogenic effects. Such chemical carcinogens are widely present in the external environment, and are commonly found to be carcinogenic polycyclic aromatic hydrocarbons, aromatic amines, nitrosamines, and the like.
3. **cancer-promoting substances, also known as tumor promoters**. Cancer-promoting substances act alone in the body without carcinogenic effects, but can promote other carcinogens to induce tumor formation. Common promotional items are croton oil (phorbol diester), saccharin and phenobarbital.

(2) Classification by the relationship chemical carcinogens and human tumors

According to the relationship between chemical carcinogens and human tumors, they can be divided into positive carcinogens, suspected carcinogens and potential carcinogens. Affirmative carcinogens are those identified by epidemiological investigations and recognized by clinicians and scientists as carcinogenic to humans and animals, and their carcinogenic effects are dose-reactive chemical carcinogens; suspicious carcinogens have in vitro ability to transform, and Contact time is related to cancer rate, animal carcinogenicity test is positive, but the results are not constant; in addition, such carcinogens lack epidemiological evidence; potential carcinogens generally get some positive results in animal experiments, but in the crowd There is no data to prove whether it is carcinogenic to people.

(3) Classified by chemical nature

Chemical carcinogens can be divided into two categories: organic chemical carcinogens and inorganic chemical carcinogens. The former is a wide variety, such as most of the compounds in the table, the latter mainly includes carcinogenic metals and metalloids, as well as crystalline silicon and asbestos. Therefore, both exogenous or endogenous chemical carcinogens are mainly organic chemical carcinogens.

4. Organic carcinogens

Organic carcinogens can be divided into seven categories: polycyclic aromatic hydrocarbons, heterocyclic amines, N-nitroso compounds, dioxins and their analogues, pesticides, azo dyes, bioalkylating agents, triazenes. Compounds, etc.

(1) Polycyclic aromatic hydrocarbons

Polycyclic aromatic hydrocarbons (PAHs) are a series of polycyclic aromatic hydrocarbon compounds produced by the pyrolysis or incomplete combustion of coal, petroleum, coal tar, tobacco, and some organic compounds, many of which are carcinogenic. It is the most widely distributed environmental carcinogen. A large number of investigations and studies in recent years have shown that air, soil, water and plants are polluted by polycyclic aromatic hydrocarbons, and modern vehicles, such as automobiles and airplanes, also contain a considerable number of multi-rings aromatic hydrocarbons. Therefore, in the streets with frequent traffic, the pollution of polycyclic aromatic hydrocarbons is also quite serious. **With the development of industry, the problem of carcinogenic polycyclic aromatic hydrocarbons has become a growing concern. It is also the closest environmental carcinogen to humans.** Certain activities and certain hobbies in human daily life are often closely related to the production of polycyclic aromatic hydrocarbons. **For example, smoking is an important way to produce polycyclic aromatic hydrocarbons. In recent years, it has been proven to be an important factor in inducing human lung cancer. For example, in the cooking, roasting, and smoking of oily foods, there are also carcinogenic polycyclic aromatic hydrocarbons. It is considered to be one of the main reasons for the increase in gastric cancer rate in some areas. Therefore, polycyclic aromatic hydrocarbons (PAHs) are the most widely distributed carcinogens that are closely related to humans and pose a great threat to human health. We must pay enough attention to them.** In 1973, the International Cancer Research Center (IARC) expert group evaluated that some polycyclic aromatic hydrocarbons are harmful to humans.

5. Sources of environmental pollution

Natural polycyclic aromatic hydrocarbons are mainly found in coal, petroleum, shale oil, tar, asphalt, and the like. Polycyclic aromatic hydrocarbons can also be produced in the combustion of hydrocarbon-containing materials.

Among the polycyclic aromatic hydrocarbon compounds, the study of benzo[a] pyrene is the most detailed and in-depth, and a relatively accurate measurement method has been established, and it is also a substance with strong carcinogenic effect in polycyclic aromatic hydrocarbons. Therefore, the following mainly uses benzene. 芘[a]芘 is an example of the environmental pollution of this type of chemical.

(1) Pollution to the atmosphere

The outdoor atmosphere can be contaminated by fixed sources of pollution (such as thermal power stations, industries, enterprises) and mobile sources of pollution (such as airplanes, automobiles, etc.). Especially for cars and trains, the level of pollutants discharged is very low, very close to the breathing zone of people, and often close to residential areas, so sometimes it causes serious pollution. Most of the polycyclic aromatic hydrocarbons adhere to the dust in a crystalline state, and a large amount of air is taken up during the measurement, and a certain amount of dust is filtered and then measured. According to historical data, **the highest concentration of benzoquinone [a] strontium in the atmosphere is London, England. <u>Exhaust gas from automobile internal combustion engines must contain polycyclic aromatic hydrocarbon carcinogens.</u>**

(2) Pollution of soil

There are many types of polycyclic aromatic hydrocarbons in the soil. For example, rural soils in the eastern United States contain benzo[a]pyrene, phenanthrene, anthracene, anthracene, and valence. Different chemical companies have different pollutions to the surrounding soil. Some people in the soil adjacent to the oil plant have measured 200 mg of polycyclic aromatic hydrocarbons per kilogram of soil, and up to 650 per kilogram in the vicinity of the coal tar plant. Mg. It has been reported in France that benzo[a]pyrene carcinogens have been isolated from limestone 50 meters below the deep formation.

(3) Pollution to water

The water environment includes surface water (rivers, rivers, lakes, reservoirs and oceans) and groundwater. The most noticeable surface water in residential areas. Dozens of polycyclic aromatic hydrocarbons have been detected from surface water, of which seven or eight are carcinogenic, such as benzopyrene, benzopyrene, dibenzopyrene, quinone, anthracene, benzo[a]pyrene.

(4) Contamination of foods

Foods also contain various polycyclic aromatic hydrocarbons such as hydrazine, benzopyrene, dibenzopyrene, benzo[a]pyrene and the like. **Since benzo[a]pyrene is an important component in tobacco, a certain amount of benzo[a]pyrene can often be detected in smoked foods.**

The main sources of benzo[a]pyrene in food are:

Bio-synthesis(synthesis In vivo)

such as benzo[a]pyrene, is detected in unpolluted marine aquatic plants in the Greenland Gulf and in terrestrial plants far from the contaminated area, and the content is sometimes similar to the contaminated area, indicating that there is the possibility of synthesis of acyclic aromatic hydrocarbons in the organism..

Absorption and enrichment from contaminated soils and water

Potatoes and wheats in contaminated soils contain higher levels of benzo[a] pyrene. The content of benzo[a]pyrene in aquatic plants and small plankton is directly related to the content of river water. The benzo[a]pyrene content of plankton in the downstream polluted river water is several times higher than that in the upstream clean area. Marine organisms have the ability to enrich polycyclic aromatic hydrocarbons, and marine fish contain benzo[a]pyrene up to 2 to 65 micrograms per kilogram.

3. XZ-C first proposed "conquer cancer and launch the general attack to cancer and create the science city of conquering cancer" in the world

How to overcome cancer I see 1 - 5

1. How to overcome cancer? In order to overcome cancer, we must create the "Innovative Molecular Oncology School"

(1) Why do you start the "Innovative Molecular Oncology Medical School"?

(2) How to create the "Innovative Molecular Oncology Medical School"?

2. How to overcome cancer? In order to overcome cancer, we must create an innovative molecular tumor hospital with the whole process of prevention and treatment during tumor occurrence and development (global demonstration of occurrence and development of cancer with full-course prevention and treatment hospitals)

(1) Why do you want to start? (2) How to create?

3. How to overcome cancer? In order to overcome cancer, we must create the Innovative Molecular Oncology Institute.

(1) Why do you want to start? (2) How to create?

4. How to overcome cancer? In order to overcome cancer, the Experimental Medicine Cancer Animal Experimental Center must be created.

(1) Why do you want to start? (2) How to create?

5. How to overcome cancer? In order to conquer cancer, we must create "Innovative Molecular Tumor Pharmaceuticals" and "Create Research Group and Laboratory of analyzing Active Components and Molecular Weight and Structural Formula and Immunopharmacology for Anticancer and Anticancer Metastatic Traditional Chinese Medication at the Molecular Level"

(1) Why do you want to start to set up?

Because it is necessary to research and develop effective drugs for anti-cancer and anti-cancer metastasis, XZ-C believes that two wheels must be used to overcome cancer:

One is the life science, biomedical (modern mediction) A wheel.

One is the clinical basis, immune regulation, anti-cancer (Chinese herbal medication) B wheel.

Its purpose is to further develop the anti-cancer, anti-metastatic and effective drugs of Chinese herbal medicines, to remove crude and to keep the essence, and to use natural medicine and Chinese herbal medicine as resources to carry out modern research and make precise medicine; further to study on the molecular level of immunomodulatory anti-cancer Chinese medicine cells; further to explore the role of anti-cancer and anti-cancer Chinese herbal medicines in the prevention and treatment of early carcinoma in situ and precancerous lesions.

4. XZ-C first proposed "conquer cancer and launch the general attack to cancer, it must establish the Cancer Research Institute and the cancer prevention system project" in the world.

It is to Conduct cancer prevention research, find cancer-causing factors, detect the source of carcinogens or carcinogenic factors, and try to prevent these carcinogenic factors from harming the human body. The Cancer Research Institute should conduct cancer prevention research, and there is a lot of need for research; it is to track the source of carcinogens or carcinogenic factors.

In the search for the cause and condition of cancer, the most prominent thing is that it was found that more than 90% of cancers are caused by environmental factors.

1. Relationship between air pollution and cancer
    Humans have developed tens of millions of tons of coal, oil and natural gas as fuel and energy. In the production and life processes such as thermal power generation, smelting steel, automobiles, airplanes, and household fuels, a large amount of tar, bituminous coal, dust and other harmful substances are discharged into the atmosphere around the clock, causing air pollution.
    Air pollution can cause many diseases, especially respiratory diseases, the most serious is lung cancer.

2. Water pollution and cancer
    The pollution of water quality is mainly caused by industrial and agricultural production and urban sewage. There are many types of pollutants in water. Pesticides and insecticides are one of the important pollutants in water. Surfactants in neutral detergents also have cancer-promoting effects.

3. Soil pollution and cancer
    A large amount of industrial waste water residue and pesticides and fertilizers are injected into the soil, which deteriorates soil quality and accumulates poisons, posing a threat to human health and a carcinogenic factor.

4. Chemistry and cancer

5. Physical factors and cancer

6. Biological factors and cancer

7. Diet and cancer

8. Life style and cancer

9. Clothing, food, housing, travel, house decoration, etc. and cancer

It should study the action way of so many carcinogens or carcinogenic factors; it should study these sources of pollution and try to stop at the source; it should study these carcinogenic mechanisms and their carcinogenic effects; it should study how to reduce or prevent these carcinogens.

Because cancer patients cover the whole world, industrial and agricultural wastewater, waste residue, and exhausted gas pollution also cover the whole world. Therefore, it is necessary to globally conquer cancer and launch the total attack to cancer together.

Professor Xu Ze suggested:

1. **All countries, provinces and states should establish cancer prevention research institutes (or institutions), carry out cancer prevention system projects, and carry out cancer prevention work for their own country, province and city.**
2. **Each country establishes cancer prevention regulations and carry out comprehensively (some should be legislated)**
3. I will use this project **to recommend the World Health Organization to hold a cancer prevention campaign, with the goal of reducing the incidence of cancer**. Conquering cancer is a frontier of science and a worldwide problem. Cancer is a human disaster. It covers the whole world. People all over the world are eager to hope that one day they can overcome cancer and benefit human being.

5. Cancer Prevention research work can not walk slowly and should run ahead to save the wounded

Cancer is a disaster for all mankind, and it must fight globally; the global people struggle together;It is an unprecedented event to conquer cancer and launch a general attack of cancer for the benefit of mankind.

Why did I propose to overcome cancer and launch a general attack? I have been working for 5-6 years because of the series of ideas and design research for cancer. We have made a complete set of basic ideas and designs, plans and blueprints to overcome cancer. In the 38th chapter of the monograph "New Concepts and New Methods of Cancer Therapy" published in 2011, a chapter on the "strategic ideas and recommendations for conquering cancer" was proposed, and the "Conquer Cancer and Launch the General Attack on Cancer" was proposed.

Later, in 2013, it was proposed "The comprehensive design for building the Science City of conquering cancer". In August 2013, it was first proposed internationally: "XZ-C Scientific Research Plan for conquering cancer and launching the General Attack of Cancer." In July 2015, it was proposed and named "Dawning C-type plan", and proposed "conquer cancer and launch the general attack of cancer" and "to build the science city of conquering cancer." This work is being reported and requested to be implemented.

Conquering cancer and launch the general attack of cancer is an unprecedented work of humanity. It is necessary to personally create experience and practice it personally.

About 8550 people in China are diagnosed with cancer every day, and 6 people are diagnosed with cancer every minute. Therefore, the research work to conquer cancer and launch the general attack of cancer can not walk slowly and should run forward so as to save the wounded.

2017.2.5 Reference message

[Effie, Geneva, February 3rd] The World Health Organization released data on the occasion of the "World Cancer Day" on February 4, saying that 8.8 million people die of cancer every year in the world, and the number of deaths from respiratory cancer is the highest, up to 1.695 million people per year.

The latest data is based on 2015 statistics, increasing the number of people dying from cancer each year from an estimated 8.1 million in 2010 to 8.8 million.

The deadliest cancers that are second only to respiratory cancer are liver cancer (788,000 deaths per year), colorectal cancer (774,000), stomach cancer (753,300) and breast cancer (571,000).

Cancers such as esophageal cancer (415,000), pancreatic cancer (358,000), prostate cancer (334,800), and lymphoma (334,300) have high mortality rates worldwide.

In terms of gender, there are nearly 5 million male deaths among 8.8 million cancer deaths. For men, the most common types of cancers are **respiratory cancer and liver cancer.** For women, the cancer with the highest mortality rate is **breast cancer and respiratory cancer**.

In terms of regional distribution, the most common cancer cases are in the western Pacific, with respiratory cancer and liver cancer accounting for the highest proportion.

Second only to the Western Pacific is Southeast Asia, where respiratory cancer, oral cancer and throat cancer account for the highest proportion.

In Europe, the most common cancer is respiratory cancer, followed by colorectal cancer.

The disaster of cancer covers the whole world. People all over the world are eager to hope to overcome cancer one day. It is hoped that the state, government, experts, scholars and scientists can find out cancer prevention measures so that people can stay away from cancer.

Professor Xu Ze has been engaged in clinical surgery for 60 years. He has been engaged in the basic research and clinical verification of animal experiments with cancer as the research direction for 30 years. He deeply understands that cancer should not only pay attention to treatment, but also should emphasize the prevention, so as to stop cancer at the source or roots or origin. Therefore, it is proposed that it should launch "conquer cancer and launch the total attack to cancer with both prevention and treatment at the same level and attention and at the same time.

1. How to overcome cancer?

Its purpose should be:
(1)
1). reduce the incidence of cancer
2). improve the cure rate of cancer, prolong the survival of cancer patients and improve the quality of life
(2) reach
1/3 can prevent
1/3 can be cured
1/3 can prolong life through treatment

2. How to improve the cure rate?

How to cure?
It should go out of a new way to cure cancer:
(1) Conquer cancer and launch a general attack

1. The general attack is to carry out the three-stage work of cancer prevention, cancer control and cancer treatment in the whole process of cancer occurrence and development, and carry out simultaneously. Three carriages go hand in hand, and drive together.
2. To Change the current mode of running a hospital—that is, change the current mode of running a hospital with a focus on treatment.

To Change the current treatment mode - that is, change the current treatment mode that focuses on the middle and late stages of treatment, and change the treatment only without prevention into prevention, control, and treatment at the same time and same level.

(2) How to implement this new mode of running a hospital?

It is necessary to establish a hospital for prevention, control and treatment according to the whole process of cancer occurrence and development.

(3) The way out for cancer treatment is "three early" (early detection, early diagnosis, early treatment), early cancer treatment is effective, **can be cured**, especially cancer lesions, well treated, can be cured.

3. How to reduce the incidence of cancer?

How to prevent?
It should go out of a new way to prevent cancer:
(1) XZ-C believes: How to prevent cancer? An anti-cancer research institute should be created and an anti-cancer system project should be created.

Study carcinogenic factors and their sources, and study to try to stop or avoid them.

(2) What to prevent?

a. What are the carcinogenic factors?
b. What are the sources of carcinogenic factors?

How to prevent it?

a. how to reduce its source
b. how to stop its source

Cancer prevention work should be blocked at the source and the source of carcinogenic factors should be prevented.

Cancer prevention is active, it is to attack

Cancer treatment is passive, it is abiding

How to prevent? What to prevent? How to prevent it? It should be studied in depth, **the evaluation goal is: reduce the incidence rate**

How to cure? What to cure? How to cure? It should be studied in depth, **the evaluation goal is: improve the cure rate**

6. How to improve the cure rate of cancer? How to prolong the survival of cancer patients, improve the quality of life and reduce complications

1. How to cure?

After more than 30 years of experimental and clinical validation studies, we have initially embarked on a new path to overcome cancer.

(1) Through experimental research, Chinese medicine immunopharmacology and molecular level Chinese and Western medicine combined with anti-cancer research, we have taken out a traditional Chinese medicine immune regulation, regulate immune activity, prevent thymus atrophy, promote thymic hyperplasia, protect bone marrow hematopoietic function, and improve immune surveillance. At the molecular level, Western medicine combines to overcome the new path of cancer.

We have initially embarked on the new path of conquering cancer with an XZ-C immune regulation and control on the molecular level of Chinese and Western medicine —— the "Chinese-style anti-cancer" new road.

   a. I am a clinical surgeon, for chest surgery work and general surgery work, why do I study cancer? This is due to the results of a petition to a group of cancer patients after surgery:

Since 1985, I have conducted a petition to more than 3,000 patients with postoperative thoracic and abdominal cancer. I found that most patients relapsed or metastasized within 2-3 years after surgery. **From the follow-up results, it was found that postoperative recurrence and metastasis were the key to affecting the long-term efficacy of surgery. Therefore, we also raised an important issue: clinicians must pay attention to and study the prevention and treatment of postoperative recurrence and metastasis, in order to improve the long-term efficacy of postoperative.**

So we established an experimental surgical laboratory to conduct experimental tumor research: the implementation of cancer cell transplantation, the establishment of tumor animal models, and a series of experimental tumor research.

   b. We conducted a full-scale clinical research work in the laboratory for 4 years, which is a basic clinical study.

<u>From the experimental results, it was found that the host thymus was acutely atrophied after inoculation of cancer cells, cell proliferation was blocked, and the volume was significantly reduced. From the above experimental studies, it is</u>

found that thymus atrophy and low immune function may be one of the causes and pathogenesis of cancer. Therefore, the principle of its (cancer) treatment must be to try to prevent thymus atrophy, promote thymocyte proliferation, and raise immunity.

In order to try to prevent thymus atrophy, promote thymocyte proliferation, and increase immunity, we look for both Chinese medicine and western medicine. The existing medicines of western medicine can improve immunity and promote the proliferation of thymus so that we changed to look for Chinese herbal medicine.

Why do you look for drugs that promote thymic hyperplasia, prevent thymus atrophy, and boost immunity from traditional Chinese medicine?

Because of the Chinese herbal medicine polysaccharides and Replenishment class **Chinese medicine, many of them have the role of regulating immunity.**

The research on anti-cancer immunity of traditional Chinese medicine polysaccharides is progressing rapidly. A large number of immunopharmacological studies have been carried out at the molecular level, and polysaccharides can improve the body's immune surveillance system.

Our laboratory has conducted a series of experimental studies to find new anti-cancer Chinese medicine of immune control and regulation with anti-cancer, anti-metastasis, anti-cancer atrophy, and increase immune.

c. **The exclusive research and development of XZ-C immune regulation anti-cancer Chinese medicine series products**

Experimental study + clinical application + typical case + case list

Self-developed XZ-C (Xu Ze - China) immunomodulation anti-cancer series of traditional Chinese medicine preparations, from experimental research to clinical verification, applied to clinical practice on the basis of successful animal experiments, after more than 20 years More than 12,000 cases of clinical validation, significant efficacy, for independent innovation.

XZ-C immunomodulation anticancer traditional Chinese medicine, from more than 200 traditional Chinese herbal medicines in China, 48 kinds of Chinese herbal medicines with good tumor inhibition rate were screened by antitumor experiments in cancer-bearing mice, and then combined with cancer The mice embody tumor inhibition experiments in vivo, and the compound tumor inhibition rate is far greater than the single tumor drug inhibition rate. Among them, XZ-C1 inhibits cancer cells 100%, does not kill normal cells, and has the effect of strengthening the body and improving the immune function of the human body.

The pharmacodynamic study of XZ-C from our experiments proves that it has a good tumor inhibition rate for Ehrlich ascites carcinoma, S180 and H22 hepatocellular carcinoma.

Acute toxicity test in mice showed no obvious side effects. In the clinical long-term oral administration for several years (2-6-8 years), no obvious side effects were observed.

Middle and advanced cancer patients, mostly weak and weak, tired and weak, loss of appetite, after taking XZ-C immunomodulation anti-cancer Chinese medicine for 4-8-12 weeks, can significantly improve appetite, sleep, relieve pain, and gradually restore physical strength.

XZ-C proposed to overcome the general attack of cancer, and must establish advice and suggestions for the Cancer Research Institute and the anti-cancer system project.

Conduct anti-cancer research, find cancer-causing factors, detect the source of carcinogens or carcinogenic factors, and try to prevent these carcinogenic factors from harming the human body. The Cancer Research Institute should conduct anti-cancer research, and there is a lot of need for research.

Track the source of carcinogens or carcinogenic factors.

In the search for the cause and condition of cancer, the most prominent thing is that more than 90% of cancers are caused by environmental factors.

How to implement the creation of this cancer research institute.

Professor Xu Ze XZ-C proposed the general design of anti-cancer and proposed anti-cancer system engineering:

The way in which so many carcinogens or carcinogenic factors should be studied

Study these sources of pollution and try to stop at the source

Study these carcinogenic mechanisms and their carcinogenic effects

Study how to reduce or prevent these carcinogens

Because cancer patients cover the whole world, industrial and agricultural wastewater, waste residue, and exhaust gas pollution also cover the whole world. Therefore, it is necessary to globally attack the cancer attack.

Professor Xu Ze suggested: 1 All countries, provinces and states should establish anti-cancer research institutes (or institutions), carry out anti-cancer system projects, and carry out anti-cancer work for their own country, province and city.

2 Countries establish anti-cancer regulations and carry out comprehensively (some should be legislated)

3 I will use this project to recommend the World Health Organization to hold an anti-cancer campaign, with the goal of reducing the incidence of cancer. Conquering cancer is a frontier of science and a worldwide problem. Cancer is a human disaster.

It covers the whole world. People all over the world are eager to hope that one day they can overcome cancer and benefit humanity.

4 advocate scientific research ethics, medical is benevolence, ethics first

Research ethics: products should have ethical standards

Standard: should be based on the standard of not damaging human health

Basic ethics: All products and people are harmless and do not harm people's health, especially for children.

(To be beautiful, living environment and living environment)

5 The health administrative department shall protect and protect health, and shall lead, lead, support, and guide anti-cancer measures, anti-cancer projects, anti-cancer tests, and anti-cancer monitoring.

7. The current is the best time, which is conducive to the proposed attack on cancer.

(1) At present, **China is building an innovative country and is prospering scientific and technological innovation. The National Science and Technology Innovation Conference deepens the reform of the science and technology system and decides to enter the ranks of innovative countries in 2020. Its goal is to achieve a major breakthrough in scientific research in key areas. The strategic high-tech field has achieved leap-forward development; new achievements in several fields have entered the forefront of the world; the scientific quality of the whole nation has generally improved and entered the ranks of innovative countries.**

How to build an innovative country? Innovative countries should not only prosper independent innovation, but also prosper original innovation. They should not only catch up with the international advanced level, but also should be at the international leading level.

Cancer is a disaster for all mankind. The complexity of cancer is beyond human imagination. This is the hottest position in the field of biomedicine, bringing together the world's largest and most elite research team and research elite.

Cancer is not a disease, but a large class of diseases with similar characteristics. Although cancer treatment has been going on for more than a century and has entered the second decade of the 21st century, "oncology" is still in the current medical sciences. The most backward subject, why? Because the etiology, pathogenesis, and pathophysiology of "oncology" are not well understood. The oncology discipline is still a scientific virgin land for scientific research, and it needs a lot of basic scientific research and clinical basic research.

That conquering Cancer become the main direction of cancer research and conducting experimental and clinical anti-cancer research should be the key area of scientific research and achieve original breakthroughs.

According to the 2012 China Cancer Registration Annual Report issued by the National Cancer Registry, there are about 3.12 million new cases of cancer each year, an average of 8550 people per day, and 6 people diagnosed with cancer every minute in the country.

There are 2.7 million cancer deaths per year in the country, with an average of 7,500 deaths per day. Such amazing data should be listed as a scientific research in key areas of technological innovation.

Human beings should not sit still, doctors should not do nothing, I think we should propose a general attack plan and basic design to overcome cancer diseases, we should launch a general attack - prevention, control, and treatment.

There are two tasks on the shoulders of our doctors. One is to treat patients and the other is to develop medicine. We should achieve leap-forward development in the strategic high-tech field of conquering cancer, and take the road of innovation in anti-cancer and anti-metastatic science with Chinese characteristics. Innovative achievements, strive to enter the forefront of the world.

My third book, "New Concepts and New Methods for Cancer Treatment," was published in October 2011 by Beijing People's Military Medical Press, Xu Ze and Xu Jie. Later, the American medical doctor Dr. Bin Wu and others translated into English, and the English version was published in Washington, DC on March 26, 2013, and was published internationally.

(2) At present, our province and the city are accelerating the construction of new breakthroughs and building Wuhan into a national central city. Under this favorable situation, we should pay close attention to the major opportunities for the implementation of the strategy of promoting the rise of the central region and the construction of a sincere new district for the comprehensive reform of the "two-oriented society" in Wuhan City Circle, and to innovate. I deeply think that in this great situation and great opportunities, it has also created good opportunities for research work on cancer prevention and cancer control.

I believe that the current energy-saving emission reduction, anti-pollution and pollution control, and creating a "two-type society" is actually a level I prevention against cancer. Its purpose and effect can achieve the level I prevention of cancer. This is a great opportunity for a once-in-a-lifetime event. We must seize this great opportunity that is once in a lifetime, and we must not lose it. **I have been engaged**

in experimental basic research and clinical medical practice in oncology surgery for half a century and deeply aware of that if the purpose of cancer prevention and control cancer be achieved, it is necessary for the government to lead and experts and scholars to work hard, the masses to participate, the mobilization of the whole people, and the participation of thousands of families. Nowadays, the in-depth implementation of the strategy of the rise of the central government in our province and the city and the construction of the national central city and the "two-oriented society" are precisely the work of the government, the masses, the mobilization of the whole people, and the participation of thousands of households, which will definitely improve the national defense. Cancer awareness, to achieve anti-cancer, cancer control, received the effect of reducing the incidence of disease in our province and the city, this is the innovative road of anti-cancer and cancer control with Chinese characteristics.

Therefore, the current is the best time for us to propose to conquer cancer and to launch the general attack of cancer - prevention, control, and treatment at the same level and attention.

(2) **At present, China is implementing the spirit of the 19th National Congress of the Communist Party of China, building a well-off society in an all-round way, and ensuring the grand goal of building a well-off society in 2008.**

Its main content is "resource-saving, environmentally-friendly society has made significant progress, the total discharge of major pollutants has decreased significantly, the stability of the ecosystem has increased, and the people's living environment has improved significantly.

Strengthen the natural ecosystem and environmental protection, adhere to prevention, comprehensive management, and focus on solving problems that harm the health of the people and highlight the environment."

Building a well-off society, people have improved their health knowledge, and effective interventions for pathogenic factors such as environmental pollution will certainly reduce the incidence of related cancers.

It is recognized that more than 90% of cancers are caused or closely related to environmental factors. Building a well-off society is closely related to cancer prevention and cancer control. Therefore, we propose to conquer cancer and launch the general attack of cancer and adhere to the innovative road of cancer prevention and cancer control with Chinese characteristics.

In the construction of a well-off society and rural urbanization work, formulate cancer prevention and anti-cancer programs, and propose and formulate cancer prevention and anti-cancer measures. Formulate prevention and control plans and measures for new towns and new rural cancers.

Recognizing that building a well-off society should be healthy for everyone, away from cancer, the way to fight cancer is prevention, carry out cancer prevention and anti-cancer work in rural urbanization, adhere to the road of cancer prevention and anti-cancer with Chinese characteristics, and propose to launch the necessity of a general attack.

Our dreams are to conquer cancer and build a well-off society. Everyone is healthy and away from cancer.

8. To avoid talk, and to work hard, no matter how far the road to conquer cancer, it always should start to walk

What should I do next? Now it is proposed to overcome cancer and launch a general attack. I hope to get support from leaders at all levels. We must work hard and start to walk. We know that in order to achieve the goal of cancer prevention and control, we must do so by government leaders, government leaders, experts, scholars, mass participation, national mobilization, and participation of thousands of families.

(1) Regardless of how far and how long the road to conquer cancer is, you should always start to walk, and the long march must always go, and the journey of a thousand miles begins with a single step. The miles long march should start to walk. As long as we move forward, the grassland will always come out of a new road. The key point is to avoid talk and to work hard and start to walk. The current status quo, attention to treatment and light defense, or just treatment should be changed. Conquer cancer should launch the general attack; cancer prevention and cancer control and cancer treatment should be the three carriages and go hand in hand, and work together, work hard, and only **work hard can produce results.**

How to do it? " Conduct scientific research on cancer control and prevention and Set up cancer control plans and measures " (see separate article)

(2) No matter how difficult it is to overcome cancer, but it should also start to walk

We have set up a research team for the Wuhan Anti-Cancer Research Society to overcome the general attack on cancer.

To Promote research and experimentation, to call for national mobilization, to promote the fight against cancer, to launch a general attack, to launch the total attack with cancer prevention, cancer control, cancer treatment at the same level and at the same attention. Appealing to the whole people, raising the knowledge of cancer prevention and cancer control is related to the vital interests of each individual. In order to achieve Conquer cancer, we must mobilize the whole people and work hard for the whole people. I know that to achieve this goal, we must arouse the people and work together. To overcome cancer, we must mobilize the whole people to mobilize, thousands of troops, government leaders, government-led, expert efforts, and mass participation.

9. To analyze the research prospects next steps and the prospective assessment of cancer treatment.

What are the next research prospects and the vision prediction evaluation of cancer treatment? There are the following sections which should be included in: a. **the molecular targeted drugs attract people's attention; b. the prospect of immunomodulatory drugs is gratifying; c. Immunotherapy opens a new era of cancer treatment; d. biological therapy and combination of Chinese and Western medications are two effective ways to prevent cancer metastasis; e. applying vaccine treatment is human hope; f. the way out for cancer treatment is "three early"; g. the way out to fight cancer is prevention. Here the first three sections are discussed as the following:**

1). Molecular targeted drug therapy attracts attention

The Philadelphia chromosome opened the door to targeted therapy. In 1960, researchers in Philadelphia, USA, found a chromosomal abnormality in patients with chronic myeloid leukemia (CML). A few years later, the researchers found that this was the result of the long arm translocation of chromosomes 9 and 22. Since this chromosomal abnormality was first discovered in Philadelphia (Phiadelphia), it was named the Philadelphia (Ph) chromosome. This chromosome has also become a target for CML targeted therapy marketed 40 years later. In 2001, the first drug that was proven to be resistant to Philadelphia molecular chromosome defects - imatinib.

The target drug trastuzumab, which targets human epidermal growth factor receptor 2 (HER2), is then used to treat HER2-positive breast cancer.

Bevacizumab, which targets VEGF, and cetuximab, which targets EGFR, treats colorectal cancer.

Gefitinib and erlotinib targeting EGFR are used for the treatment of non-small cell lung cancer.

Molecularly targeted drugs are cell stabilizers, and most patients cannot achieve complete remission (CR) or partial remission (PR), but rather stable

disease and improved quality of life. In addition to gefitinib, erlotinib, imatinib, more need to be combined with chemotherapy drugs.

Molecularly targeted drugs represent a new class of anticancer drugs, and Gleevec is a classic example of **controlling cancer by inhibiting abnormal molecules that cause cancer without damaging other normal nuclear tissues**. More and more molecularly targeted drugs have been used in cancer treatment. For example, rituximab (Trastuzumab) for treating breast of Rituximab for treating B cell lymphoma, Gifitinib for treating lung cancer, Erlotinib, and the like. Targeted therapy brings anti-tumor hope.

2). The prospect of immunomodulatory drugs is gratifying

Regardless of the complexity of the mechanisms behind cancer, immune suppression is the key to cancer progression. Removal of immunosuppressive factors and restoration of the recognition of cancer cells by immune system cells can effectively prevent cancer.

More and more research evidence shows that by regulating the body's immune system, it is possible to achieve cancer control. Treating tumors by activating the body's anti-tumor immune system is an area that is currently exciting for researchers. The next major breakthrough in cancer is likely to stem from this.

In order to explore the etiology, pathogenesis and pathophysiology of cancer, our laboratory has carried out a series of animal experiments in the laboratory for 4 years, and obtained new findings from the experimental results. New inspirations: thymus atrophy, low immune function is cancer One of the causes and pathogenesis, Xu Ze (Zu Ze) proposed at the International Oncology Society in 2013: one of the causes of cancer and one of the pathogenesis may be thymus atrophy, low immune function, decreased immune surveillance ability and immune escape.

Therefore, the treatment principle must be to prevent progressive atrophy of the thymus, promote thymic hyperplasia, protect bone marrow hematopoietic function, improve immune surveillance, and provide experimental basis and theoretical basis for cancer immune regulation treatment.

Through the above four years to explore the basic experimental research on the mechanism of recurrence and metastasis, after 3 years from the natural medicine Chinese herbal medicine internal laboratory through the cancer-bearing animal experiment screening, 48 kinds of Chinese medicines were screened out of 48 kinds of good tumor inhibition rate, and then The cancer-bearing animals were screened to form XZ-C1-10 anti-cancer immune regulation Chinese medicine.

After 20 years of clinical application of more than 12,000 patients with advanced cancer in the oncology clinic, the clinical observation and verification confirmed that the principle of immune regulation and treatment of "chest lifting" is reasonable and the curative effect is satisfactory. The application of immunomodulatory Chinese medicine has achieved good results, improved the quality of life, and significantly prolonged the survival period.

3). Immunotherapy opens a new era of cancer treatment

ASCO Announces: <u>the Major Progress in Clinical Oncology in 2015</u>

On February 4, 2016, the American Society of Clinical Oncology (ASCO) announced the "**2016 Annual Report: ASCO Clinical Oncology Progress**" on Capitol Hill, Washington, DC. The contents of this report **Detailed and in-depth Summarized the research on global clinical oncology in 2015, at the same time, looking forward to the future research and development direction. ASCO rated the 2015 progress <u>as "tumor immunotherapy"</u>.**

ASCO President Professor Julie M. Vose believes that the most important development in 2015 is the discovery of immunotherapy. She wrote in the foreword: "We are no longer determined by tumor type and staging as we have in the past. Treatment, in the era of precision medicine, we select or exclude treatment based on each patient and tumor genetic data. No other major advances, like immunology can be translated into clinical practice, so ASCO decided that the biggest progress in 2015 is immunotherapy."

The chairman of the committee, Professor Don Dizon, also believes that the annual research results are increasing, but from the perspective of being able to benefit patients, **<u>the most important development this year should be immunotherapy</u>**.

CHAPTER 10

XZ-C proposed that cancer prevention research work cannot walk slowly and should run ahead to save the wounded

TABLE OF CONTENTS

The Status of Cancer Treatment XZ-C Document

Cancer is a disaster for all mankind. It must fight globally and the people of the world will work together.

Conquering cancer and launching a general attack is an unprecedented event that benefits mankind.

1. XZ-C proposed: cancer prevention research work can not walk slowly and should run ahead to save the wounded

Why did I propose to overcome cancer and launch a general attack? I have been working for 5-6 years because of the series of ideas and design research for cancer. We have made a complete set of basic ideas and designs, plans and blueprints to overcome cancer. In the 38th chapter of the monograph "New Concepts and New Methods of Cancer Therapy" published in 2011, a chapter on the "strategic ideas and recommendations for conquering cancer" was proposed, and the "General Attack on Cancer Attack" was proposed.

Later, in 2013, he proposed "To build a comprehensive design for the Cancer Science City." In August 2013, it was first proposed internationally: "XZ-C Scientific Research Plan for Overcoming the General Attack of Cancer." In July 2015, it was proposed and named "Dawning C-type plan", and proposed "to overcome the general attack of cancer" and "to build a science city to overcome cancer." This work is being reported and requested to be implemented.

Conquering the general attack of cancer is an unprecedented work of humanity. It is necessary to personally create experience and practice it personally.

About 8550 people in China are diagnosed with cancer every day, and 6 people are diagnosed with cancer every minute. Therefore, research and research work to overcome the general attack of cancer, can not walk slowly, should run forward, save the wounded.

2. XZ-C proposes: Cancer is a disaster for all mankind, it must fight with the world, and the people of the world work together.

1). The disaster of cancer covers the whole world (Figure 1.1)

Worldwide cancer incidence

Publication on the incidence of cancer in five continents. The 2002 volume of the publication, co-published by the International Agency for Research on Cancer (IARC) and the International Association for Cancer Registration, contains data on 50 cancers from 215 populations in 55 countries.

The IARC Special Report brings together findings from a cross-disciplinary panel of experts from different regions of the world on retrospective analysis of different potential carcinogenic risk factors. These panels evaluated a number of factors (including chemical factors, complex mixtures, occupational exposure factors, physical and biological factors, and lifestyle habits) to increase the risk of cancer risk.

Since 1971, the panel has evaluated more than 900 factors, of which nearly 400 have been identified as carcinogenic or potential carcinogenic factors. The full catalogue and classification of these factors is regularly updated and can be found at http://monographs.iarc.fr/. This catalogue is the scientific basis for public health, other disciplines, and national health authorities to take steps to avoid exposure to potential carcinogenic factors.

Worldwide cancer incidence

There is a large regional difference in the morbidity and mortality of cancers around the world as well as some special organ sites. The WHO Cancer Mortality Database and the GLOBOCAN 2002 database provide data on the incidence, prevalence and mortality of 27 different cancers in each country in 2002.

In 2002, there were an estimated 10.9 million new cancer patients (53% male and 47% female), of which 5.1 million occurred in developed countries and 5.8 million occurred in less developed countries.

The number of cancer deaths was 6.7 million (57% male and 43% female), 2.7 million in developed countries and 4 million in less developed countries. An estimated 24.5 million patients are still alive with various cancers (not including skin non-melanoma cancer within 5 years after diagnosis).

According to population standardization, cancer incidence and mortality in different regions of the world are shown in Figure 1.1.

2). The mortality rate and current status of cancer patients worldwide

2017.2.5 Reference message

[Effie, Geneva, February 3rd] The World Health Organization released data on the occasion of the "World Cancer Day" on February 4, saying that 8.8 million people die of cancer every year in the world, and the number of deaths from respiratory cancer is the highest., up to 1.695 million people per year.

The latest published data is based on 2015 statistics, increasing the number of people dying from cancer each year from an estimated 8.1 million in 2010 to 8.8 million.

The deadliest cancers that are second only to respiratory cancer are liver cancer (788,000 deaths per year), colorectal cancer (774,000), stomach cancer (753,300) and breast cancer (571,000).

Cancers such as esophageal cancer (415,000), pancreatic cancer (358,000), prostate cancer (334,800), and lymphoma (334,300) have high mortality rates worldwide.

In terms of gender, there are nearly 5 million male deaths among 8.8 million cancer deaths. For men, the most common types of cancers are respiratory cancer and liver cancer.

For women, the cancer with the highest mortality rate is breast cancer and respiratory cancer.

In terms of regional distribution, the most common cancer cases are in the western Pacific, with respiratory cancer and liver cancer accounting for the highest proportion.

Second only to the Western Pacific is Southeast Asia, where respiratory cancer, oral cancer and throat cancer account for the highest proportion.

In Europe, the most deadly cancer is also respiratory cancer, followed by colorectal cancer.

The disaster of cancer covers the whole world. People all over the world are eager to hope to overcome cancer one day. It is hoped that the state, government, experts, scholars and scientists can find out anti-cancer measures so that people can stay away from cancer.

3). Current status of global cancer 5-year survival rate

Today, the current state of cancer 5-year survival rate is still at a lower level.

It can be said that there are more and more methods and means available to clinicians today in the clinical diagnosis and treatment of cancer. However, we have to face up to a reality. A large number of clinical epidemiological analysis shows that the maturity and development of the ability and means of diagnosis and treatment, and the improvement of the overall treatment effect of the tumor do not seem to be completely synchronized. According to the data distributed by The American Cancer Society (pictured), the diagnosis and treatment of various malignant tumors has been greatly improved in the past ten years, but its 5-year survival rate is still in one. Lower level. For example, the 5-year survival rate of global colon cancer in 2004 was 62%. Although the diagnostic techniques and surgical treatment of colon cancer have made great progress, it has only increased to 65% and no breakthrough has been made. The etiology, epidemiological studies and various treatment techniques of liver cancer have been greatly improved, but the current 5-year survival rate is only 18%, which is only 11 percentage points higher than 10 years ago. How to improve the prognosis of patients is still a problem. The problem of hepatobiliary surgeons. The mortality rate of gastric cancer has remained high. Although the level of surgical technology has been continuously improved, the 5-year survival rate of gastric cancer has only increased from 23% 10 years ago to 29%. In addition, the 5-year survival rate of pancreatic cancer is not much changed from 10 years ago, and it is 5%; the 5-year survival rate of esophageal cancer has been maintained at 14%; the 5-year survival rate of breast cancer has been 87% from 10 years ago. Down to the current 79%, cervical cancer has dropped from 71% to 69%, and the 5-year survival rate of lung cancer has dropped from 15% to the current 14%.

CHAPTER 11

XZ-C proposed that scientific research ethics should be promoted and doctor is benevolence and the first thing which should be done is to build up ethics

TABLE OF CONTENTS

1. Research ethics

2. standard

3. Basic ethics

About "The steps, plans, programs and the overall design of how to achieve to conquer cancer and to launch the general attack to cancer" the XZ-C has been developed and published in a book, distributed worldwide.

Why publish English books worldwide? Because cancer patients cover the whole world, industrial and agricultural wastewater, waste residue, and exhaust gas pollution also cover the whole world. Therefore, it is necessary to globally conquer cancer and to launch the total cancer attack.

The above-mentioned plan, planning, general design, and blueprint for conquering cancer and launching the general attack of cancer can be applied to a country, a province, a state, and a market reference application to conquer cancer and even win cancer.

1. How to implement the creation of this cancer prevention research? XZ-C proposed the cancer prevention general design and cancer prevention system engineering

Professor Xu Ze suggested:

(1) All countries, provinces and states should establish cancer prevention research institutes (or institutions) to carry out cancer prevention system projects and carry out cancer prevention work for their own country, province, state and city. (Because there are a large number of cancer patients in various countries, provinces and cities)

(2) Countries should establish cancer prevention regulations and comprehensively carry out (some should be legislated)

(3) I will use this project to recommend the World Health Organization to hold a cancer prevention campaign, with the goal of reducing the incidence of cancer. Conquering cancer is a frontier of science and a worldwide problem. Cancer is a human disaster. It covers the whole world. People all over the world are eager to hope that one day they can overcome cancer and benefit humanity.

Professor Xu Ze XZ-C proposed:

<u>(4) Scientific ethics should be advocated, medicine is benevolence, and ethics is the first</u>

<u>Research ethics: Products, achievements, and patents should all have ethical standards.</u>

<u>**Standards: The bottom line should be based on standards that do not harm human health. In particular, it must not contain carcinogens.**</u>

<u>**Basic ethics: All products, achievements, patents, goods and people are harmless and do not harm people's health, especially for children. Do not contain carcinogens.**</u>

<u>**(5) XZ-C proposes scientific ethics, and it should recommend to WHO that all products, achievements, and patents should be the bottom line of moral standards that do not harm human health, especially the carcinogens. For example:**</u>

1. Women's cosmetics, hair dyes, children's toys... should be tested without carcinogens, without damaging human health
2. house decoration, materials ... should be tested without carcinogens
3. food additives, preservatives, food processing packaging ... should be tested without carcinogens
4. .leather products, cloth dyes ... should be tested, no carcinogens
5. **The feed of collectively fed pigs should not contain hormones, auxins, vegetarian meat, growth-promoting hormones... all should be tested without carcinogens.**
6. **group feed chicken, duck feed must not contain hormones, auxin ... should be tested without carcinogens**

(6) The health administrative department shall protect and protect health, and shall lead, lead, support, and guide anti-cancer measures, anti-cancer projects, anti-cancer tests, and anti-cancer monitoring.

(7) XZ-C proposes to establish the "Anti-Cancer Research Institute" and carry out anti-cancer system engineering:

- The way in which so many carcinogens or carcinogenic factors should be studied
- These sources of pollutants should be studied and managed to stop at the source
- These carcinogenic mechanisms should be studied, their carcinogenic effects, and environmental factors leading to genetic mutations.
- It is necessary to study the "two-type society" resource-saving and environment-friendly community to prevent cancer (to achieve a green living environment and a living environment where birds and flowers are fragrant).

CHAPTER 12

The Past and Future of Tumor Development

TABLE OF CONTENTS

1. Prospects and predictive assessment for cancer treatment

1).Analyzing the next research prospects and the prospective assessment of cancer treatment. They are the following sections:

——Molecular targeted drugs attract people's attention
——The prospect of immunomodulatory drugs is gratifying
——Immunotherapy opens a new era of cancer treatment
——Biological therapy and combination of Chinese and Western medicine are two effective ways to prevent cancer metastasis
—— Applying vaccine treatment is human hope
——The way out for cancer treatment is "three early"
——The way out to fight cancer is prevention

(1). Molecular targeted drug therapy attracts attention

The Philadelphia chromosome opened the door to **targeted therapy**. In 1960, researchers in Philadelphia, USA, found a chromosomal abnormality in patients with chronic myeloid leukemia (CML). A few years later, the researchers found that this was the result of the long arm translocation of chromosomes 9 and 22. Since this chromosomal abnormality was first discovered in Philadelphia (**Phiadelphia)**, it was named the Philadelphia (**Ph**) chromosome. This chromosome has also become a target for CML targeted therapy marketed 40 years later. In 2001, the first drug that was proven to be resistant to Philadelphia molecular chromosome defects - imatinib.

Later the target drug trastuzumab, which targets human epidermal growth factor receptor 2 (HER2), is then used to treat HER2-positive breast cancer.

Bevacizumab which targets VEGF and cetuximab which targets EGFR are used to treat colorectal cancer.

Gefitinib and erlotinib targeting EGFR are used for the treatment of non-small cell lung cancer.

Molecularly targeted drugs are cell stabilizers, and most patients cannot achieve complete remission (CR) or partial remission (PR), but rather stable disease and improved quality of life. In addition to gefitinib, erlotinib, imatinib, more need to be combined with chemotherapy drugs.

Molecularly targeted drugs represent a new class of anticancer drugs, and Gleevec is a classic example of controlling cancer by inhibiting abnormal molecules that cause cancer without damaging other normal nuclear tissues. More and more molecularly targeted drugs have been used in cancer treatment. For example, rituximab

(Trastuzumab) for treating breast of Rituximab for treating B cell lymphoma, Gifitinib for treating lung cancer, Erlotinib, and the like. Targeted therapy brings anti-tumor hope.

(2). The prospect of immunomodulatory drugs is gratifying

Regardless of the complexity of the mechanisms behind cancer, immune suppression is the key to cancer progression. Removal of immunosuppressive factors and restoration of the recognition of cancer cells by immune system cells can effectively prevent or stop cancer.

More and more research evidence shows that by regulating the body's immune system, it is possible to achieve cancer control. Treating tumors by activating the body's anti-tumor immune system is an area that is currently exciting for researchers. The next major breakthrough in cancer is likely to stem from this.

In order to explore the etiology and pathogenesis and pathophysiology of cancer, our laboratory has carried out a series of animal experiments in the laboratory for 4 years, and obtained new findings from the experimental results. New inspirations: thymus atrophy, low immune function is one of cancer causes and pathogenesis, Xu Ze proposed at the International Oncology Society in 2013: one of the causes of cancer and one of the pathogenesis may be thymus atrophy, low immune function, decreased immune surveillance ability and immune escape.

Therefore, the treatment principle must be to prevent progressive atrophy of the thymus, promote thymic hyperplasia, protect bone marrow hematopoietic function, improve immune surveillance, and provide experimental basis and theoretical basis for cancer immune regulation and control treatment.

Through the above four years to explore the basic experimental research on the mechanism of recurrence and metastasis and after another 3 years of the screening experiments from the natural medication and Chinese herbal medication in cancer-bearing animals in the laboratory, 48 kinds of medications which have better tumor inhibition rate were screened out from 200 Chinese herbs, then selected in cancer-bearing animal experiments, it constitutes XZ-C1-10 anti-cancer immune regulation and control Chinese medication. After 20 years of clinical application in the more than 12,000 patients with advanced cancer in the oncology clinic, the clinical observation and verification confirmed that the principle of treatment with immune regulation and control "protection of thymus and increase of immune function " is reasonable and the curative effect is satisfactory. The application of immunomodulatory Chinese medication has achieved good results, improves the quality of life, and significantly prolong the survival period.

(3). ASCO Announces Major Progress in Clinical Oncology in 2015

Immunotherapy opens a new era of cancer treatment

On February 4, 2016, the American Society of Clinical Oncology (ASCO) announced the "2016 Annual Report: ASCO Clinical Oncology Progress" on Capitol Hill, Washington, DC. <u>The report details the global clinical oncology in 2015. The research is summarized and at the same time, the future research direction is forecasted. ASCO rated the 2015 progress as "tumor immunotherapy"</u>.

ASCO President Professor Julie M. Vose believes that the most important development in 2015 is the discovery of immunotherapy. She wrote in the foreword: "We are no longer determined by tumor type and staging as we have in the past. Treatment, in the era of precision medicine, we select or exclude treatment based on each patient and tumor genetic data. No other major advances, like immunology can be translated into clinical practice, so ASCO decided that the biggest progress in 2015 is immunotherapy."

The chairman of the committee, Professor Don Dizon, also believes that the annual research results are increasing, but from the perspective of being able to benefit patients, the most important **development this year should be immunotherapy.**

2. The past and future of oncology development

(1) Two leaps in the treatment of malignant tumors in the last two centuries

Looking back over the past 100 years, human beings have been deeply worried about cancer. So far, there is still no essential comprehensive understanding of cancer formation, that is, what factors control normal cell proliferation, and how they lose the control of proliferation and become malignant cells.

In the last two centuries, there have been two leaps in the treatment of malignant tumors:

The first was in 1890, Hals tad proposed the concept of tumor radicalization.

The second time was in the 1970s, Fish integrated chemotherapy into radical surgery (adjuvant chemotherapy or neoadjuvant chemotherapy).

Since then, malignant tumor treatment has been faltering.

Fish is a systemic intravenous route. After half a century, it has not been able to reduce mortality, and it has not stopped recurrence, metastasis, and mortality.

Now we have questioned and reformed the traditional doctrine, the traditional method of drug administration, and changed the idea into the target organ intravascular administration, combined with the establishment of XZ-C comprehensive treatment and XZ-C immunomodulation therapy (ie immunization) Chemotherapy) will probably help drive currently not squatting status quo.

(2) In 1971, President Nixon issued the "Anti-Cancer Declaration" and proposed an anti-cancer slogan in the UN speech.

In 1971, the US Congress passed a "National Cancer Regulations" and President Nixon issued the "Anti-Cancer Declaration", so he invested considerable human and financial resources to overcome cancer in one fell swoop.

In December 1971, President Richard Nixon presented an anti-cancer slogan in a message from the United Nations.

42 years have passed, and now Nixon has made a lot of progress, and has made many significant advances in cancer research, such as the discovery of tumor suppressor genes, the advent of monoclonal antibodies, the use of CT and magnetic resonance imaging, and the improvement of ultrasound and endoscopic techniques and the innovation of various treatment methods.

However, in the second decade of the 21st century, the mortality rates of lung cancer and colon cancer, which constitute the greatest threat to human beings, are still basically the same as those of 50 years ago. Cancer deaths are still the leading cause of death for urban and rural residents in China.

Then the experts in medicine, biology, and related disciplines began to reflect. **Most scientists believe that the prevention and treatment of cancer should start from the most basic problems, namely, the nature of cancer cells, the mechanism of disease, the metabolic characteristics of cancer cells, and their signal transduction etc to understand the "face of the mountain" of cancer which is the only way to prevent and treat cancer most effectively.**

It should conduct interdisciplinary collaborative research, promote cooperation between basic research and clinical medical research, and attach importance to clinical research.

Clinical basic research must be carried out, and without breakthroughs in basic research, clinical efficacy is difficult to improve.

(3) In 1982, Oldham founded **the theory of biological response regulation. On this basis, he proposed the fourth mode of cancer treatment in 1984: Biotherapy. According to the theory of biological response regulation, under normal circumstances, the dynamic balance between tumor and body defense, tumor occurrence and even invasion, metastasis, is completely caused by this imbalance of dynamic balance. If the state of the disorder has been artificially**

adjusted to a normal level, the growth of the tumor can be controlled and allowed to subside.

Biotherapy is supplemented, induced or activated the cellular activity and the biological cell (or) factor possessed by the inherent biological response regulation system in vivo from outside the body to adjust this biological response.

Biotherapy differs from the previous three treatment modes, namely surgery and radiation therapy and chemotherapy with the goal of directly attacking tumors. The scope of biotherapeutics clearly exceeds the traditional concept of immunotherapy because the dynamic balance between the body and the tumor is not limited to immune responses, but also involves various regulatory genes and cytokines involved in tumor proliferation.

Biological response modifiers (BRMs) have opened up new areas of cancer biotherapy. At present, BRM is widely regarded in the medical community as the fourth program of tumors.

(4) As more and more cancer patients, the incidence rate is rising, the mortality rate remains high, recognizing that cancer should not only pay attention to treatment, but also pay attention to prevention, in order to stop the source. The research aims to focus on the prevention and treatment of the whole process of cancer occurrence and development.

Xu Ze put forward the **"Strategic of Way Out and Suggestions for Conquering Cancer" in the book "New Concepts and New Methods of Cancer Treatment" published in October 2011. In June 2013, XZ-C proposed to "the basic idea and design of conquering cancer and launching the general attack on cancer" in an attempt to reduce the incidence of cancer, reduce mortality, improve cure rate and prolong survival terms.**

The general attack means "cancer prevention + cancer control + cancer treatment" and the troika goes hand in hand.

Cancer prevention: Class I prevention of cancer can be achieved by building a "two-oriented society" and building a well-off society to carry out "ride research".

Control cancer: through the "three early" clinic, precancerous lesion treatment, screening.

Treatment of cancer: surgery + immune regulation + biological therapy + differentiation induction therapy + integrated Chinese and Western medicine treatment as the main methods and supplemented by radiotherapy and chemotherapy.

The near-term goal: to curb the momentum of cancer development, reduce its incidence, and gradually improve the cure rate, gradually realizing three one-thirds.

CHAPTER 13

XZ-C proposed that people work together to conquer cancer

The Main Concepts
Cancer Prevention and Anti-Cancer
Conquer cancer and launch a general attack
New Moon Plan (US) and Dawning C Plan (China)

Moving forward together, heading for the science hall to overcome cancer
How to conquer? XZ-C proposed that cancer is a disaster for all
human beings. It must work together for the people of the world,
and China and the United States will jointly tackle the problem.

TABLE OF CONTENTS

1. The history record of proposing "conquer cancer" plan internationally In the past 100 years

There are three persons: the two presidents have proposed the National Plan for Conquering Cancer and A Chinese doctor Xu Ze –C who **proposed a blueprint for designing, planning, and planning a series of cancers, and published a monograph (a full-English version, globally distributed).**

(1) In 1971, the US Congress passed a "National Cancer Regulations" and President Nixon issued the "Anti-Cancer Declaration." So he invested a lot of manpower and financial resources to overcome cancer in one fell swoop.

In December 1971, President Richard Nixon presented an anti-cancer slogan in a message from the United Nations.

(2) On January 12, 2016, US President Barack Obama announced a national plan to "catch cancer" in his annual State of the Union address speech, which was under the responsibility of Vice President Biden.

The name of the program: "**Cancer moon Shot**"

Goal: **Conquer cancer**

On June 29, 2016, US Vice President Vice President Biden convened a summit to broadcast the National Cancer Month Plan to the United States from 9 am to 6 pm in the White House. There are dozens of cancer centers and the doctors, nurses, scientists, volunteers, patients, family members, cancer survivors, and rehabilitators in the communities organization across the country who participated in this mission to overcome cancer and encourage scientists to condense wisdom to conquer cancer.

The White House called on Americans to join them to host community events.

Immunotherapy opens a new era of cancer treatment and announces $1 billion a year to overcome cancer research.

(3) In 2011, Chinese physician Xu Ze put forward the "strategic ideas and suggestions for conquering cancer" in his published monograph. In August 2013, he first proposed at the International Congress of Oncology: "XZ-C Research plan to overcome cancer and launch the general attack of cancer."

In July 2015, he proposed the "Dawning C-type plan" to overcome cancer and launch the general attack on cancer.

The Chapter 38 in Xu Ze's third monograph "The New Concepts and New

Methods of Cancer Therapy". In a chapter of the chapter, "strategic ideas and suggestions for conquering cancer"

How to overcome cancer I see one: the road of scientific research lies in exploring the experimental basis of cancer etiology, pathogenesis and pathophysiology

How to overcome cancer I see two: the road of scientific research lies in the scientific research on the prevention and treatment of cancer occurrence and development

How to overcome cancer I see three: the road to scientific research lies in the development of multidisciplinary research, the establishment of cancer-related research groups, special in-depth clinical basic and clinical research

The book was translated into English in 2013 under the title "New Concept and New Way of Treatment of Cancer".

The full English version was published in Washington, DC in March 2013 and is distributed worldwide.

- Xu Ze's fourth book, "On Innovation of Treatment of Cancer"

——(Cancer treatment innovation theory)

Full English version, published in Washington, DC in December 2015, with electronic version, global distribution

The brief introduction to this book: the experimental research, Chinese medicine immunopharmacology and molecular level Chinese and Western medicine combined with anti-cancer research, has initially formed the theoretical system of XZ-C immune regulation and treatment of cancer.

Walked Out of a new Chinese medicine with immune regulation, regulate immune activity, prevent thymus atrophy, promote thymic hyperplasia, protect bone marrow hematopoietic function, improve immune surveillance, and combine Western medicine at the molecular level to overcome cancer.

- Xu Ze's fifth book, The Road To Overcome Cancer

- (to overcome the road to cancer)

Full English version, published in Washington, DC on December 6, 2016, with electronic version, global distribution

Chapter 11 of this book, an initiative to overcome the general attack on cancer

——The overall strategic reform of cancer treatment

The first section is necessary to launch the general attack

Section 2 Feasibility of launching the general attack

Section III XZ-C Plan to Overcome the General Attack of Cancer

Chapter 12 Strengthening research on anti-cancer prevention and treatment, changing the status of re-treatment and prevention

The first section must recognize the current problems and clarify the research direction.
The second quarter, the victory over cancer prevention, treatment effect in the "three early"

Chapter 13 Suggestions on the Cultivation of Scientific and Technological Innovation Talents and the Transformation of Scientific Research Achievements

The first section to overcome cancer, technology talent is the key
Section 2 Establishing a good laboratory

Chapter 14 Adhere to the new anti-cancer road with Chinese characteristics

This book has been published in English for more than two years. Therefore, China, Hubei, and Wuhan should catch up with conquering cancer research. Because conquer cancer and launch the general attack to cancer was proposed by professors in China and Wuhan, and has published the monographs, it should be carried out in the domestic work to overcome cancer and launch the general attack on cancer to catch up and should report to the province and city.

Contemporary, now, to overcome the research work of cancer, Chinese physicians have done the most, the earliest, published monographs, experimental research, theory, and clinical practice.

It was originally hoped that our country's leadership suggest or report "conquer cancer and launch the general attack to cancer "to the United Nations. However, the President of the United States has announced" the national plan for conquering cancer and called on all American and global scientists to unite wisdom to overcome cancer.

I should remember the story of smallpox and cowpea in the Ming Dynasty of China! The kind of cowpea was invented by Chinese doctors, but after being passed to France, it was reported by French doctors.

How to do? You should apply to open an international oncology conference in Wuhan: "To overcome the peak of the cancer attack general academic forum, the first batch of scientific research results have been achieved by the international announcement that China has overcome the general attack on cancer."

2. Why do you say that you can move forward together? What are in common together?

(1) The 38 chapter in the monograph "The New Concepts and Methods of Cancer Therapy" published in Beijing in 2011 (Chinese version), followed by the third edition of Xu Ze, published in Washington in 2013 (English version) was

"Strategic ideas and suggestions for conquering cancer" proposed: "Collecting cancer"

How to overcome cancer I see one: the road to scientific research lies in exploring the etiology, pathogenesis, pathophysiology of cancer

How to overcome cancer I see two: the road to scientific research lies in the study of cancer occurrence, the development of prevention and treatment of the whole process

How to overcome cancer I see three: the road to scientific research lies in the development of multidisciplinary research, the establishment of relevant specialist groups, special in-depth basic and clinical research

The book was translated into English by Dr. Bin Wu, an American medical scientist. The English book titled "New Concept and New Way of Treatment of Cancer" was published in Washington, June 2013, and published in Europe and America.

This book focuses on: attacking the general attack of cancer

(2) **Xu Ze's fourth monograph** "On Innovation of Treatment of Cancer" - (English version of cancer treatment innovation) published in Washington, DC in December 2015, electronic version, global distribution

This book focuses on: immune regulation and treatment of cancer

Experimental research, Chinese medicine immunopharmacology and molecular level Chinese and Western medicine combined with anti-cancer research, has initially formed a theoretical system of immune regulation and treatment of cancer.

Stepped out of a traditional Chinese medicine immune regulation, regulate immune activity, prevent thymus atrophy, promote thymic hyperplasia, protect bone marrow hematopoietic function, improve immune surveillance, and combine Western medicine at the molecular level to overcome cancer.

The above two books:
the former focuses on: conquering cancer
The latter focuses on: immune regulation and treatment of cancer

(3) On January 12, 2016, US President Barack Obama proposed a national cancer plan to overcome cancer in his State of the Union address: conquering cancer.

The name of the program is: "Cancer moon shot", which was carried out by Vice President Biden. Biden proposed to focus on immunotherapy, immune prevention, and immunotherapy to open a new era of cancer treatment.

On June 29, 2016, Vice President Vice President convened a summit to broadcast the National Cancer Lunar Plan to the United States from 9 am to 6 pm in the White House to encourage scientists to concentrate on conquering cancer and announce 10 per year. Billions of dollars are used to overcome cancer research.

The above goal: overcome cancer
The methods and pathways: immune treatment and immune prevention of cancer

In short, Chapter 38 in the above-mentioned Xu Ze's third monograph puts forward: **conquer cancer and how to overcome cancer**; the fourth monograph of the whole book focuses on: **immune regulation and control of treatment of cancer, walked out of a new path to overcome cancer.**

The goal of "Cancer Moon Shot" with the United States is to overcome cancer, and the method and route are immunotherapy.

Both of the above goals are to overcome cancer. The methods and pathways are immunotherapy, immune regulation, and immune prevention. The goals, methods, and approaches of the two are consistent.

Therefore, it is proposed to move forward together. Going to the science hall to overcome cancer.

3. how to overcome cancer? XZ- C proposed that it needs two wheels: A wheel and B wheel

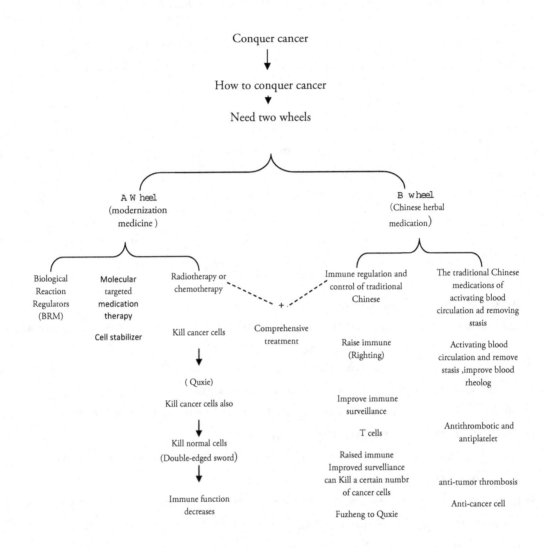

Conquer cancer

↓

How to conquer cancer

↓

Need two wheels

A W heel
(modernization
medicine)

B wheel
(Chinese herbal
medication)

Biological
Reaction
Regulators
(BRM)

Molecular
targeted
medication
therapy

Cell stabilizer

Radiotherapy or
chemotherapy

Kill cancer cells

↓

(Quxie)

Kill cancer cells also

↓

Kill normal cells
(Double-edged sword)

↓

Immune function
decreases

Comprehensive
treatment

Immune regulation and
control of traditional
Chinese

Raise immune
(Righting)

Improve immune
surveillance

T cells

Raised immune
Improved survelliance
can Kill a certain numbr
of cancer cells

Fuzheng to Quxie

The traditional Chinese
medications of
activating blood
circulation ad removing
stasis

Activating blood
circulation and remove
stasis ,improve blood
rheolog

Antithrombotic and
antiplatelet

anti-tumor thrombosis

Anti-cancer cell

A+B
The combination of
chinese and western
medications

4. How to overcome cancer? XZ-C proposes the need for A-wheel, A-runway and B-wheel, B-runway

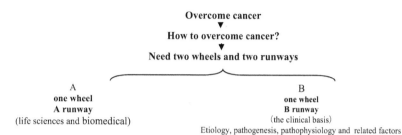

Overcome cancer
▼
How to overcome cancer?
▼
Need two wheels and two runways

A	B
one wheel	**one wheel**
A runway	**B runway**
(life sciences and biomedical)	(the clinical basis)
	Etiology, pathogenesis, pathophysiology and related factors

The A wheel and A runway are :

a. the DNA found
Under a variety of internal and external factors the body occurs the mutation or error, causing DNA structure and function changes, resulting in cancer.

b. the gene mutation
1928 it was considered that gene mutation is the root cause of cancer and tumor occurrence and the development is involved in genes and the basic life activities such as the cell proliferation, differentiation, apoptosis and other etc, therefore, it is now recognized as a disease of the tumor.

c. the Philadelphia chromosome opens targeted therapy
In 1960, the researchers in Philadelphia found that there was a chromosomal abnormality in patients with chronic myeloid leukemia (CML), and that years later it was found to be the result of chromosomes of chromosome 9 and chromosome 22. The chromosome became the target of CML targeted therapy for 40 years. In 2001 it was the first time confirmed to the drug of being against Philadelphia chromosome molecular defects - imatinib.

°

The B wheel and B runway are :
a. The virus
• 1951 it was found that virus can transmit the mice leukemia.
• In 1960 the African sub-Saharan region reported that Hodgkin's lymphoma was thought to be caused by a virus and later confirmed as an AIDS virus.
• 1983 human papillomavirus infection is one of the factors of cervical cancer.
• Preventive vaccines for cervical cancer in 2006 were approved by the US FDA.
b. the immune
• in 2001 in the Animal experiments it was found that removal of thymus can produce a mouse model of mice.
Mouse thymus had the acute progressive atrophy after inoculated with cancer cells and cell proliferation was blocked and the immune function was low, the volume was significantly reduced, thymus atrophy, immune function was slow and it could promote cancer metastasis.
c. the hormones
• in 1916 it was found that removal of ovaries can reduce the incidence of breast cancer, suggesting that ovarian can promote the occurrence of breast cancer.
• in 1941 the hormone dependence of the prostate cancer was confirmed and the injection of androgen could promote metastasis.

d. the environmental pollution

• In 1907, the sun exposure was associated with skin cancer
• in 1978 the nitrosamines in tobacco leaves were confirmed to be carcinogens in cigarettes and were found to be carcinogenic in animal models

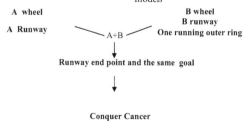

A wheel **B wheel**
A Runway **B runway**
A+B **One running outer ring**
▼
Runway end point and the same goal
▼
Conquer Cancer

5. For the first time in the world, how to overcome cancer? XZ-C proposes to overcome the three targets A, B and C

Treatment must be based on the cause, pathogenesis, pathophysiology

Anti-cancer and cancer treatment must also prevent and treat the cause, pathogenesis and cancer metastasis mechanism.

How did the tumor happen?

Research should be carried out according to each target or "target" in the process of tumorigenesis.

The occurrence of tumors is caused by genetic and environmental factors, mutations, abnormal expression or deletion, resulting in a common feature of tumor cells - uncontrolled infinite reproduction

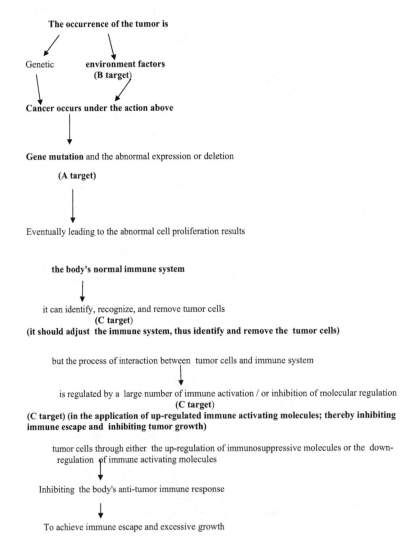

The occurrence of the tumor is

Genetic   **environment factors**
                 (B target)

Cancer occurs under the action above

Gene mutation and the abnormal expression or deletion

(A target)

Eventually leading to the abnormal cell proliferation results

the body's normal immune system

it can identify, recognize, and remove tumor cells
(C target)
(it should adjust the immune system, thus identify and remove the tumor cells)

but the process of interaction between tumor cells and immune system

is regulated by a large number of immune activation / or inhibition of molecular regulation
(C target)
(C target) (in the application of up-regulated immune activating molecules; thereby inhibiting immune escape and inhibiting tumor growth)

tumor cells through either the up-regulation of immunosuppressive molecules or the down-regulation of immune activating molecules

Inhibiting the body's anti-tumor immune response

To achieve immune escape and excessive growth

According to the process of the occurrence of tumors as described above, XZ-C proposes that the target or target for conquering cancer should be:

A target: should be directed to genetic mutations, abnormal expression or deletion

However: genetic mutations, abnormal expression or deletions are the cause of cancer? Or is it fruit?

Why is it a mutation? What causes it to mutate? What are the consequences of the mutation?

Is an environmental factor that causes genetic mutations

B target: should be for environmental factors

B target is the target of anti-cancer

Environmental factors: external environment - air, water, soil, physical, chemical, biological factors, clothing, food, housing, travel

Internal environment - micro, ultra-micro, immune, endocrine, neurohumoral

Is the environment (internal and external) → causing genetic mutation

Therefore, it is necessary to create the "Anti-Cancer Research Institute" to carry out anti-cancer system engineering.

C target: should be: • adjust the normal immune system to remove tumor cells

- A large number of immune activations, up-regulation, and balance of tumor and immune system interactions
- Immune activating molecules should be up-regulated to suppress immune escape and inhibit tumor growth
- Immunization prevention, immunotherapy, vaccines are human expectations

6. XZ-C proposes that several treatments of traditional Chinese medicine can be applied to the treatment of tumors.

Professor Xu Ze (XZ-C) proposed several treatments for traditional Chinese medicine, which can be applied to the treatment of tumors and the combination of Chinese and Western medicine. Experimental research and clinical basic research on the combination of Chinese and Western medicine should be carried out, as well as clinical application verification observation.

A. The rule of Chinese medicine: Fuzheng Guben and A' Western medicine treatment principles: improve immunity, immune regulation, and immunity

Epidemiological reconstruction
Anti-cancer immunological pharmacology research and immune regulation of traditional Chinese medicine
The mechanism of action of anticancer traditional Chinese medicine should be carried out at the molecular level.
Experimental study on the combination of Chinese and Western medicine

B. TCM treatment: blood stasis and B' western medicine treatment principles: anti-cancer metastasis, anti-cancer, anti-micro-transfer

The movement of anti-cancer plugs must resist blood clots and improve blood rheology.
Live blood can be paralyzed to avoid the formation of cancerous plugs
Eliminate cancer cells on the way to metastasis, must resolve cancerous plugs and micro-cancers
Bolt to prevent cancer cell metastasis

C. TCM treatment: detoxification and C' western medicine treatment principles: some cancers and chronic inflammation, stubborn

Sexual ulcers may be related, such as chronic atrophic gastritis, chronic
Pelvic inflammatory disease, cervicitis, chronic hepatitis, etc., some are cancer
Pre-lesion, can be treated with heat-clearing and detoxifying Chinese medicine to control

D. TCM treatment: soft and firm dispersal and D' western medicine treatment principle: current physical examination CT, sometimes reported in a certain

Organs have multiple small nodules, small, only a few millimeters, both
Can not be operated, can not put chemotherapy, can be used to soften the Chinese medicine
Treatment, dynamic observation, often have a good effect.

7. "New Moon Plan" (USA) and Dawning C Plan (China)

- Moving forward together, heading for the science hall to overcome cancer

1).The time of proposed to the "moon shot"

On January 12, 2016, US President Barack Obama announced in his last State of the Union speech during his tenure a national plan to conquer cancer, the "new moon landing plan that Vice President Biden called in 2015. ", the plan will be handled by Biden. In May 2015, Biden's son died of brain cancer, only 46 years old. Since then, Biden has announced that he will not participate in the 2016 presidential election and will join the anti-cancer career during the remaining vice presidential term.

Biden will visit the Abramson Cancer Center at the University of Pennsylvania School of Medicine next week to discuss the plan. He said that the "new moon landing plan" is a commitment to overcome cancer in the world and will inspire a new generation of scientists to explore the scientific world.

Obama did not mention the specific plan of the plan in his speech, but he mentioned that the expenditure and tax bill passed by Congress in December 2015 has raised the financial budget of the National Institutes of Health (NIH).

The United States has just recently established a national immunotherapy alliance consisting of pharmaceutical companies, biotechnology companies and academic medical organizations. The alliance is trying to develop a vaccine immunotherapy by 2020 to overcome cancer and complete cancer. Monthly plan."

The American Society of Clinical Oncology (ASCO) issued a statement on its website to welcome Obama's "New Moon Plan" and support Biden's leadership, arguing that the "New Moon Plan" will reduce the pain and reduce the risk of cancer for humans. Death caused by cancer. The statement mentions that "all effective treatments should be transformed from the laboratory to the clinic"; the application of "big data" technology, such as ASCO's "CancerLinQ" rapid learning system, can accelerate the pace of cancer. Enable physicians to better develop individualized treatment options for each patient and understand which areas are urgently needed to invest more research (Liu Quan).

(January 21, 2016, China Medical Tribune)

2) The proposed time of the dawn of the C-type plan

1. Before January 12, 2016, the progress of the scientific research plan "to overcome the general attack of cancer"

2. Before January 12, 2016, we have carried out scientific research and scientific innovation series with the research direction of cancer.

3. Dawning C-type plan C. Racing with moon shot

1. Before January 12, 2016, we proposed the research work that has been carried out to "conquer the general attack of cancer." Proposing "to overcome the general attack of cancer" is unprecedented work. XZ-C (Xu Ze-China, Xu Ze-China) has been running for the first 3-4 years.

(1) Chapter 38 of the monograph "New Concepts and New Methods of Cancer Treatment" published by Xu Ze in October 2011 uses a chapter to propose "strategic ideas and suggestions for conquering cancer".

(2) In June 2013, Xu Ze proposed to "conquer the basic concept and design of the general attack on cancer" in an attempt to reduce the incidence of cancer, reduce cancer mortality, improve the cure rate, and prolong the survival period. The total attack is anti-cancer + cancer control + Governing cancer, the troika goes hand in hand

(3) Xu Ze first proposed in the international exhibition in August 2013: "XZ-C Scientific Research Plan for Overcoming the General Attack of Cancer" - The overall strategy and development of cancer treatment in China

(4) In July 2015, Professor Xu Ze submitted to the government the following four application reports for the feasibility report for the general attack on cancer.

"XZ-C proposes a scientific research plan to overcome the general attack of cancer"
——The overall strategic reform and development of cancer treatment in China

1. first proposed internationally:
   "Necessity and Feasibility Report on Overcoming the General Attack of Cancer"
2. First proposed at the international level:
   "Preparing to build cancer, develop and prevent the whole hospital"
   (Global Demonstration Prevention and Treatment Hospital)
   "Implementation of the plan for the prevention and treatment of cancer in the whole process of anti-cancer and feasibility report"

—— Explain the necessity and feasibility of establishing a full-scale prevention and treatment hospital

3. first proposed at the international level:

"To build a general plan to overcome cancer and the basic vision and feasibility report of Science City"

- Equivalent to designing an overall framework for Chinese characteristics to overcome cancer design

4. first proposed at the international level:

"In the construction of a well-off society, it is recommended to "catch the car scientific research" - the necessity and feasibility report of medical research and cancer prevention and treatment for cancer prevention and cancer control" - adhere to the road of anti-cancer and cancer control with Chinese characteristics

- Our dreams, conquer cancer, build a well-off society, everyone is healthy, stay away from cancer
- These four scientific research projects were first proposed internationally. They are the first international initiative and internationally leading. They have opened up new fields of anti-cancer research and will open up a new era of anti-cancer research.
- Raise the general attack to overcome cancer, this is unprecedented work

(5) Xu Ze applied to the Hubei Provincial Government in August 2015 to establish a preliminary plan and design for the experimental area of the Cancer Working Group (Station) in Hubei and Wuhan.

(6) In July 2015, reported to the Provincial Department of Science and Technology the scientific research achievements in the field of cancer research, the scientific and technological innovation series and the research plan that outlined the general attack on cancer (reporting outline) and the initiative of cancer treatment reform, innovation and development. 4 application reports in the letter

(7) In July 2015, reported to the Provincial Department of Education the scientific research achievements and scientific and technological innovation series to overcome cancer research.

(8) Professor Xu Ze's fourth book, "Only Theology" - "On Innovation of Treatment Of Cancer" was published in Washington in December 2015, published in English, published globally, and distributed electronically. Edition, introduction of new books

Introduction to the new book: experimental research, Chinese medicine immunopharmacology and molecular level Chinese and Western medicine combined with anti-cancer research, has initially formed the theoretical system of XZ-C immune regulation and treatment of cancer.

Step out of a traditional Chinese medicine immune regulation, regulate immune activity, prevent thymus atrophy, promote thymic hyperplasia, protect bone marrow hematopoietic function, improve immune surveillance, and combine Western medicine at the molecular level to overcome cancer.

(9) Xu Ze's fifth "Monograph" new book: "Collecting the Road to Cancer"

—— Reform, innovation and development of cancer treatment
New book preview for the first quarter of 2016

2. Before January 12, 2016, we have carried out research and development of science and technology innovation series with the focus on cancer research.

(1) New findings from experimental research:

In January 2001, Xu Ze published a new discovery from laboratory experimental tumor research in his monograph "New Understanding and New Models of Cancer Therapy":

1. Excision of the thymus (Thymus) can be used to create a model of cancer-bearing animals. Injection of immunosuppressive agents can help establish animal models of cancer.
2. After the host thymus was inoculated with cancer cells, it showed acute progressive atrophy, cell proliferation was blocked, and the volume was significantly reduced. The laboratory was observed in a laboratory model of cancer-bearing animals for more than 6,000 years. The experimental results showed that the tumor progressed even if the thymus Progressive atrophy.

(2) In the second chapter of "New Concepts and Methods of Cancer Treatment" published by Xu Ze in October 2011, the new findings of experimental research on cancer etiology, pathogenesis and pathophysiology are proposed:

"Thymus atrophy, immune dysfunction is one of the causes and pathogenesis of cancer", and in Chapter 3, based on the enlightenment of animal experiments, its treatment principle should protect, regulate, and activate the anti-cancer immune system in the human body. Proposed: "The theoretical basis and experimental basis of the "Zhang-Climb-up" of XZ-C immunomodulation therapy.

(3) Report cancer research papers at the American Society of International Oncology:

1. Received an invitation letter from the American Association for Cancer Research AACR to Xu Ze, who reported "XZ-C immunomodulation anticancer therapy" at the International Cancer Society in Washington, USA in September 2013, which has attracted extensive attention from the international oncology community. And highly valued.

2. From October 27 to 30, 2013, attending the 12th International Conference on Cancer Research of the American Association for Cancer Research (AACR) in Washington, DC, reported: "Thymus atrophy, low immune function is the cause of cancer, one of the pathogenesis", and The academic report on the theoretical basis and experimental basis of the principle of "protecting the thymus and protecting the thymus" (protecting the thymus and improving immunity) and protecting the bone marrow from the blood stem cells has been warmly welcomed and highly valued by the participants.

(4) Publishing monographs

In the above experimental research, basic research, and clinical verification with conquering cancer as the research direction, we have gone through 28 years and obtained a series of scientific research achievements and scientific and technological innovation of anti-cancer, anti-cancer metastasis and recurrence research. The research papers on innovation or independent innovation are published in my series of monographs.

1. in January 2000 the first book o<<new recognition and new model of cancer treatment>> was published by Hubei Science and Technology Press, the author is Prof. Xu Ze.

2. in January 2006 the second monograph "new concepts and new methods of cancer metastasis therapy" was published by Beijing People's Medical Publishing House, the author was Xu Ze, in April 2007 the People's Republic of China issued the certificate of the original book publication of "Three of one hundred"

3. In October 2011 the third monograph "new concepts and new methods of cancer treatment" was published in Chinese version by Beijing People's Military Publishing House and Xu Ze, Xu Jie are the authors.

4. In March 2013 the fourth monograph <<New concepts and new ways of cancer treatment>> was published in the English version

5. In 2015, the fifth monograph "On Innovation Of Treatment Of Cancer" was published in English version (Cancer Treatment Innovation on the first volume) by Washington, the United States, the global distribution, and the issue of electronic Edition

6. In 2016 the sixth monograph "the road to overcome cancer " was published.

7. In 2017 the seventh monograph "condense wisdom and conquer cancer for the benefit of mankind ——how to conquer cancer? how to prevent cancer?" was published in English version in the United States, the global distribution, and the issue of electronic Edition.

8. In 2018 the eighth monograph" condense wisdom and conquer cancer for the benefit of mankind——how to conquer cancer? How to treat cancer? Was published in English version in the Unite States, the global distribution, and the issue of electronic Edition.

9. In 2018 the ninth monograph" New progress of cancer treatment" was published in English version in the Unite States, the global distribution, and the issue of electronic Edition.

These nine monographs are the results of four different levels of research, four hardships, hard progress, four different scientific research stages, and four different levels of research. (I published my first monograph at the age of 67, the second monograph at the age of 73, the third monograph at the age of 78, the third monograph in English and the English version at the age of 80, Washington Publishing, International Distribution, At the age of 82, the fourth monograph was published, in English, published in Washington, and distributed worldwide. At the age of 83, the fifth monograph was published in the first quarter of 2016.)

The results of these four different levels, if compared to a scientific building:

The first monograph is: three floors

The second monograph is: five floors

The third monograph is: eight floors

The fourth and fifth monographs are: ten floors

It is the top design, it is the golden dome, it is the way to overcome cancer.

(These nine monographs will be a reference for the compulsory courses of the Innovative Molecular Oncology School)

(5) Visiting the Stirling Cancer Institute in Houston, USA

In order to strengthen the exchanges and cooperation of international scientific and technological organizations, on December 10, 2009, we were invited to visit the Stirling Cancer Institute in the United States. We were warmly welcomed and warmly treated by the colleagues of the Institute. The 86-year-old director and professor and A number of professors, researchers, and the principal of the nude animal model laboratories and anti-cancer drug analysis laboratories participated in the discussion and exchanges, and reported the latest scientific research results with slides.

We presented the color map of the Institute of Cancer Metastasis and Recurrence in our institute to the Institute of Oncology in US which these paper introduces the experimental research on the tumor-free technique in radical surgery and the experimental study on the removal of thymus to produce cancer-bearing animal models and the related information of the exclusive development of Z-C immune regulation and control of anti-cancer, anti-metastasis Chinese medicine series Z-C1-10 and presented the monograph "New Concepts and New Methods for Cancer Metastasis Treatment" published by me, which is the three hundred original books that won the book award in China, and was warmly welcomed and appreciated by the researchers.

(6) Innovation: The basic and clinical research on anti-cancer and anti-cancer metastasis for more than 30 years has preliminarily embarked on a road of "Chinese-style anti-cancer" and Chinese and Western medicine combined with immune regulation and treatment of cancer. We have accumulated more than 12,000 cases in 30 years. The clinical application experience can be pushed to the whole country and can go to the world. It can connect with the "Belt and Road" to make Chinese medicine go to the world, so that "Chinese-style anti-cancer" and Chinese and Western medicine can combine cancer with immune regulation and control, which not only develops and enriches immunity. The content of studying cancer has brought China's medical modernization into line with the international market and is at the forefront of the world.

It makes cancer therapy of "Chinese-style anti-cancer" and the combination of Chinese medications and Western medications not only develops and enriches the content of cancer immunology treatment, but also brings China's medical modernization into line with international standards and is at the forefront of the world.

3)."New Moon Plan" (US) and "Dawning C Plan" (middle)

A. The New moon landing plan
United States

> Plan Name: "New Moon Plan"
> Objective: To overcome cancer
> Sexuality: National Plan to Conquer Cancer
> Announcement: Announced in the State of the Union Address
> Announcer: President Obama
> Announced: January 12, 2016
> The person in charge of the plan: Vice President Biden
> The specific plan of the plan: unknown
> National Institutes of Health: increased financial budget
> (NIH)
> Recently formed: pharmaceutical company
> Biotechnology company
> Academic medical organization

The alliance is trying to develop a vaccine therapy by 2020 to overcome cancer and complete a new cancer landing program.

B. Dawning C plan ——China

> Plan name: "Dawning C-type plan"
> Objective: To overcome cancer
> Nature:
> Advocate and

The total designer: Professor Xu Ze proposed in 2011 to "conquer cancer and launch a general attack", and in 2013 proposed "to build a comprehensive design for cancer science city". In 2013, he proposed "XZ-C to overcome the scientific research plan for cancer attack". In July 2015, the "Dawning C-type plan" was proposed. In July 2015, four application reports for the feasibility report for the general attack on cancer were launched. In August 2015, the application for the government was established in Hubei and Wuhan. Conquer the initial vision and design of the cancer working group test area.

8. What is Dawning C-type plan No. 1 - No. 6

A. Why should "Dawning C-type plan" be used?

The dawn is the morning light, it is the dawn, it is the morning sun.

Vigorous, vigorous, original innovation, independent innovation

C=China

Type C = Chinese mode

About 8550 people in China are diagnosed with cancer every day, and 6 people are diagnosed with cancer every minute. Therefore, the research work to overcome the general attack of cancer, can not walk slowly, should run forward, save the wounded.

Time is money, time is money = one inch of time, one inch of gold

Time is life, time is life

Time flies, time flies

Empty talk about mistakes, hard work

Avoid talk, work hard, start off

No matter how far the road to cancer is, you should always start.

This research plan is the original innovation, it is time to declare war on cancer, and the general attack should be launched.

Our dreams, conquer cancer, build a well-off society, everyone is healthy, away from cancer

B. The main points of Dawning C

1. Dawning C-type plan No. 1: "Collecting cancer, launching the general attack"
——The overall strategic reform and development of cancer treatment in China
Proposed a general plan, plan, design, blueprint and rules for conquering cancer
Avoid talk, work hard, start off
No matter how far the road to cancer is, you should always start.
(see separate article)

2. Shuguang C-type plan No. 2: "Preparation of the whole process of prevention and treatment of hospitals"
(Global Demonstration Prevention and Treatment Hospital)
——Strategic reform, changing the mode of running a hospital
Reforming treatment mode

3. Dawning C-type plan No. 3: "Building a science city to overcome cancer"

——XZ-C proposes the overall design, planning and blueprint of Science City to overcome the general attack of cancer

- This is the only way to overcome cancer

This is the "high-speed rail" to overcome cancer, "high-speed" channel)

(see separate article)

4. Shuguang C-type plan No. 4: "Building a multidisciplinary research group and laboratory"

- for the cause, pathogenesis, pathophysiology, metastasis, recurrence mechanism of cancer...

Study anti-cancer, anti-recurrence, anti-metastatic measures to improve the overall level of medical care

Benefit

——The standard of efficacy evaluation is: long life expectancy, good quality of life, complications

No or less, each school group is a provincial key laboratory.

(see separate article)

5. Dawning C-type plan No. 5: "The vaccine is human hope, immunological prevention"

—— Today's immunology prevention and treatment has become an extremely important in clinical medicine and preventive medicine

Required field

——△△学组+△△学组+△△学组→Scientific Alliance, Joint Group

(see separate article)

6. Shuguang C-type plan No. 6: A "The prospect of immunomodulatory drugs is gratifying"

- Regardless of the complexity of the mechanisms behind cancer, immune suppression is the progression of cancer

The essential

- From the analysis of experimental results, to obtain new discoveries, new inspirations:

Thymus atrophy, immune function, immune surveillance ability and immune escape are one of the causes and pathogenesis of cancer, so the treatment principle should be to prevent thymus atrophy, promote thymic hyperplasia, and improve immune surveillance.

——XZ-C immune regulation Chinese medicine, is from the traditional Chinese traditional Chinese herbal medicine,

In the animal model of cancer mice, 48 kinds of Chinese herbal medicines with good cancer suppression rate were screened by in vivo anti-tumor experiments, and 26 of them had better immune regulation.

(see separate article)

Shuguang C-type plan No. 6: B "XZ-C immunomodulation anti-cancer Chinese medicine active ingredient, molecular level analysis research group and laboratory"

—— Further research and development of XZ-C immunomodulation anti-cancer Chinese medicine active ingredients, molecular weight, knot

Construction, molecular level analysis

——Methods, steps: animal experiment, molecular level experiment; gene level experiment, first

Separating the active ingredients first makes the precious heritage of traditional Chinese medicine modern and scientific.

(see separate article)

"Collect Cancer Science City" to establish the following genetic testing research groups:

(1) Establish genetic testing and cancer research groups and laboratories

(2) Establish HPV anti-cancer research group and laboratory

(3) Establish genetic testing and immunology and cancer research groups and laboratories

(4) Establish genetic testing and endocrine hormone and cancer research groups and laboratories

(5) Establish genetic testing and pathological sections, and related studies on immunohistochemistry

(6) Establish correlation analysis and research on gene detection and tumor markers

(7) Establish HPV treatment, exploration research groups and laboratories

Expected results:

Using modern science and technology and analytical testing methods, the study of traditional Chinese medicine, the material basis of the efficacy of traditional Chinese medicine in clinical practice is the chemical composition contained therein. To study the anti-cancer work of traditional Chinese medicine and its mechanism, it is necessary to conduct in-depth research and analysis. The active ingredients in it make the precious heritage of traditional Chinese medicine more modern and scientific.

After 28 years of experimental research, basic research and clinical verification, a series of "Chest Enhancement" immunomodulatory anticancer Chinese medicine XZ-C1-10 has been screened. After 20 years of clinical observation, more than 12,000 cases have been verified. Prolong life, improve symptoms, improve quality of life, how to know, evaluate can prolong survival? Some surgical explorations can not be cut down (all pathological sections confirmed diagnosis), or have been widely transferred, it is estimated that only 3-6 months, or 6-12 months of cases, XZ-C immune regulation and anti-cancer, For patients with anti-metastasis and recurrence, some patients can still survive for 4 to 5 years to 8 years, with original data and complete data as well as follow-up data.

After a rehabilitation teacher, after a heart attack, calm down, hide in a small building, self-reliance, hard work, adhere to anti-cancer, anti-cancer metastasis, recurrence of animal experiment basic research and outpatient clinical validation research, from the year of the flower (60 years old)→To the age of the ancients (70s)→To the age of 耄耋(80s), still perseverance, persevere in scientific research to overcome cancer, because he has retired, failed to apply for projects, projects, so no research Funding is to fight alone, to fight alone, to be self-reliant, to work hard, no one cares, no one knows, nowhere to report, no support, hard work for more than 20 years, has achieved a series of scientific and technological innovations, scientific research results, due to retirement In the past 20 years, no one cares, no one supports, retired professors, I don't know where to manage, where to support, so where the scientific research results are reported, I have to make a "monograph" for the benefit of mankind, but published a series of monographs, and then Report to the Provincial Department of Science and Technology and the Provincial Department of Education: 1 hope to open an international high-end academic forum; 2 report to the government to apply for cancer, launch a general attack; 3 report to the province, the provincial government The city has conquered the cancer test area (station) and tried it first. Hope: Apply to establish the "National Science City to overcome the general attack of cancer" in Hubei and Wuhan, which is the "World's first science city to overcome the general attack of cancer."

How to implement this unprecedented event in human history?

(1) Reporting to the government, requesting instructions
(2) Report to the province and city, request instructions
(3) Make recommendations to the city to build in Wuhan: "The first national cancer science city"

"The world's first to overcome Cancer Science City"

C. The detail of Dawning C plan

1. **Dawning C-type plan No. 1**: "Collecting cancer, launching the general attack"

Anti-control + treatment and treatment, and drive together, put forward the general idea and design of conquering cancer

——The overall strategic reform and development of cancer treatment in China

Turn treatment-oriented to focus on prevention and treatment (see separate article)

Avoid talk, work hard, start off

No matter how far the road to cancer is, you should always start.

2. Shuguang C-type plan No. 2: "Preparation of the whole process of prevention and treatment of hospitals"

(Global Demonstration Prevention and Treatment Hospital)

Strategic reform, changing the mode of running a hospital

Reforming treatment mode

Target: three early, precancerous lesions, carcinoma in situ

Research early diagnostic methods, reagents, techniques, theory

Research on early methods, techniques, and theories

Study chemical anti-cancer, endocrine and cancer prevention

Research to promote cancer prevention, "hold your mouth" to prevent cancer (see separate article)

3. Dawning C-type plan No. 3: "Building a science city to overcome cancer"

Preparing an innovative molecular tumor medical school

Innovative molecular level integrated Chinese and Western medicine hospital

Innovative Molecular Oncology Institute

Innovative Environmental Protection and Health Cancer Research Institute

Innovative molecular tumor nano preparations

Cancer Animal Experimental Center

This is the only way to overcome cancer

This is the "high-speed rail" and "high-speed" channel for cancer (see separate article)

4. Dawning C-type plan No. 4 "Building a multi-disciplinary research group"

(For the cause, pathogenesis, pathophysiology, metastasis, recurrence mechanism of cancer...

Anti-cancer, anti-metastasis, recurrence measures)

Form:

A, Immunology and Cancer Research Group and Laboratory

B, virus and cancer research groups and laboratories

C, (endocrine) hormone and cancer research groups and laboratories

D. Environmental and Cancer Research Group and Laboratory

E, fungal and cancer research groups and laboratories

F, Molecular Biology and Cancer Research Group and Laboratory

G, Genetic Engineering and Cancer Research Group and Laboratory

H, Chinese Medicine and Cancer Research Group and Laboratory

I, Three Early and Cancer Research Groups and Laboratories

J, precancerous lesions and cancer research groups and laboratories

The objectives, tasks, planning, implementation, coordination of projects, projects, and goals of the above research groups, research institutes, and research institutes; scientific research achievements, scientific and technological innovation. To overcome the cancer research direction, to benefit patients with the overall level of medical treatment, the criteria for efficacy evaluation are: long survival time, good quality of life, and no or no complications. Each school group is a provincial key laboratory.

(see separate article)

5. Dawning C-type plan No. 5 "vaccine is the hope of human beings Immunological prevention"

With the development of immunology theory and technology, human application of immunological control methods has successfully eliminated smallpox and effectively controlled the spread of many infectious diseases. Immunology prevention has made tremendous contributions in the history of medical development. (A case of rabies, whooping cough, tetanus, influenza, hepatitis B, measles, water beans, etc.), today's immunological prevention has become an extremely important field in clinical medicine and preventive medicine.

Form:

Immunology group + virology group + $^{\triangle\triangle}$ group + $^{\triangle\triangle}$ group → scientific alliance, science conquer cancer group, alliance

A, anti-hepatitis B vaccine → further suppression of cirrhosis → anti-hepatocellular vaccine

B. Development of EB virus vaccine for prevention and treatment of nasopharyngeal carcinoma

C, research and treatment of viral lymphoma

D. Studying virus particles in breast milk to prevent breast cancer vaccine

E. Studying herpes simplex type 2 virus to prevent cervical cancer vaccine

F. Study on the relationship between type C virus and leukemia, sarcoma and sputum gold lymphoma

Study vaccines to prevent their occurrence and control their prevalence

composition:

Immunization and Cancer Research Group

Virus and Cancer Research Group

Goal: Immunization prevention

Specific immunization target (target): development of cancer vaccine

Possibility: Hepatitis B vaccine + Dawning C plan → Liver cancer vaccine

Milk Ca vaccine

Ovarian Ca vaccine

Prostate Ca vaccine

Lymphoma vaccine

Leukemia vaccine

The experimental center is located in Huangjiahu, Science City, Cancer Experimental Animal Center.

It is required to start from the city, the municipal science association, and the Wuhan University, accelerate the formation, and implement the plan.

Implementation and completion methods:

1 graduate student 100; 2 city and province combination

3 Wuhan Anti-Ca Research Association collaborates with universities and research institutes

The chief conductor and chief designer are Professor Xu Ze and academic committee member:

a laboratory building, a single column, and the United States

Hurry: than: super

Experiment first - you can get a batch of papers, results

Post-clinical - based on the above success

Establishing an immunology laboratory

Immunological test

Immunomolecular detection: complement determination

Immunoglobulin assay

Cytokine detection

Immune cells and their function tests
Basic technology of immunology experiment

Research and prospects of new vaccines
(see separate article)

6. Shuguang C-type plan No. 6 "Immune regulation drug prospects gratifying"

Defects in abnormal immune function can lead to a variety of diseases, such as autoimmune diseases, immunodeficiency diseases and tumors.

Immunotherapy consists of two aspects: immune regulation and immune reconstitution.

Immunomodulators can be divided into synthetic drugs, microbial preparations, immune molecules, immune cells and Chinese herbal medicines according to their sources.

With the development of immunology and penetration with other disciplines, a large class of biologically active substances with immunomodulatory effects have been discovered. They have a wide range of biological activities and anti-tumor activities, collectively referred to as biological response modifiers (BRM). The research and application of BRM is an important advancement in modern immunotherapy.

Regardless of the complexity of the mechanisms behind cancer, immune suppression is the key to cancer progression. By removing immunosuppressive factors and restoring the recognition of cancer cells by systemic cells, it is effective against cancer.

In order to explore the etiology, pathogenesis and pathophysiology of cancer, we conducted a series of animal experiments. From the analysis of experimental results, we obtained new findings and new enlightenments: thymus atrophy and low immune function are one of the causes and pathogenesis of cancer. Therefore, Professor Xu Ze proposed one of the causes and pathogenesis of cancer at international academic conferences, which may be thymus atrophy, central immune organ damage, immune dysfunction, decreased immune surveillance, and immune escape.

As a result of the above laboratory experiments, it was found that the cancer-bearing animal model had progressive thymus atrophy and low immune function. Therefore, the treatment principle must be to prevent progressive atrophy of the thymus, promote thymic hyperplasia, protect bone marrow hematopoietic function, improve immune surveillance, and provide theoretical basis and experimental basis for immune regulation and treatment of cancer.

XZ-C immunomodulatory Chinese medicine is a traditional Chinese herbal medicine from China. It has screened 48 kinds of Chinese herbal medicines with good cancer suppression rate in mice with cancer-bearing mice. After compounding, it inhibits tumor growth in mice. The compound tumor inhibition rate is much higher than that of single drug inhibition. Among them, XZ-C1100% inhibits cancer cells from killing 100% of normal cells, XZ-C4 promotes lymphocyte transformation, enhances cellular immune function, inhibits cancer cells, and prevents thymus atrophy. It promotes thymic hyperplasia and is a promising immunomodulatory anticancer drug in clinical practice. It should be further researched and developed to benefit the majority of cancer patients.

D. How to carry out Dawning C-type plan No. 6?

To build anti-cancer, anti-cancer metastatic active ingredients, analytical research groups and laboratories
aims:
(1) Further research and clinical application and clinical application of XZ-C immunomodulation anti-cancer Chinese medicine cell molecular and molecular levels.

(2) Further research on the prevention and treatment of early cancer in situ and precancerous lesions by anti-cancer and anti-cancer Chinese herbal medicines and its clinical application.

(3) Further research and development of the effective components, molecular weight and structural formula of XZ-C immunomodulation anticancer Chinese medicine.

(4) Further research and development of the XZ-C1-10 series of drugs to carry out the following studies one by one:

1Z-CA→Z-CB→Z-CC→......→Z-CZ
A total of 26 kinds, divided into 6 batches, 4 in each batch, each batch takes 4 months
2 For example, Z-CA steps and content:
A, Z-CA phytochemical study: extraction and identification
B, Z-CA immunopharmacology:
a, toxicity
b. Changes in immune organs in mice (thymus, spleen, brain, liver, kidney)
c, the effect on the peripheral cells of mice
d, the effect of mouse peritoneal autophagic cells (MΦ) function
e, the effect on mouse T lymphocytes

C, main components, chemical structure

D, pharmacological effects

E, preparation of preparation

purpose:

In-depth development of Chinese herbal medicine anti-cancer, anti-cancer metastasis is indeed an effective drug, to crude storage, to the false truth, natural medicine Chinese herbal medicine as a resource, modern research, so that become a precise medicine.

Method steps:

(1) Animal experiment: a, in vitro experiment screening

b, in vivo experimental screening

c, experimental tumor model

(2) Experimental study at the molecular level: screening of Chinese herbal medicine for anti-cancer and anti-cancer metastasis

Induction of differentiation of precancerous lesions

(3) Gene level experimental study of anti-cancer, anti-cancer transfer Chinese herbal medicine screening

Topic selection and selection: Firstly, the Chinese herbal medicine which is effective in clinical application will be further studied, and the active ingredients will be separated first.

laboratory:

(1) Equipment: equipment for pharmaceutical composition analysis

(2) Personnel: Scientific and technical personnel who can conduct drug composition analysis

(3) Topic selection and material selection

Expected results:

Using modern science and technology and analytical testing methods, the research on traditional Chinese medicine, the material basis of the efficacy of traditional Chinese medicine in clinical practice is the chemical composition contained therein. To study the anticancer effect and mechanism of traditional Chinese medicine, it is necessary to conduct in-depth research and analysis. The active ingredients in it make the precious heritage of traditional Chinese medicine more modern and scientific.

(see separate article)

After 7 years and 28 years of experimental research, basic research and clinical verification, the series of "Chest Enhancement" immune regulation anti-cancer Chinese medicine XZ-C1-10 has been screened. After 20 years of clinical observation, more than 12,000 cases have been verified. Can prolong life, improve symptoms, improve quality of life, how to know, evaluate can prolong survival? Some surgical explorations can not be cut down (all pathological sections confirmed diagnosis), or have been widely transferred, it is estimated that only 3-6 months, or 6-12 months of cases, XZ-C immune regulation and anti-cancer, For patients with anti-metastasis and recurrence, some patients can still survive for 4 to 5 years to 8 years, with original data and complete data as well as follow-up data.

8. A retired professor, after rehabilitation of the heart attack, calm down, hide in a small building, self-reliance, hard work, adhere to the basic research of animal experiments and clinical validation of anti-cancer, anti-cancer metastasis, recurrence, by the flower Year → to the age of ancient times → to the year of 耄耋, still perseverance, persevere in scientific research, because he has retired, failed to apply for projects, projects, so no research funding, is alone, fighting alone, no one cares, hard work For more than 20 years, he has obtained a series of scientific and technological innovations and scientific research achievements, published a series of monographs, and then reported to the Provincial Science and Technology Department and the Provincial Department of Education: 1 hope to open an academic council or high-end academic forum; 2 report to the government to apply for cancer And launch the general attack; 3 report to the provinces and departments to set up the province and the city to overcome the cancer test area (station), and try first.

9, preparation for publishing work: anti-Ca, anti-Ca

Wuhan Anti-Cancer Research Society will publish the following publications and monographs

1. Popularize anti-Ca scientific research and popular science maps
2. the publication of anti-Ca, anti-Ca science reading "People's Medicine" quarterly
3. published magazine publication "Clinical recurrence, metastasis based and clinical" bimonthly
4. Publish the monograph on "The Road to Conquer Cancer"
5. the publication of "tumor-free technology" - how to do a good radical cancer surgery, intraoperative anti-recurrence, anti-metastasis monograph
6. Publication of "Three Early" and "Precancerous Lesions" publications
7. Publication of the journal "From clothing, food, housing, and anti-cancer knowledge", quarterly

Collaborative publishing house to be invited:

- **Hubei Science and Technology Press**
- Huazhong University of Science and Technology Press
- Wuhan University Press

E. The Request of " Dawning C-type plan (China)

Hope: Apply to incorporate the "Dawning C-type plan" into the National Cancer Program

To the Party Central Committee and the State Council
Provincial Party Committee, Provincial Government

Goal: Conquer cancer
Mission: Prepare a science city to overcome the general attack on cancer

President of Science City, General Director, President of the General Academic Committee: Professor Xu Ze
(former director of the Institute of Experimental Surgery, Hubei University of Traditional Chinese Medicine)
Science City Innovative Oncology Medical College
Innovative Cancer Research Institute Chief Dean:
Innovative Tumor Hospital Integrated Traditional Chinese and Western Medicine Hospital Leadership Team:
Innovative Environmental Protection and Cancer Research Institute

9. Annex 2 provides a brief description of the research environment and recent international research situation:

First, "New Moon Plan" (Cancer Moon Shot) (US)
(Introduction)

On January 12, 2016, US President Barack Obama announced a national plan to overcome cancer in his annual State of the Union speech. The plan is under the responsibility of Vice President Biden.
The name of the program: "New Moon Plan"
Goal: Conquer cancer

Nature: National plan to overcome cancer

Announced: Announced in the State of the Union Address

Announcer: President Obama

Announced: January 12, 2016

The person in charge of the plan: Vice President Biden

The specific plan of the plan is unknown

National Institutes of Health: increased financial budget

Recently composed:

Pharmaceutical company

Biotechnology company

Academic medical organization

The alliance is trying to develop a vaccine therapy by 2020 to complete the new cancer landing program. "Dawning C-type plan" (middle)

(Introduction)

Plan name: "Dawning C-type plan"

The main content of the plan is:

"Overcoming the general attack on cancer" and

"Building a science city to overcome cancer"

Goal: Conquer cancer

nature:

Advocate and chief designer:

(1) Chapter 38 of the monograph "New Concepts and New Methods of Cancer Therapy" published by Xu Ze in October 2011 uses a chapter to propose "strategic ideas and suggestions for conquering cancer."

(2) In June 2013, at the International Academic Conference, "Basic Ideas and Designs for Overcoming the General Attack of Cancer Attack"

(3) In the international exhibition for the first time in August 2013, the "XZ-C Scientific Research Plan for Overcoming the General Attack of Cancer" – the overall strategy and development of cancer treatment in China

(4) Xu Ze proposed in July 2015 "four reports on the feasibility of attacking the general attack on cancer"

"Xu Ze proposes a scientific research plan to overcome the general attack of cancer"
——The overall strategic reform and development of cancer treatment in China

1. first proposed internationally:

"Necessity and Feasibility Report on Overcoming the General Attack of Cancer"

2. First proposed at the international level:

   "Preparing to build cancer, develop and prevent the whole hospital"

   (Global Demonstration Prevention and Treatment Hospital)

   "Implementation of the plan for the prevention and treatment of cancer in the whole process of anti-cancer and feasibility report"

   —— Explain the necessity and feasibility of establishing a full-scale prevention and treatment hospital

3. first proposed at the international level:

   "To build a general plan to overcome cancer and the basic vision and feasibility report of Science City"

   - Equivalent to designing an overall framework for Chinese characteristics to overcome cancer design

4. first proposed at the international level:

   "In the construction of a well-off society, it is recommended to "catch the car scientific research" - the necessity and feasibility report of medical research and cancer prevention and treatment for cancer prevention and cancer control" - adhere to the road of anti-cancer and cancer control with Chinese characteristics

(5) Before January 12, 2016, we have been conducting research work for "to overcome the general attack on cancer" for 3-4 years. It is unprecedented to propose scientific research work to "conquer the general attack of cancer."

1. On January 12, 2016, President Obama announced in the State of the Union address a national plan to overcome cancer, which was under the responsibility of Vice President Biden.

   The name of the program: "New Moon Plan"

   Goal: Conquer cancer

   Nature: National plan to overcome cancer

2. In the second week of the program's announcement, Vice President Biden visited the Abramson Cancer Center at the University of Pennsylvania School of Medicine and discussed the plan. He said that the "new moon landing plan" is a commitment to overcome cancer in the world and will inspire a new generation of scientists to explore the scientific world.

3. On February 4, 2016, the American Society of Clinical Oncology (ASCO) announced the "2016 Annual Report: ASCO Clinical Oncology Progress" on Capitol Hill, Washington, and reviewed the 2015 progress, "Tumor

Immunology Treatment". ASCO Chairman Julie M. Vose believes that the most important development in 2015 is the discovery of immunotherapy. She said in the foreword: "We no longer decide treatment based on tumor type and stage as in the past. In the era of precision medicine, we select or exclude treatment based on each patient and tumor genetic data. No other major advances can be translated into clinical practice like immunology, so the biggest advance in 2015 is immunotherapy." Immunotherapy opens tumor treatment New Era.

4. On April 28, 2016, a policy luncheon was held at the US Capitol to discuss Vice President Biden's "Cancer Moon Shot", "Cancer Moon Plan" and the price structure of the drug. Presided over by former US Senator Tom Coburn. The fourth author of my fourth book, On Imovation of Treatment of Cancer, and translator, Wu Wu, were invited to the meeting and to discuss.

(Note: Xu Ze's fourth monograph: "On Inmovation of Treatment of Cancer" - published on December 25, 2015 in Washington, English, globally distributed, and electronically distributed Introducing a new book. Dawning C-type plan

China

Before January 12, 2016, we have carried out research and development of science and technology innovation series with the focus on cancer research.

(1) New findings from experimental research:

In January 2001, Xu Ze published a new discovery from laboratory experimental tumor research in his monograph "New Understanding and New Models of Cancer Therapy":

1. Excision of the thymus (Thymus) can be used to create a model of cancer-bearing animals. Injection of immunosuppressive agents can help establish animal models of cancer.
2. After the host thymus was inoculated with cancer cells, it showed acute progressive atrophy, cell proliferation was blocked, and the volume was significantly reduced. The laboratory was observed in a laboratory model of cancer-bearing animals for more than 6,000 years. The experimental results showed that the tumor progressed even if the thymus Progressive atrophy.

(2) In the second chapter of "New Concepts and Methods of Cancer Treatment" published by Xu Ze in October 2011, the new findings of experimental research on cancer etiology, pathogenesis and pathophysiology are proposed:

"Thymus atrophy, immune dysfunction is one of the causes and pathogenesis of cancer", and in Chapter 3, based on the enlightenment of animal experiments, its treatment principle should protect, regulate, and activate the anti-cancer immune system in the human body. Proposed: "The theoretical basis and experimental basis of the "Zhang-Climb-up" of XZ-C immunomodulation therapy.

(3) Report cancer research papers at the American Society of International Oncology:

1. Received an invitation letter from the American Association for Cancer Research AACR to Xu Ze, who reported "XZ-C immunomodulation anticancer therapy" at the International Cancer Society in Washington, USA in September 2013, which has attracted extensive attention from the international oncology community. And highly valued.
2. From October 27 to 30, 2013, attending the 12th International Conference on Cancer Research of the American Association for Cancer Research (AACR) in Washington, DC, reported: "Thymus atrophy, low immune function is the cause of cancer, one of the pathogenesis", and The academic report on the theoretical basis and experimental basis of the principle of "protecting the thymus and protecting the thymus" (protecting the thymus and improving immunity) and protecting the bone marrow from the blood stem cells has been warmly welcomed and highly valued by the participants.

New moon landing plan
United States

Introduction to the new book:
Experimental research, Chinese medicine immunopharmacological research and molecular level Chinese and Western medicine combined with anti-cancer research have initially formed the theoretical system of XZ-C immunomodulation and cancer treatment.

Step out of a traditional Chinese medicine immune regulation, regulate immune activity, prevent thymus atrophy, promote thymic hyperplasia, protect bone marrow hematopoietic function, improve immune surveillance, and combine Western medicine at the molecular level to overcome cancer.

Xu Ze, Xu Jie (China)

Bin Wu (United States)

(The former senator Tom and many members of the conference have an electronic version of our new book, all of which read our book.

5. On June 3, 2016, the annual meeting of the American Society of Clinical Oncology was held in Chicago. This is one of the highest level clinical cancer conferences in the world. The theme of the conference focused on "concentrating wisdom and conquering cancer." Vice President Biden reported on the US's anti-cancer "moon Shot" plan at the conference. A total of 50,000 people attended the conference, which was unprecedented and attracted worldwide attention.

6. On May 25, 2016, Vice President Biden visited Hopkins University and Cancer Research Journal to report on the "New Moon Plan", saying that in the future, mainly immunotherapy will conquer cancer, and immunotherapy will control cancer. This new discovery strongly supports immunotherapy and is worth $1,2 million in research funding from Hopkins University. The cover of the magazine featured photos of Vice President Biden's visit.

7. On June 29, 2016, US Vice President Vice President Biden convened a summit to broadcast the National Cancer Month Plan to the United States from 9 am to 6 pm in the White House. Dozens of cancer centers and community organizations around the world organize doctors, nurses, scientists, volunteers, patients, families, cancer survivors, and rehabilitators to participate in this mission to overcome cancer and encourage scientists to focus on cancer.

The American Cancer Society's Cancer Action Network and the Chief Cancer Officer and Chief Medical Officer and President of the American Cancer Society (ACS) are present at this historic summit event.

The White House called on Americans to join them to host community events.

Immunotherapy opens a new era of cancer treatment and announces $1 billion a year to tackle cancer research. Dawning C plan

China

(4) Publishing monographs

In the above experimental research, basic research, and clinical verification to overcome cancer research, we have gone through 28 years and obtained a series of scientific research achievements and scientific and technological innovation series of anti-cancer, anti-cancer metastasis and recurrence research. The research papers on innovation or independent innovation are published in my series of monographs.

1. In January 2001, the first monograph "New Understanding and New Model of Cancer Treatment" was published.
   Hubei Science and Technology Press, Xu Ze
2. In January 2006, the second monograph "New Concepts and New Methods for Cancer Metastasis Treatment" was published.
   Beijing People's Military Medical Press, Xu Ze
   In April 2007, the General Administration of Press of the People's Republic of China issued the "Three One Hundred" Original Book Publishing Engineering Certificate.
3. In October 2011, the third monograph "New Concepts and New Methods for Cancer Treatment" was published.
   Beijing People's Military Medical Publishing House, Xu Ze, Xu Jie / Zhu
4. The fourth monograph was published in December 2015. The English version of "On Innovation Of Treatment Of Cancer" - (Therapeutic Innovation of Cancer - Volume I) was published in Washington, DC, distributed worldwide, and distributed electronically. Ze, Xu Jie
5. The fifth monograph "The Road To Overcome Cancer" <Overcoming Cancer Road> Full English version published in Washington in December, globally distributed

(5) Innovation - The basic and clinical research on anti-cancer and anti-cancer metastasis in the past 28 years has preliminarily embarked on a "Chinese-style anti-cancer", Chinese and Western medicine combined with immune regulation and treatment of cancer, we have accumulated more than 12,000 cases in 20 years The clinical application experience can be pushed to the whole country and can go to the world. It can connect with the "Belt and Road" to make Chinese medicine go to the world, so that "Chinese-style anti-cancer" and Chinese and Western medicine can combine cancer with immune regulation and control, which not only develops and enriches immunity. The content of studying cancer has brought China's medical modernization into line with the international market and is at the forefront of the world.

10. The Current Situation Analysis

A. Situation analysis (1)

a. Analyzing their respective technological advantages

The United States

China

Advantages: (+)

Advantage:(-)

1, life science   originated from
                         the United States
Molecular biology   extremely high
Genetic engineering   patent, invention
Proteomics Group   Precision medicine

1, Life Sciences   learn from
                         the United States
Molecular biology
Genetic engineering
Proteomics Group

2, cancer targeting   originated
   Treatment, drug s   from the United States
                         patent, invention

2, cancer targeting   imports from
   Treatment   the United States
   the drugs   it did not have
                         (in 2015 had a self-roduced)

3, cancer treatment   originated
   equipment   from the United States

Precision instrument   patent, invention

3, cancer treatment   imports and
   equipment   learn from
                         the United States
Precision instrument   almost no patent

4, molecular level   cancer diagnostic techniques
   detection   mostly derived from
Genetic level tests   the United States
Tumor marker   patent, invention

4, new surgery   learn from
   Innovative new   the Unite States
   Surgery Technique   no self patent
                         Invention

6, minimally invasive   derived from
   technology   the United States
States,
minimally invasive   and Europe
equipment
Well-equipped   patent, invention

6, minimally invasive   imported from
   technology   the Unite

minimally invasive   Europe
equipment   without patent
                         and invention

United States

Advantages: (+) China

Advantage:(-)

1, life sciences from the United States

Molecular biology

Genetic engineering patent, invention

Proteomics Group Precision Medicine 1. Life Science

Molecular biology learned from the United States

Genetic engineering, studying and studying in the United States

Proteomics group

2, cancer targeted treatment from the United States

Treatment, drug patent, invention 2, cancer targeted treatment imported from the United States

Treatment, drugs, not (self-produced in 2015)

3, cancer diagnosis and treatment equipment mostly from the United States

Precision instrument patent, invention

3, cancer diagnosis and treatment equipment imported from the United States, from the United States

Precision instruments, training, training, almost no patent

4, molecular level detection cancer diagnosis technology,

Gene level detection

Tumor markers Patent, invention 4, new surgery or study and study from the United States

Innovative new hands, no patents, inventions

Technique

6, minimally invasive technology are from the United States

And minimally invasive equipment

Excellent equipment, patents, inventions 6, minimally invasive technology imported from the United States and Europe

And minimally invasive equipment, learning and studying from the United States

Equipment does not have a patented invention

In short, modern medicine originated from Europe and the United States. In the past 100 years, the modern American medicine has developed and advanced and has been far ahead. It has developed into microscopic → ultra-micro → precision medicine and nanotechnology. However, modern medicine in China is still far behind and depends on imported Medication an follows behind to learn. There are 39 cancer research centers in the United States, and the Anderson Cancer Center is one of the first three comprehensive cancer treatment centers designated by the US National Cancer Action Program in 1971. It is also one of the 39 comprehensive cancer treatment centers designated by the Oncology Medical Association. The Anderson Cancer Center is recognized as the best cancer hospital in the world, ranking first in the field of cancer treatment and scientific research. The MD Anderson Cancer Center has more than 20,000 employees, including nearly 2,000 doctors and more than 500 beds. Each year, more than 19,000 inpatients in the United States and other countries are admitted, and the number of outpatients per day is 1,800.

As mentioned above, China's modern medicine is still far behind the United States. In cancer treatment, it relies more on imported medicine, and its own inventions, patents, and intellectual property rights are small.

What is the race against people? Is there any comparison? What do you want to compare?

Because our country's advantages are:

1. Traditional Chinese medications, anti-cancer traditional Chinese medications, immune-regulating and controlling traditional Chinese medication, promoting blood circulation and removing blood stasis medications with anti-thrombosis
2. Combination of Chinese and Western medication, combined with innovation

The advantage of the United States is:

Modern medicine, advanced treatment technology, targeted drugs.

It should play our country's advantages, potential, and should increase efforts to develop, and to explore the advantages of Chinese herbal medicine.

Situation Analysis:

Western medicine: the United States>China

Chinese medicine: China > the United States

Surgery: the United States and China are the same (the United States can do the surgery, China can do and also has more cases)

Diagnostic technology equipment: The United States and China are the same (large hospitals have equipments)

Radiology therapy and chemotherapy: China and the United States are the same

Chinese medication: China >the United States [the majority can improve symptoms, improve physical fitness, prolong survival, increase immunity (lesions do not shrink, but can survive with tumors, live a long time), can be used as adjuvant therapy of surgery, can develop and dig.

Experimental research, innovation, patents, inventions, new drugs, targeted drugs: The United States>China

B. Analyzing the current status

1. The current Status: Please look at the current situation: (currently the 21st century)

(1) Status of cancer incidence

The more patients are treated, the more new cases of cancer in China each year are 3.12 million cases, with an average of 8550 new cancer patients per day, and 6 people diagnosed with cancer every minute in the country.

(2) Status of cancer mortality:

It stays the high level without decreasing. It is the highest cause of death in urban and rural areas in China. The number of deaths due to cancer is 2.7 million per year, and an average of 7,500 people die every day from cancer.

(3) Status of treatment:

Despite the application of traditional three major treatments for nearly a hundred years, thousands of cancer patients have been exposed to radiotherapy and chemotherapy, but what is the result? So far, cancer is still the leading cause of death. Although regular, systematic radiotherapy and/or chemotherapy, or radiotherapy and chemotherapy, have not stopped cancer metastasis and recurrence, the results have been minimal.

(4) Current status of the hospital model of the oncology hospital or oncology:

1. Fully focused on treatment, focusing on the middle and late stages, poor efficacy, exhausted human and financial resources, and failed to achieve lower mortality, improve cure rate, and reduce morbidity.
2. only treatment without prevention, or attention to treatment with little prevention, the more treatment the more patients.
3. ignored the "three early" and ignored precancerous lesions.
4. Many large-scale cancer hospitals and university affiliated hospitals have no laboratories (or centers) to establish basic research or clinical basic research on cancer, because without the breakthrough of basic research, clinical efficacy is difficult to improve. "Oncology" is still the most backward discipline in the current medical sciences. Why? Because the etiology, pathogenesis, pathophysiology of oncology are still unclear, people still lack sufficient understanding of its pathogenesis and cancer cell metastasis mechanism, and still lack sufficient understanding of the complex biological behavior of cancer cells, so the current treatment plan is still It is quite blind, so it is necessary to establish a laboratory for basic research and clinical basic research.
5. The road that has passed in a century is to attention to treatment with little prevention. Prevention cancer and anti-cancer are human career and causes, but for many years we have only been working on cancer treatment, and we have done very little on cancer prevention work, and almost never done it.

2. What to do:

(1) Conducting scientific research on cancer is an urgent need of the current oncology discipline.

1. It must know the current problems of oncology
2. It must know the problems in the current treatment

(2) How can we reduce the incidence rate, improve the cure rate and reduce the mortality rate?

1. How to improve cancer cure rate and reduce mortality
    ——The way out for cancer treatment is "three early" (early detection, early diagnosis, early treatment), early cancer treatment is effective and can be cured.
    In particular, precancerous lesions are well treated and can be cured. One-third of cancers can be cured by early treatment.
2. How to reduce the incidence of cancer
    ——The way to fight cancer is prevention, and more than 1/3 of cancer can be prevented.

C. Analyzing the next research prospects

1. Analyzing that we should develop our advantages in areas where China has advantages.

China also has our advantages. We should give full play to our advantages in areas where our country has advantages. In the field of cancer research, traditional Chinese medication is an advantage of China. To play the role of this advantage in the field of cancer research, to explore and develop cancer prevention and anti-cancer herbal medications, the study of this advantage should be a strategic vision of international significance.

The combination of Chinese and Western medicine is the characteristics and advantages of Chinese medicine. The goal of combining Chinese and Western medicine should be to combine innovation, and the goal of combining innovation should be to improve the treatment effect. The standard of efficacy of cancer patients should be: patients have a long survival time, good quality of life, and fewer complications.

The combination of Chinese and Western medicine, it comes from Chinese medicine, higher than Chinese medicine; it comes from Western medicine, higher than Western medicine, the combination of the goal is to combine innovation, combined with the results of innovation should be innovative "Chinese medicine", innovation "Chinese-style anti-cancer."

At present, in addition to research on synthetic drugs, countries around the world are also studying herbs in the region and the country. Scientists have returned to nature to find new anticancer drugs and study the immunotherapeutic capabilities of biological response modifiers. There are many natural medicines in this field in China, such as lentinan, ginseng polysaccharide, ganoderma lucidum polysaccharide, and polysaccharides of Hericium erinaceus. Many natural plant herbs contain various histones, polysaccharides, etc., and all have good effects of biological response modifiers., have immunomodulatory effects. It is necessary to conduct further in-depth research in the experiments with experimental tumor research conditions, using modern science and technology, strictly, scientifically, objectively, and realistically, and carry out in-depth and modern research on traditional Chinese medicine immunopharmacology.

Many Chinese herbal medicines are immune enhancers, biological response modifiers, and nourishing drugs. Many of them can strengthen the body's immunity and anti-cancer power. Trying to improve the body's immunity is an important measure to prevent cancer and cancer. How to improve immunity? Chinese herbal medicine is an extremely important advantage.

2. The research work we have carried out in 30 years:

(1) New findings in anti-cancer and anti-cancer metastasis research

① it was found from the results of follow-up:
A. The postoperative recurrence and metastasis are the key to long-term efficacy of surgery

B, suggesting that clinicians must pay attention to and study of postoperative recurrence, metastasis prevention and control measures

② it was found from the experimental tumor study
A, the experimental results suggest that: animal model can be made after the removal of thymus

B, the experimental results suggest that: the first low immunization, and then easy to occur the occurrence of cancer, development

C, the experimental results suggest that: metastasis is immune-related, and immune dysfunction may promote cancer metastasis

D, the experimental results suggest that: the host thymus immediately showed acute atrophy after inoculated cancer cells, cell proliferation was blocked, the volume was significantly reduced.

E, the experimental results suggest that some experimental mice are not vaccinated, or the tumor is very small, the thymus is not obvious atrophy, in order to study the relationship between tumor and thymus atrophy, cancer cells were inoculated in mice after the tumor grows to the thumb size and then removed them, after a month anatomical findings are that thymus is no longer atrophy.

F, the above experimental results show that: the progress of the tumor makes the thymus atrophy, then, we can use some ways to prevent the host thymus atrophy, so that the use of mice fetal liver, fetal spleen, fetal thymocyte transplantation to reconstruct immunization reconstruction The results showed that: S, T, L three groups of cells combined transplantation, the recent tumor complete regression rate was 40%, long-term tumor complete rate of regression was 46.6%, the group of complete regression of the tumor were long-term survival.

In summary, from the above series of experimental studies, it is found that thymus atrophy and immune dysfunction may be one of the causes and development mechanisms of cancer.

③ XZ put forward to : " one of the cancer etiology, pathogenesis may be thymus atrophy and immune function" in the monograph and at the International Conference on Oncology. After investigation, it is the first time that it was reported in the international community.

④ XZ put forward to: "XZ-C immunomodulation therapy - the theory Basic and experimental basis of the principle of treatment " protect thymus and increase immune "(to protect the thymus, increase immune, protect marrow and produce blood (to protect bone blood stem cells) " in the monograph and at the International Conference on Oncology, which is the first time to be proposed in the international.

⑤ XZ proposed in the monograph: " the goals or targets of cancer treatment must be for both the tumor and the host, the establishment of a comprehensive treatment concept," the current domestic and foreign hospitals, chemotherapy is only to kill cancer cells, we think this is a one-sided treatment concept, not only did not protect the patient's immune system, but also a large number of killing the host immune cells and bone hematopoietic cells, resulting in the more chemotherapy the lower immune function; while chemotherapy is done, the metastasis is occurring.

⑥ XZ initiatives in the monograph: the establishment of a multi-disciplinary comprehensive treatment program

Whole course of treatment is as the main axis: to surgery-based + biological therapy, immunotherapy, integrated traditional Chinese and Western medicine treatment, XZ-C immunoregulation treatment … …

Short-term treatment for the auxiliary axis: to radiotherapy, chemotherapy-based, not a long course of treatment, cannot be excessive, and it should change the current treatment of over-treatment status quo in some hospitals.

⑦ XZ in the book put forward the new concept of cancer anti-metastasis therapy, that: in the human body there are three manifestations of cancer: the first for the primary cancer; the second for the metastasis cancer cells; the third is the cells on the metastasis way

The annihilation, blocking or interference of the cancer cells on the metastasis way to cut off the new pathways of metastasis is the key to anti-cancer metastasis.

⑧ **It initially formed a theoretical system of XZ-C treatment cancer: immune regulation therapy.**

1. Resection of thymus can be made to produce animal model
    Laboratory animal found
    experiments found disease
2. With the progress of cancer, thymus was progressive atrophy

Due to: thymus atrophy, immune dysfunction → put forward the theoretical basis of treatment: XZ-C immunoregulation "protect thymus and increase immune function" → exclusive development products : XZ-C1-10 → clinical validation: 20 years outpatient observation was followed up with advanced cancer patients more than 12,000 cases, can improve the quality of life, and extend the survival period.

(2) Overview of XZ-C immunomodulation anticancer Chinese medications

① the experimental study of finding a new anti-cancer and the external anti-recurrence new drugs from the natural drug.

The existing anti-cancer drugs kill both cancer cells and also the normal cells and have the adverse reactions. We searched the new drugs which only inhibit cancer cells without affecting the normal cells through the cancer-bearing mice in vivo tumor inhibition test from the natural drug.

A, the use of cancer cells in vitro culture method, the screening experimental study of Chinese herbal medicine screening effect - in vitro screening test

B, the manufacture of animal models, the experimental study of Chinese herbal medicine on the tumor in vivo tumor inhibition rate - in vivo tumor suppression screening test

We spent a total of three years, the commonly used traditional anti-cancer prescription and reported anti-cancer prescription in the use of 200 kinds of Chinese herbal medicine, taste flavor of the tumor in vivo tumor inhibition test. A total of nearly 6,000 tumor-bearing animal models were obtained. After each mouse died, the anatomy of the liver, spleen, lung, thymus and kidney was performed. 48 kinds of them were screened out with having anti-tumor effect, meanwhile there are better immune regulation traditional Chinese medication.

②<u>clinical validation work</u>

Through the above four years to explore the recurrence and metastasis of the basic experimental study, and after 3 years from the natural drug screening in the experimental study to find a group of XZ-Cl-10 immune regulation of traditional Chinese medicine, and then through 30 years in more than 12,000 cases in the late or Postoperative metastatic cancer patients with clinical validation, the application of XZ-C immunomodulatory anti-cancer traditional Chinese medications have achieved good results and can improve the quality of life of patients, improve patient symptoms, significantly prolong the survival of patients.

(3) The experiment study and clinical observation of XZ-C immunoregulation anti-cancer traditional Chinese medicine in the treatment of malignant tumors

① XZ-C immunoregulation anti-cancer traditional Chinese medication is the result of the modernization of traditional Chinese medication

② XZ-C immunoregulation anti-cancer Chinese medication treatment of cancer cases and typical cases

<u>(4) to study the traditional Chinese medication anti-cancer effect must carry out modern scientific research, analyze active ingredients, and purify and do modern immunopharmacology experiments and research.</u>

Although we should play the advantages of our country with our country has the dvantage in our country, in the field of cancer research, Chinese drugs and Chinese medicine, the combination of Chinese and Western medicine is the advantage of our country, play this advantage in the field of cancer research, it should conduct scientific research, and conduct experimental research, active ingredient analysis, purification and modern pharmacological experiments to study the traditional Chinese medicine anti-cancer effect and its mechanism, we must study the active ingredients so as to Chinese medicine to become modern and scientific.

But it must be aware of the strengths of traditional Chinese medicine, what weaknesses are, and whether there is no toxicity or not, the application should be considered for the patient's "long", "short", "get", "lost", it must conduct modern scientific research, it should be scientific research, analysis, clinical validation, should be scientific, authenticity, safety, doctors in scientific research, clinical application must be both ability and political integrity, medical is benevolence, legislation and morals for the first.

(5) Analysis of the next step of the study prospects and the prospective assessment of cancer treatment:

- Molecular targeted drug therapy is eye-catching
- Immunomodulatory drugs are promising
- Immunotherapy opens a new era of cancer therapy
- Application of vaccine to cancer is a human hope
- The way out of cancer treatment is three early
- The way out of cancer is preventing

3, the initial work that we have been in the fight against cancer:

(1) Xu Ze published in October 2011, "the new concept of cancer treatment and new methods" monograph of Chapter 38 with a chapter of the length of "to overcome the strategic thinking and suggestions of cancer"

(2)In June 2013 Xu Ze also proposed "to overcome the cancer to start the general idea and design", in an attempt to reduce the incidence of cancer, reduce cancer mortality, improve the cure rate, prolong survival, the total attack is anti- Cancer, three carriages go hand in hand

(3) Xu Ze put forward in August 2013 for the first time in the international community that : " the XZ-C research program to overcome the cancer and to launch a total attack " - the overall strategy and development of cancer treatment in China

4. in July 2015 Xu Ze proposed the feasibility report from the following four aspects to conquer cancer and launch a total attack

"XZ-C proposed the research program to attack the cancer and launch a total offensive " - China's cancer treatment of the overall strategic reform and development

1. in the international it is the first time proposed:

"the feasibility the need of the report to capture the total attack of cancer"

② in the international community for the first time it was put forward :

"To build the hospital with the prevention and the treatment of cancer during the development and occurrence of cancer of the whole process"

(the Global Demonstration Prevention and Treatment Hospital)

"the hospital vision and feasibility report of building anti-cancer and treatment of cancer throughout the prevention and treatment"

- Describe the necessity and feasibility of establishing a complete prevention and cure hospital

③ in the international it was the first time proposed:

"the basic vision and feasibility report To build the general idea of conquering cancer and the science city"

- is equivalent to the framework of the design of conquering cancer with China characteristic.

④ in the international it was the first time proposed:

"the necessity and feasibility report of building a moderately society at the same time, it was proposed" ride research "- perform ing the medicine research and cancer prevention and cancer control and cancer prevention and treatment " — adhere to walk on the new way with the Chinese characteristics of anti-cancer and control cancer.

These four research projects in the international community were put forward for the first time and opened up a new field of anti-cancer research.

To propose to capture the total attack of cancer is unprecedented work.

(5) Xu Ze's fourth monograph book ": "On Innovation Of Treatment Of Cancer" - (Cancer Treatment Innovation Theory) was published in Washington, DC in December 2015, in English, published worldwide, and also released electronic version to Introduce the new book.

Introduction to the new book: the experimental study of Chinese medicine immunopharmacology of traditional Chinese and Western medicine combined with anti-cancer research at the molecular level has formed XZ-C immune regulation of the theoretical system of cancer.

Walking out the new path of an immune regulation with traditional Chinese medications which regulate immune activity, prevent thymus atrophy, promote thymic hyperplasia, protect bone hematopoietic function, improve immune surveillance at the molecular level of the combination of western and Chinese medications to overcome cancer.

How to overcome the cancer I see:

- To avoid empty talking, to focus on hard work, no matter how far away it is from the cancer, it should always start.
- To attack cancer should start to launch the total attack, what is the total attack against cancer?

The total attack is to conduct work and to develop in full swing simultaneously for three stages of cancer prevention, cancer control and cancer treatment during the whole process of the occurrence and development of cancer,.

That is:

To prevent cancer - before the formation of cancer

To control cancer - malignant transformation of precancerous lesions

To treat cancer - has formed a lesion or metastasis

The main target of launching the cancer attack: to reduce cancer lesions, reduce cancer mortality, improve the cure rate, prolong survival, improve quality of life, reduce complications.

- What should I do next? Now it is proposed to overcome cancer and to launch a total attack. It is hoped to get leadership support at all levels. I know that to achieve the purpose of cancer prevention, cancer control and treatment of cancer must be government leadership, government-led, experts, scholars efforts, the masses to participate in the mobilization of all, thousands of households to participate in order to do.

- Because cancer patients are getting more and more, the morbidity is on the rise, the mortality rate is high, it is recognized that in order to stop at the cancer source it should not only pay attention to treatment, but also pay attention to prevention; the research goal and focus should be on the study of prevention and treatment of cancer during the whole process of the occurrence and development of cancer.

D. "Dawning C-type plan" scientific and technological innovation, realization of outlines, avoiding empty talk, heavy work, starting

1. Combination of Chinese and Western medicine
   Comprehensive (Chinese and Western) anti-cancer strength
   From Chinese medicine - higher than Chinese medicine
   From Western medicine - higher than Western medicine
   (see separate article)
2. I would like to invite Hubei University of Traditional Chinese Medicine, Wuhan Association for Science and Technology
   Co-organized by Wuhan Anticancer Research Association under the leadership of the province and city
   (see separate article)
3. Hubei and Wuhan four collaborations, lead
   Hubei University of Traditional Chinese Medicine
   Tongji
   Concord
   Wu Da
   (see separate article)

4. Organize the combination of Chinese and Western forces, four collaborations, and lead
   Hubei·Wuhan—Hubei University of Traditional Chinese Medicine
   Shanghai - Fudan University
   Tianjin - Nankai University
   Shanghai - Shanghai University of Traditional Chinese Medicine
   (see separate article)
5. Division of labor, each with a focus on achieving goals and achievements, achievements
   Jiangxi
   Shanxi
   Liaoning
   (see separate article)
6. the task

1. overcome the general attack of cancer
2. Establish a global demonstration of prevention and treatment hospitals (the combination of Chinese and Western medicine at the molecular level, prevention and treatment)
3. Prepare to "conquer the Cancer Science City"
4. Establish multidisciplinary research institute
5. Preparation for Environmental Protection and Cancer Research Institute
6. Establish a cancer animal experiment center (all above are provincial)
   (see separate article)
7. Hope: In Hubei and Wuhan, the country will establish the first "Science City to overcome the general attack of cancer" and establish the world's first "Science City to overcome the general attack of cancer."
   Why is it set up in the university town of Huangjiahu?
   Because it depends on Hubei University of Traditional Chinese Medicine (Chinese medicine, Chinese and Western medicine combined)
   Wu Da
   Huake University
   invite:
8. Chairman of the General Design and Academic Committee of Science City: Professor Xu Ze (Chinese Medicine)
   Secretary-General: Professor Zou Shengquan (Tongji)
   Chief Dean: Professor Hong Guangxiang (Concord)
   (see separate article)

invite:

9. "Conquering Cancer Science City" Chinese and Western Medicine combined with academic leaders: Academician Wu Xianzhong (Tianjin)
Academician Tang Wei (Shanghai)
Professor Xu Ze (Wuhan)
(see separate article)

B. The Situation Analysis (2)

1. Why is it not to be led by the Oncology, Cancer Center or Provincial Cancer Hospital of some famous university affiliated hospitals in China or our province? They have superior equipment conditions and superb medical technology, but are led by the University of Chinese Medicine?

Because the current status of modern medicine in the oncology and cancer centers of the affiliated institutions of higher education institutions in China and our province is:

- Life sciences, molecular biology, genetic engineering, and protein science groups are all studied and advanced from the United States, and they have no innovative patent inventions;
- Targeted therapeutic drugs and monoclonal antibody drugs are imported from the United States, and they have no innovative patents or inventions;
- Cancer diagnosis and treatment equipment and precision instruments are imported from the United States. They have studied and studied from the United States, and they have almost no innovation patents or inventions.
- New surgery for tumors or innovative new surgical techniques, from the United States to further study and study, without their own innovative patents, inventions;
- Minimally invasive technology and minimally invasive equipment, all imported from the United States, studied and studied from the United States, and have no innovative patents or inventions.

In short, the source of modern medicine has come from Europe and the United States. In the past 100 years, the modern medicine in the United States has developed and advanced, and has developed into precision oncology medicine. Our oncology lacks innovative medicine, medicine and technology in our own oncology, innovative academics, theories, innovative patents and inventions.

We must be self-reliant, independent innovation, original innovation, and breakthrough medical and scientific achievements. Only then can we have our own medical, pharmaceutical, and scientific achievements, and we can have our own doctors, medicines, and scientific and technological achievements to compete with others and race with others.

Innovation is not only technology, product innovation, but also basic theoretical innovation, and theoretical innovation is the biggest achievement. Scientific development is based on the innovation of basic theory, which is the biggest invention.

2. Why is it led by the University of Chinese Medicine?
because:

(1) We should give full play to China's advantages in areas where China has advantages. In the field of cancer research, traditional Chinese medicine is an advantage of China. We should play this advantage in cancer research and discover and develop effective anti-cancer and anti-cancer effects. Chinese herbal medicine.

In-depth research should be carried out to analyze and purify the active ingredients; to carry out research on the immunological pharmacology of traditional Chinese medicine; to carry out research on molecular level and gene level, so that the modernization of Chinese herbal medicines is in line with international standards.

(2) The combination of Chinese and Western medicine is the characteristic and advantage of Chinese medicine. It comes from Chinese medicine, higher than Chinese medicine. It comes from Western medicine, higher than Western medicine, and is a combination of Chinese medicine and Western medicine. 1+1=2,2>1, which makes the treatment of cancer combined with Chinese and Western medicine more perfect and reasonable, and improves the curative effect. Because traditional cancer therapy (surgery, radiotherapy, chemotherapy) reduces the body's immune function, and immune regulation and anti-cancer Chinese medicines increase the body's immune function, and become a comprehensive treatment, post-operative + immunity, radiotherapy + Chinese medicine immunity (immunotherapy) Chemotherapy + Chinese medicine immunization (immunotherapy) will inevitably improve its efficacy.

1. Why is Chinese herbal medicine the advantage of China in cancer research? Because treatment must be directed to the cause, pathogenesis, pathophysiology The following multidisciplinary and cancer-related relationships should be sought for treatments, drugs

a. cancer and immunity have a positive relationship, should look for immunomodulatory drugs;

b. some cancers have a positive relationship with the virus, should look for antiviral drugs;

c. some cancers have a positive relationship with endocrine hormones, should look for drugs that regulate endocrine hormones;

d. some cancers are related to fungi, and anti-fungal drugs should be sought;

e. Some cancers are associated with chronic inflammation and should be searched for drugs that are resistant to chronic inflammation.

These immune regulation, adjustment of endocrine hormones, anti-virus, etc., are rare in modern medicine and western medicine. However, China's Fuzheng Guben and Buxu Chinese herbal medicines are rich in resources, and have immune regulation, hormone adjustment, and anti-virus. Good function, and has a long history and clinical application experience and works. In recent years, some researchers and graduate students have carried out some experimental analysis and research on the molecular level of Chinese herbal medicine. It should be said that in the study of cancer, the richness of Chinese herbal medicine resources is an advantage.

2. Why is Chinese herbal medicine the advantage of China in the field of cancer research? Our experiment has the following experimental basis and accumulated data of our own clinical verification.

Because our laboratory has screened out 48 Chinese herbal medicines that have a good anti-tumor rate.

Existing anticancer drugs not only kill cancer cells but also normal cells, and have large adverse reactions. We have tried new cancer drugs in cancer-bearing mice to find new drugs that inhibit cancer cells without affecting normal cells. We spent a full three years on the anti-tumor screening experiments of cancer-bearing animals in 200 kinds of Chinese herbal medicines used in traditional anti-cancer prescriptions and anti-cancer agents reported in various places. As a result, 48 strains were screened for better tumor inhibition.

Looking for Chinese herbal medicine, screening anti-cancer, anti-metastatic new drugs:

The purpose is to screen out new anti-cancer, anti-metastatic, anti-recurrent and anti-cancer drugs that have no drug resistance, no toxic side effects, and high selectivity.

To this end, we conducted an experimental study in the laboratory for screening anticancer and anti-metastatic drugs from traditional Chinese medicine for three years:

a. Using the method of in vitro culture of cancer cells, screening experiments on the inhibition rate of Chinese herbal medicine.

b. Manufacture of animal models of cancer-bearing animals, and conduct experimental research on the rate of cancer suppression in cancer-bearing animals by Chinese herbal medicine.

Experimental results:

Among the 200 Chinese herbal medicines screened by animal experiments in our laboratory, 48 strains were selected to have certain or even excellent inhibitory effects on cancer cell proliferation, and the tumor inhibition rate was 75-90%. However, there are also some commonly used traditional Chinese medicines that are generally considered to have anti-cancer effects. After screening for animal tumors in vitro and in vivo, there is no anti-cancer effect. In this group, 152 kinds of anti-cancer effects were eliminated by animal experiments.

The 48 kinds of traditional Chinese medicines with good tumor inhibition rate were selected by this experiment, and then the anti-tumor experiments were carried out in vivo by optimizing the combination. Finally, the XU ZE China preparation with immunomodulation and anti-cancer Chinese medicine with Chinese characteristics was developed (XZ). —C1-10).

XZ-C1 can significantly inhibit cancer cells, but does not affect normal cells; XZ-C4 can promote thymic hyperplasia and increase immunity; XZ-C8 can protect the marrow from hematopoiesis and protect bone marrow hematopoietic function.

3 Why is Chinese herbal medicine the advantage of China in cancer research?

Because our laboratory finds from the Chinese herbal medicine to promote thymic hyperplasia, prevent thymus atrophy, and improve the immune regulation of traditional Chinese medicine.

We conducted a full 4 years of oncology research work in the laboratory. Our laboratory experimental results showed that the thymus of the cancer-bearing mice showed progressive atrophy, the volume was reduced, the cell proliferation was blocked, and the mature cells were reduced. By the end of the tumor, the thymus is extremely atrophied and the texture becomes hard.

From the above experimental studies, it is found that thymus atrophy and low immune function may be one of the pathogenic factors and pathogenesis of tumors, so it is necessary to try to prevent thymus atrophy, promote thymocyte proliferation, and increase immunity. The immune function of the body, especially cellular immunity, the function of T lymphocytes, and the immune regulation function of the thymus should be explored at the molecular level, and methods for immune regulation and effective drug research should be sought.

How should we find new ways to regulate immune therapy?

In order to prevent thymus atrophy, promote thymocyte proliferation, and increase immunity, we look for both Chinese medicine and western medicine. The existing medicines of western medicine can improve immunity and promote the proliferation of thymus. So we changed to look for Chinese herbal medicine.

Why do you look for drugs that promote thymic hyperplasia, prevent thymus atrophy, and boost immunity from traditional Chinese medicine?

Because Chinese medicine's tonic drugs generally contain the role of regulating immunity. Chinese medicine has Chinese medicine and polysaccharide Chinese medicine.

a. tonic Chinese medicine, have the role of regulating the body's immune function. When the animal is at a low level of immune activity (such as dethymus, aging animals, or chemotherapy drugs cyclophosphamide inhibition and tumor animals), the tonic drugs improve the body's immunity is more significant.

b. Anti-cancer immunity of traditional Chinese medicine polysaccharides is progressing rapidly. A large number of immunopharmacological studies have been carried out at the molecular level. Polysaccharides can improve the body's immune surveillance system, including natural killer cells (NK), macrophages (MΦ), and killer T cells. (CTL), T cells, LAK cells, tumor infiltrating lymphocytes (TIL), interleukin (IL) and other cytokines are active to kill tumor cells.

Traditional Chinese medicine and western medicine have their own strengths, each with its own shortness. Compared with Western medicine immunopharmacology, traditional Chinese medicine immunopharmacology has its own characteristics and advantages, and each has its own shortcomings. The advantage of traditional Chinese medicine immunology is that a large number of Chinese medicines have the effect of regulating the body's immune function. Chinese medicine is rich in source and is an effective medicine for long-term clinical treatment. After extraction, it may obtain active ingredients and obvious pharmacological effects (including immunomodulatory effects). The research process saves people time and has high efficiency.

3. Why is the race proposed by our Institute of Experimental Surgery, Hubei University of Traditional Chinese Medicine?

(1) For 28 years, we have achieved scientific research results and technological innovation series of cancer research:

Can participate in competitions, participate in learning, and inspire us to move forward

The goal of the competition is: 1 to prolong the survival time of cancer patients (long live), good quality of life, and fewer complications.

2 reduce the incidence of cancer, improve the cure rate and reduce the mortality rate.

(2) In the past 28 years, we have obtained research and research achievements in anti-cancer and anti-cancer metastasis, and scientific and technological innovation series:

A. New findings in experimental research, new theory, new theory

a. "thymus atrophy, low immune function is one of the causes and pathogenesis of cancer"
   - propose a new concept of cancer treatment principles
b. "Theoretical Basis and Experimental Basis of XZ-C Immunomodulation Therapy"
   ——Proposed the theoretical basis and experimental basis of cancer immune regulation therapy

B. Propose new concepts and new initiatives for cancer treatment

a. "Cancer treatment should change the concept, establish a comprehensive treatment concept"
   - propose a new concept of cancer treatment principles
b. "A new model for the combination of multidisciplinary treatment of cancer"
   - Proposing a new concept of a combination of cancer treatment models

C, cancer metastasis research, theoretical innovation

a. "There are three main forms of cancer in the human body"
   ——Proposed theoretical innovation of cancer metastasis treatment
b. "Two Points and One Line" in the Whole Process of Cancer Development
——Proposed theoretical innovation of cancer metastasis treatment
c. "Three Steps of Anticancer Metastasis Treatment"
   ——Proposed theoretical innovation of new concept of cancer metastasis treatment

——Incorporate the "eight steps" of cancer cell transfer into "three stages" and try to break through

d. "Open up the third field of anti-cancer metastasis treatment"

——Proposed the theoretical innovation of cancer metastasis treatment, and found and proposed the third field of human anti-cancer metastasis treatment

——The circulatory system has a large number of immune surveillance cells, and the "main battlefield" of cancer cells on the way to annihilation is in the blood circulation.

D, exclusive research and development products: XZ-C immune regulation anti-cancer Chinese medicine product series

a. "Overview of XZ-C Immunoregulation of Anticancer Traditional Chinese Medicine"

——Adopting the method of in vitro culture of cancer cells to conduct screening experiments on the inhibition rate of Chinese herbal medicine

——Manufacturing a cancer animal model and conducting an experimental study on the cancer suppression rate of Chinese herbal medicines in cancer-bearing animals

b. "XZ-C immunomodulation anticancer Chinese medicine treatment of malignant tumors experimental study and clinical efficacy observation"

——Animal experiment research and clinical application

——XZ-C immunomodulation Chinese medicine is the result of the modernization of traditional Chinese medicine

c. "XZ-C immunomodulation anticancer Chinese medicine treatment of cancer cases list and some typical cases"

E. Propose cancer treatment reform and innovation

a. "Cancer Treatment Reform and Innovation Research"

——Adhere to the road of scientific research and innovation of anti-cancer transfer with Chinese characteristics

——1-8 of cancer treatment reform and innovation research

b. "Get out of a new road to overcome cancer"

——The theoretical system of XZ-C immunomodulation therapy has been initially formed, and it is undergoing clinical application and observation verification.

——There are exclusive research and development products, XZ-C immunomodulation anti-cancer Chinese medicine series, there have been a large number of clinically validated cases

——In the past 20 years, a new road to overcome cancer has been preliminarily

Now is the fourth stage of our research work, which is being carried out and carried out, research work, step by step, positioning the research target or "target" to reduce the incidence of cancer, improve the cure rate and prolong the survival period.

At present, the tumor hospital or oncology hospital model is fully focused on treatment. For the middle and late patients, the curative effect is poor, the human and financial resources are exhausted, and the incidence rate is not reduced, and the more patients are treated. The status quo is: the road that has passed in a century is to rectify the light, or to cure it. For many years we have only been working on cancer treatment. However, work on cancer prevention has been done very little and almost nothing has been done. As a result, the incidence of cancer continues to rise.

In short, anti-cancer has not been taken seriously, and prevention has not been taken seriously. The prevention of the old-fashioned talks is mainly based on failure to pay attention.

How to do? How to reduce the incidence of cancer? How to improve the cure rate of cancer? How to reduce cancer mortality? How to prolong the survival period? How to improve the quality of life?

Should be launched to overcome the general attack of cancer, prevention and treatment are equally important.

The goal of conquering cancer should be: reduce morbidity, increase cure rate, reduce mortality, prolong survival, improve quality of life, and reduce complications.

At present, the global hospitals and hospitals in China are all devoted to treatment, re-treatment and light prevention, or only cure.

XZ-C believes that this mode of hospitalization or cancer treatment is unlikely to overcome cancer and it is impossible to reduce the incidence. Global hospitals and hospitals in China must carry out overall strategic reforms on cancer treatment, focusing on treatment and focusing on prevention and treatment.

Therefore, we propose to launch a general attack plan and design to overcome cancer. XZ-C (Xu Ze-China) proposed to launch a general attack, that is, the three stages of anti-cancer, cancer control and cancer treatment were carried out in full swing.

Application report for "Necessity and Feasibility Report for Overcoming the General Attack of Cancer Attack"

Application report for "XZ-C Scientific Research Plan for Overcoming Cancer Attack"

In short, as mentioned above, China's modern medicine relies on imported medicine for cancer treatment, and its own inventions, patents, and intellectual property rights are small.

So how do you race? What to take to the game?

As mentioned above, in the field of cancer treatment, Chinese herbal medicine is China's advantage. In the past 28 years, the experimental research of our Experimental Surgery Institute and the clinical validation of a large number of cases in the oncology clinic for 20 years have confirmed that in the treatment of cancer, Chinese herbal medicine is China. The advantages can go international and benefit patients. Many cancer patients have significantly prolonged their survival.

Therefore, our country's advantages are:

1. Traditional Chinese medicine, anti-cancer traditional Chinese medicine, immune control traditional Chinese medicine, blood stasis anti-cancer suppository Chinese medicine
2. Combination of Chinese and Western medicine, combined with innovation
   $1+1=2$
   $2>1$

The advantages of the United States are:

Modern medicine, advanced diagnosis and treatment technology, targeted drugs

Should give full play to China's advantages, we should increase efforts to develop and explore the advantages of Chinese herbal medicine

Therefore, I think: should be the game, should race

Chinese and Western medicines have their own strengths and shortcomings. The two should complement each other and combine advantages. One runs in the inner circle, one runs in the outer circle, and one main attack cancer.

Running with the "New Moon Plan" is not a challenge or a challenge, but to motivate yourself to achieve the "Dawning C-type plan" and move forward together to reach the scientific hall of cancer.

C. The Situation Analysis (3)

Conquering cancer, where is the road? - Where to go? How to go?

Analysis of the existing roads, how is the prospect? What is the future?

1.Analyzing how the occurrence and development of cancer has occurred in the past century.

I am a medical worker who has been a medical practitioner for 60 years. What I have seen in Wuhan for 65 years is that I feel that the incidence of cancer is rising. When our Central South Tongji moved from Shanghai to Wuhan in 1951, at that time, we were looking for a lung cancer patient to show the students for teaching. Even if it was a week earlier to call each hospital, it was hard to find a cancer patient. In the past, there were no cancer departments in all hospitals, only tuberculosis. Today (65 years later) is a common disease, frequently-occurring disease, each hospital has an oncology department, and some large hospitals have cancer centers, the more treatment and the more patients.

It should be analyzed, why?

It should be analyzed, what should we do? Where is the way out?

I am deeply aware that cancer should not only pay attention to treatment, but also pay attention to prevention, in order to stop at the source. The way out for cancer treatment is "three early" (early detection, early diagnosis, early treatment), and the way to fight cancer is prevention.

It should analyze, what should Wuhan do? How can we reduce the incidence? Improve the cure rate?

How can we have "three early"? It is necessary to establish a full-range hospital with control cancer + prevention cancer + treatment cancer, change the hospital mode, and change the treatment mode.

How can I prevent it? A science city should be established to overcome cancer

We will establish the first "Science City for Cancer Prevention" in Hubei and Wuhan, which will be the world's first science city to overcome cancer.

2. Analyzing the prospects of the current three traditional treatments? What is the future?

Can you rely on three major treatments to win cancer and even control and conquer cancer?

Traditional cancer therapy (surgery, chemotherapy, radiotherapy) for nearly a century, should review, reflect, summarize the lessons of success and failure.

The traditional concept holds that cancer is the continuous division and proliferation of cancer cells, and its therapeutic goal must be to kill cancer cells.

After more than half a century, what is the result of the treatment? The more patients are treated, the higher the mortality rate is. Therefore, the above three major treatment methods must be further studied and improved. The problems and shortcomings of surgery, radiotherapy and chemotherapy should be analyzed and reviewed separately.

One evaluation for chemotherapy:

Comment on the **problems and drawbacks of systemic intravenous chemotherapy for solid tumors**

The current status of cancer chemotherapy, mainly systemic intravenous chemotherapy, the route of administration of this systemic intravenous chemotherapy is:

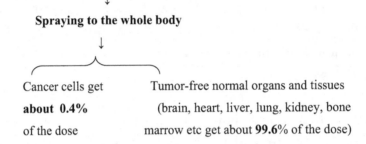

Chemotherapy cell poison → elbow vein → superior vena cava → right heart → left heart → aorta

↓

Spraying to the whole body

↓

Cancer cells get **about 0.4%** of the dose

Tumor-free normal organs and tissues (brain, heart, liver, lung, kidney, bone marrow etc get about **99.6%** of the dose)

However, the route of administration of systemic intravenous chemotherapy for such solid tumors, although it has been used in the world for decades, should we consider and analyze whether it is reasonable? Is it scientific? Does it harm the patient? Does it cause toxic side effects?

Should be analyzed and commented:

Review 1: Evaluation of the route of administration of systemic intravenous chemotherapy for solid tumors

This route of administration is not a targeted drug delivery, but a heart pump is used to administer the cytotoxic drug to the whole body with blood, so that the cytotoxic drug is distributed throughout the whole body so that each normal organs of the body (brain, heart, liver, The lungs, kidneys, and bone marrow) all obtained chemotherapy cell toxic drugs, which were damaged by them and caused toxic side effects. It is very unreasonable and very unscientific, the result is:

1. The cancer has very few drugs, only about 0.4%, and the curative effect is very small (because the cancerous area accounts for a small proportion of the total body surface area)

2. 99.6% of the cytotoxic drugs were killed to the normal proliferating cells of the whole body, causing toxic side effects of brain, heart, liver, lung, kidney, bone marrow, gastrointestinal system, hematopoietic system, immune system and endocrine system.

3. The current hospital chemotherapy drug selection has not been tested for drug susceptibility, if the drug is resistant, the chemotherapy is to kill normal tissue cells! Especially inhibit bone marrow hematopoietic cells and immune cells! It has no effect on the cancerous spot! (It was white to do a chemotherapy!)

4. So does chemotherapy kill cancer cells each time? I don't know; how much has it killed? It doesn't know, it can only say that a chemotherapy has been done once.

Therefore, this route of administration is unreasonable, unscientific, and easily leads to iatrogenic side effects.

How to do? The route of administration should be changed to the route of intravascular chemotherapy of the target organ tissue, and the drug should be directly delivered to the **"target organ"**. The drug amount is small, the curative effect is certain, and there is no toxic side effect, which is beneficial to the patient.

Review 2: Evaluation of the dose of systemic intravenous chemotherapy for solid tumors

This is to extend the experience and methods of leukemia treatment to the treatment of solid tumors. The guiding ideology is to administer according to the whole body surface area. This is not sensible and unreasonable.

why?

Because leukemia cells are distributed in the systemic blood circulation system, the "target" of treatment is also present in the systemic blood circulation system, so systemic intravenous chemotherapy is reasonable, sensible, and also in line with targeted therapy.

However, solid tumors are limited to only one organ, and the "target" of treatment should be an organ with cancer, and targeted administration should be targeted by intravascular administration of the target organ. It is not wise and unreasonable to use the leukemia treatment experience to calculate the total body surface area.

However, solid tumors are now systemic intravenous chemotherapy, and the dose is calculated according to the body surface area. In order to achieve the goal of shrinking the tumor, it is necessary to increase the amount of chemotherapy cells, which will lead to more toxic side effects and complications, and damage the patient.

How to do?

Should change the route of administration, and change to the intravascular chemotherapy route of the target organ, the drug volume is small, the curative effect is certain, and there is no toxic side reaction.

Comment 3: Analysis and evaluation of evaluation criteria for systemic intravenous chemotherapy of solid tumors

1. Why is the efficacy evaluation standard determined as relief?

At present, the clinical use of chemotherapy drugs can reduce the tumor, but the effect is usually temporary, and can not significantly extend the life of patients. Therefore, the standard of efficacy evaluation is called "alleviation." - Generally calculated by day, week or month, if complete remission is only the tumor completely disappears, lasting for more than 4 weeks, that is to say, there may be recurrence and progression after 4 weeks.

Relief is only a temporary effect and cannot be cured.

2. **Why can it only be alleviated?**

a. the patient's chemotherapy to effectively kill cancer cells only 3-5 days of intravenous infusion, there is a role in killing cancer cells, and then there is no role in killing cancer cells, it is only a short time to kill (3-5 Days), can't be done once and for all,

   After 3-5 days, the cancer cells continue to divide and proliferate, so it can only be relieved for a short time and cannot be cured.

b. Chemotherapy cell toxic drugs can only kill the differentiated mature cancer cells and cannot kill stem cells that have not yet matured, this time Chemotherapy kills matured cancer cells. After some time, those stem cells that have not yet matured gradually mature and continue to division, proliferation, divided into two, two divided into four clones, so the geometrical value added, so that the cancer is "wild fire burned, spring breeze is born again", recurrence and metastasis and progress.

Therefore, chemotherapy cannot be cured, only relieved. Can only cure the symptoms, can not cure the disease, can not rely on chemotherapy to overcome cancer.

Comment 4: What is the adjuvant chemotherapy for abdominal solid tumors that failed to prevent recurrence and metastasis?

After abdominal solid tumor surgery, why failed to prevent recurrence and metastasis? Because of systemic intravenous chemotherapy cytotoxic drugs, it is not easy to reach the portal vein by the superior vena cava. The vena cava system is generally not Interlinked with the portal system. This route of administration is unreasonable and unscientific.

Where are the cancer cells of solid tumors of the abdomen (gastric cancer,

colorectal cancer, liver cancer, biliary tract cancer, pancreatic cancer, abdominal cavity, etc.)? It is mainly in the portal system, but the current global and domestic hospitals in the abdominal solid tumor postoperative adjuvant chemotherapy from the elbow vein → **superior vena cava** → right heart → double lung → left heart → aorta → spray to the whole body organs, but not directly into the portal system **because the vena cava system is generally connected with the portal system.**

Therefore, for the abdominal malignant tumors (stomach, intestine, liver, gallbladder, pancreas, abdominal cavity and other cancers), adjuvant chemotherapy after the abdominal tumors surgery from the venous vein → **vena cava is unreasonable, unscientific, does not conform to anatomy Physiology and pathology, which does not conform to the actual path of cancer metastasis, because this route of administration cannot directly enter the portal system where cancer cells exist.**

For half a century, thousands of cancer patients all over the world and all over China have suffered huge pain from the widespread killing of normal cells by chemotherapy cell poisons. Clinicians should seriously think about, analyze, reflect, and evaluate this.

What should it be done?

The route of administration should be changed to the intravascular chemotherapy route of the target organ, so that the drug can be directly introduced into the vein. For the above solid tumor, it should not be administered by the elbow vein, but should be changed to the intravascular administration of the target organ to give the drug so as to target cancers which will greatly reduce the dose and improve the efficacy, will inevitably reduce or eliminate the toxic side effects of chemotherapy, **so that thousands of cancer patients are free from the pain and risk of adverse reactions to chemotherapy, and benefit patients.** Reducing or eliminating the side effects of chemotherapy, it will greatly reduce the medical expenses, and will save more medical expenses for the country and patients, which will help solve the problem of difficult medical treatment and expensive medical treatment. This reform will benefit millions of cancer patients.

Comment 5: There are some important misunderstandings and drawbacks in current chemotherapy

a. **chemotherapy inhibits immune function, inhibits bone marrow hematopoietic function, and reduces overall immune function.** When the cancer is inhibited, the thymus is inhibited, and chemotherapy inhibits the bone marrow. It is like "adding frost", which damages the entire central immune organ and promotes further decline in immune surveillance. It may lead to chemotherapy, metastasis, and more chemotherapy.

b. chemotherapy target kill cancer cells, is a one-sided treatment, **neglecting the body's own anti-tumor ability, neglecting the host anti-cancer system anti-cancer system (NK cells, K cells, macrophages, LAK cells)**, anti-cancer cells Factor system (IFN, IL2, TNF, LT and other factors), anti-oncogene system (Rb gene, P53 gene), neglecting the role of anti-cancer institutions and their influencing factors in the human body, ignoring the inherent factors of the body's own anti-cancer Not activated, mobilized, but only blindly killing cancer cells, this one-sided treatment concept is very unreasonable, which does not meet the biological characteristics and biological behavior of cancer cells.

Second evaluation for radiotherapy:

Comment 1: Radiation therapy can kill a large number of normal tissue cells while killing cancer cells, causing patients to suffer from radiotherapy complications, and the quality of life is declining. The toxicity and damage of radiotherapy are generally persistent and irreversible. Therefore, we must pay attention to the prevention and treatment of complications of tumor radiotherapy.

Comment 2: The main problem of cancer treatment is how to resist metastasis. If it can't solve the problem of cancer metastasis, cancer treatment can't make progress.

Radiotherapy is a local treatment, and cancer metastasis is a systemic problem. This is a major contradiction. How to play its role in anti-metastasis treatment must be seriously considered and studied in depth.

Three evaluations for surgical treatment:

Comment 1: Surgical operation is an effective and effective method for the treatment of malignant tumors. Even if cancer treatment is developed into multidisciplinary comprehensive treatment, surgery is still one of the most important and commonly used methods for the treatment of malignant tumors. It is a multidisciplinary treatment. An important part of.

Comment 2: Surgical treatment is the main treatment for solid tumors, but the design of "radical surgery" needs further research and improvement to reduce postoperative recurrence and metastasis. Attention should be paid to the "tumor-killing technique" in the operation to reduce or prevent the cancer cells from falling off, planting and metastasizing. Should pay attention to the operation of light, stable, accurate, to reduce intraoperative promotion of cancer cell metastasis and reduce the spread of cancer cells from the tumor vein. To prevent postoperative recurrence and metastasis, it must be started from the surgery. Must pay attention to the technology of tumor suppression to prevent the transfer of the incision and the drainage port.

Comment 3: Surgical treatment of solid tumors, after centuries of century history evaluation, remains the most important and reliable, the main treatment that can be relied upon, is the main scientific technology and main treatment method to overcome cancer in the future.

In short:

As mentioned above, there are problems and drawbacks in radiotherapy and chemotherapy. It is difficult to overcome cancer, and it is necessary to find another way to overcome cancer.

Recognizing the problems and drawbacks of radiotherapy and chemotherapy, it is difficult to overcome the situation of cancer. We have taken a different approach and propose: building a science city of overcoming cancer to overcome cancer and launch a general attack.

3. Analyzing the next research prospects, the evaluation of the prospective assessment of cancer treatment.

——Molecular targeted drugs attract people's attention

——The prospect of immunomodulatory drugs is gratifying

——Immunotherapy opens a new era of cancer treatment

——Biological therapy and combination of Chinese and Western medicine are two effective ways to prevent cancer metastasis

- Applying vaccine treatment is human hope

——The way out for cancer treatment is "three early"

——The way out to fight cancer is prevention

1). Molecular targeted drug therapy attracts attention

The Philadelphia chromosome opened the door to targeted therapy. In 1960, researchers in Philadelphia, USA, found a chromosomal abnormality in patients with chronic myeloid leukemia (CML). A few years later, the researchers found that this was the result of the long arm translocation of chromosomes 9 and 22. Since this chromosomal abnormality was first discovered in Philadelphia (Phiadelphia), it was named the Philadelphia (Ph) chromosome. This chromosome has also become a target for CML targeted therapy marketed 40 years later. In 2001, the first drug that was proven to be resistant to Philadelphia molecular chromosome defects - imatinib.

Later the target drug trastuzumab, which targets human epidermal growth factor receptor 2 (HER2), is then used to treat HER2-positive breast cancer.

Bevacizumab, which targets VEGF, and cetuximab, which targets EGFR, treats colorectal cancer.

Gefitinib and erlotinib targeting EGFR are used for the treatment of non-small cell lung cancer.

Molecularly targeted drugs are cell stabilizers, and most patients cannot achieve complete remission (CR) or have the partial remission (PR), but rather stable disease and improved quality of life. In addition to gefitinib, erlotinib, imatinib, more need to be combined with chemotherapy drugs.

Molecularly targeted drugs represent a new class of anticancer drugs, and Gleevec is a classic example of controlling cancer by **inhibiting abnormal molecules that cause cancer without damaging other normal nuclear tissues.** More and more molecularly targeted drugs have been used in cancer treatment. For example, rituximab (Trastuzumab) for treating breast of Rituximab for treating B cell lymphoma, Gifitinib for treating lung cancer, Erlotinib, and the like. Targeted therapy brings anti-tumor hope.

2). The prospect of immunomodulatory drugs is gratifying

Regardless of the complexity of the mechanisms behind cancer, immune suppression is the key to cancer progression. Removal of immunosuppressive factors and restoration of the recognition of cancer cells by immune system cells can effectively prevent cancer.

More and more research evidence shows that by regulating the body's immune system, it is possible to achieve cancer control. Treating tumors by activating the body's anti-tumor immune system is an area that is currently exciting for researchers. The next major breakthrough in cancer is likely to stem from this.

In order to explore the etiology, pathogenesis and pathophysiology of cancer, our laboratory had carried out a series of animal experiments in the laboratory for 4 years, and obtained new findings from the experimental results. The new inspirations: thymus atrophy, low immune function is cancer Cause.

In order to explore the etiology, pathogenesis and pathophysiology of cancer, our laboratory has carried out a series of animal experiments in the laboratory for 4 years, and obtained new findings from the experimental results. The new inspirations or findings : thymus atrophy, low immune function is one of the causes and pathogenesis of cancer. Therefore, Xu Ze proposed at the International Oncology Society in 2013: the cause of cancer, one of the pathogenesis, is thymus atrophy and immune function is low and immune surveillance ability is reduced and immune escape.

Therefore, the principle of treatment must be to prevent progressive atrophy of the thymus, promote thymic hyperplasia, protect bone marrow hematopoietic function, and improve immune surveillance. It provides experimental basis and theoretical basis for the immunomodulatory treatment of cancer.

Through the above 4 years to explore the basic experimental research on the mechanism of recurrence and metastasis and followed by 3 years of which it was screened from the internal laboratory of natural medications and Chinese herbal medication through the cancer-bearing animal experiment, 48 out of 200 Chinese medications were screened for better tumor inhibition rate. After screening by cancer-bearing animal experiments, it constitutes XZ-C$_{1-10}$ anti-cancer immune regulation and control Chinese medication.

After 20 years of clinical application and clinical observation and verification in more than 12,000 patients with the advanced cancer patients in the oncology clinics, it confirmed that the treatment principle of immune regulation and control "protecting Thymus function and increase the immune function " is reasonable and the curative effect is satisfactory. The application of immunomodulatory Chinese medication has achieved good results, improved the quality of life, and significantly prolonged the survival period.

3. ASCO Announces Major Progress in Clinical Oncology in 2015

Immunotherapy opens a new era of cancer treatment

On February 4, 2016, the American Society of Clinical Oncology (ASCO) announced the "2016 Annual Report: ASCO Clinical Oncology Progress" on Capitol Hill, Washington, DC. The report details the global clinical oncology in 2015. The research is summarized and at the same time, the future research direction is forecasted. ASCO rated the 2015 progress as "tumor immunotherapy". **The content of this report detailed and in-depth summarized the research on global clinical oncology in 2015; simultaneously looked forward the direction of the future research and development. ASCO rated the progress of 2015 as "tumor immunotherapy"**

ASCO President Professor Julie M. Vose believes that the most important development in 2015 is the discovery of immunotherapy. She wrote in the foreword: "We are no longer determined by tumor type and staging as we have in the past. Treatment, in the era of precision medicine, we select or exclude treatment based on each patient and tumor genetic data. No other major advances, like immunology can be translated into clinical practice, so ASCO decided that the biggest progress in 2015 is immunotherapy."

The chairman of the committee, Professor Don Dizon, also believes that the annual research results are increasing, but from the perspective of being able to benefit patients, **the most important development this year should be immunotherapy.**

D. The Situation Analysis (4)

1. **The goal of conquering cancer: reduce the incidence of cancer, improve the cure rate, and prolong the survival period.**
   Reach:
   1/3 can be prevented
   1/3 can be cured
   1/3 can be treated to relieve pain, is a chronic disease
   Survival with tumor, prolong survival
2. **The road to conquer cancer**
   The road:
   (1) Conquer cancer and launch a general attack
   What is the total attack?
   That is, anti-cancer + cancer control + cancer treatment, and at the same time,
   (2) Prepare a science city to overcome cancer:
   1.Innovative Molecular Oncology Medical College
   - and modern high-tech experimental talents
   2.Innovative molecular tumors for prevention and treatment of Chinese and Western hospitals
   3. Innovative Molecular Oncology Institute
   4. innovative molecular tumor nano preparations pharmaceutical factory
   5. Innovative Cancer Research Institute
   6. Cancer Animal Experimental Center
   (The following are provincial key disciplines or subjects)
3. **How to prevent it? Specific measures, feasible solutions (not empty talk), pragmatic**
4. **How to do it? Avoid talk, work hard, start to go**
5. **How to get started?**
   1 First, prevent, control, and treat hospitals → establish various disciplines → establish each group
   (Department) (Study Group)
   2 First, run a doctor, education, research (section, group) one-stop, with emphasis, basic, clinical, three basic, three strict, theory, technology, experience
   Cultivate all-round talents: learn, experience, technology, and theory, change the current status quo, have points, and have
   3 first run a graduate school, talent training methods, ways;
   a, first run a graduate tutor class, training classes, training talents, seeds, training and guiding talents, put forward learning, how to overcome the general attack content of cancer, discussion

b. Talent seed plan: recruit talents, experts, seeds, and educated experts and professors as seeds

Cultivating talent is seeding:

Recruit graduate students (shuo, Bo) to cultivate seeds, work while studying, 100 people, all stay as new seeds, so generations of training, requires results, achievements, achievements (not only papers), that is, three years and five years later, The talents are very good and the results are numerous.

6. **How to carry out anti-cancer and anti-cancer work in Wuhan**:

(1) Department of anti-cancer surgery in hospitals of more than dimethyl

Each of the top three hospitals is responsible for three community cancer prevention efforts.

Each of the top three hospitals' cancer prevention or prevention departments needs to develop responsibilities and scope.

Not only to take vaccination, but to go deep into the community to carry out anti-cancer work

(2) The city's dimethyl and tertiary hospitals will formulate the scope of anti-cancer and anti-cancer duties, and the division of labor will be responsible for the work.

1 The top three hospitals in each province of the province are responsible for the prevention, control and treatment of the two regions.

The top three hospitals in each province are responsible for group medical treatment in two regions, consultation, solution, treatment, training, training, graded diagnosis and treatment of difficult medical problems, and resolving the quality and level of technical problems.

The quality, level, talents and technology of the top three hospitals in the province must meet the quality level of the top three hospitals. It must be true, and it is necessary to solve the personnel training and technical level of the lower-level hospitals.

3 Establish a consultation system, brainstorm ideas, improve medical standards, solve difficult problems, and conduct inter-disciplinary consultations and inter-disciplinary consultations.

4 Tongji, Xiehe, People, Central South, and subordinate hospitals must solve the referral and consultation of the subordinate hospitals and solve the difficult problems.

5 Tongji Health System Training for the province's cancer prevention department, general practitioners, senior and intermediate health and epidemic prevention pre-scientific talents

6Each community has anti-cancer, anti-cancer, anti-cancer, supervision, mission group, responsibilities, tasks, division of labor

7 Provincial and Municipal Health Planning Commissions set up anti-cancer and cancer control offices to organize missions, guidance, and supervision.

7. **How to carry out anti-cancer and cancer control work in the community**

Demonstration areas for cancer prevention, control and treatment in several communities

Establish a system of prevention, control and governance, "China mode"

(1) Through the standardization of the "three early" information early warning system

The history of the following patients in the community is checked on time

1. The history of blood in the stool, history of hemorrhoids, that is, colonoscopy

2. The patients with a history of hematuria, that is, cystoscopy

3. Lumps, sarcoidosis, that should be percussion + surgery

4. Hepatitis B, cirrhosis, half a year or once a year check

(2) Standardized community anti-cancer training

(3) Community registration, timely assessment

(4) Focus on "three early", precancerous lesions

Will greatly reduce the funds for the use of three early examinations, different cancers, for prevention, early diagnosis, early treatment

Pathfinding and footprinting

(scientific footprints)

(To conquer cancer, where is the footpath or the direction?
Where is the road? Where to go? How to go?)

TABLE OF CONTENTS

1. Preface

1). The path of cancer research

Finding the problems and ask the questions from follow-up results
(Hint: Study how to prevent postoperative recurrence and metastasis is the
key to improve long-term outcomes after surgery)

Pathfinding (to overcome cancer, where is the road? How do you find it?)

Pathfinding and footprint (anti-cancer, anti-cancer metastasis research and scientific research results, scientific and technological innovation series)

Published cancer monographs (3 Chinese editions are exclusively distributed nationwide, 7 full English editions are published worldwide)

Participate in the International Congress of Oncology (AIACR Academic Conference, Washington)

Visiting the Stirling Cancer Institute in Houston, USA (2009)

Basic and clinical research on anti-cancer and anti-cancer metastasis in the past 30 years

More than 12,000 clinical application experience in 20 years

Walk out of a new road of cancer treatment on the molecular level of an immune regulatory and control with combination of Chinese and Western medication

1). Walked out of a new road to conquer cancer and to treat cancer with "Chinese-style anti-cancer", combination of Chinese and Western medication with immune regulation and control

2) Published the English monograph "The Road to Overcome Cancer" on December 6, 2016 in America, worldwide.

3) Published the English monograph "Condense Wisdom and Conquer Cancer"; Published in December 2017 (volume 1), published in February 2018 (the next volume), published in USA, full English version, globally distributed.

2. Pathfinding and footprinting

(scientific footprints)

1. Causes:

(1) Why do I study cancer? I am a clinical surgeon, why do you study cancer? This is due to the results of a petition to a group of cancer patients after surgery. In 1985, I conducted a petition with more than 3,000 patients who underwent radical surgery for various cancers outside the chest (all according to the operating room registration list). It was found that most patients relapsed and metastasized 2 to 3 years after surgery. This made me realize that although the operation is successful, the long-term efficacy is not satisfactory. Postoperative recurrence and metastasis are the key factors affecting the long-term efficacy of the operation. It also reminds us that prevention and treatment of postoperative recurrence and metastasis is the key to prolonging postoperative survival. Therefore, clinical basic research must be carried out. Without breakthroughs in basic research, clinical efficacy is difficult to improve, so we established the Institute of Experimental Surgery and conducted a series of experimental studies and clinical acceptance work.

(2) From the results of follow-up, it was found that:

1)postoperative recurrence and metastasis are the key factors affecting the long-term efficacy of surgery;

2) prompt clinicians must pay attention to and study the prevention and treatment of postoperative recurrence and metastasis, in order to improve the long-term effect of surgery

2. To find the way:

(1) Why do we look for the road to conquer cancer? How to find this way? To conquer cancer, where is the road? - Where is the direction or path? Where to go? How to go?

For more than a hundred years, many people with lofty ideals and scientific research elites are looking for them.

(2) How to find a path?

The research we conduct is based on the following research routes:
1)).

The problem was found

Through high-volume patient follow-up, it was found that the key factors affecting long-term postoperative outcome were postoperative recurrence and metastasis.

↓

The questions were proposed

It was proposed that it is necessary to study the recurrence and metastasis to improve the long-term efficacy of the operation, and it was proposed the the goal or "target" of solving the problem should be how to resist or stop the metastasis

↓

The Problems were researched

It was established a research institute to carry out a series of projects, experiments, explore the transfer mechanism and find anti-recurrence and metastasis techniques and new drugs, screen 200 kinds of Chinese medicines, and find out that 48 kinds have certain anti-cancer effects.

↓

The problems were solved

It was carried out clinical verification and clinical research, explore the law of cancer metastasis and find a new model of anti-metastasis treatment, and rise to the theory of independent innovation and the new anti-metastatic treatment model and new scheme

2)). From clinical → experimental → clinical → re-experiment → re-clinical, return to the clinical to solve the problem.

3)). Theory and practice are closely combined. The topics are all from the clinical, to find the focus of clinical problems and clinical breakthroughs, after experimental research and clinical verification, and then applied to the clinic to solve clinical practical problems.

4)). Take the road of combining Chinese and Western medicine → macroscopic combination → molecular level combination, using modern cancer cell molecular transfer mechanism and the latest theory of "eight steps" and "three stages" to find and screen anti-metastatic drugs from 200 ancient Chinese medicines. It protects immune organs, activates cytokines and immune factors, modernizes ancient Chinese medications, and integrates with the international community, enabling modern medications to combine with ancient Chinese herbal medications at the molecular level and BRM level.

5)). The establishment of the Experimental Surgery Institute conducted a series of experimental studies and clinical basic research of cancer. Without the breakthrough of basic research, the clinical efficacy is difficult to improve.

6)). Establish a Dawning tumor specialist clinic:

(a) Establish an outpatient medical record database, keep outpatient medical records, follow-up throughout the whole process, long-term follow-up for many years, call at any time to answer questions, guide rehabilitation and dietary precautions;

(b) Establish detailed medical records (including epidemiological data of patients) to analyze in depth the successful experience and failure lessons of each treatment and the particularity of the disease (eg, analytical data);

(c) A summary of the stage of the 6-month-to-year follow-up visit, and the cases of more than 3 years of follow-up were extracted from the medical records, the medical records were summarized, and the treatment experience and lessons were analyzed (eg, summary medical records). The Twilight Oncology Clinic has been in existence for 33 years and the outpatient medical records have remained intact.

7)) Through the laboratory of the Institute of Experimental Surgery to establish animal models of various cancers, a series of experimental studies were carried out; explore the etiology, pathogenesis, recurrence and metastasis mechanism of cancer, and conduct experimental research on effective measures to control cancer invasion, recurrence and metastasis. Experimental research, obtained a series of experimental research new findings.

(3) How to find this road? It should be based on clinical actual problems and experimental research findings:

The road we have been looking for 30 years has come step by step:

1) Through the findings of follow-up results: the postoperative recurrence and metastasis are the key factors affecting the long-term efficacy of surgery, **thus revealing: it must look for ways to prevent and treat cancer after recurrence and metastasis (method, medicine, technology, basic theory)**

2) Through the results of animal experiment research: As the cancer progresses, the thymus is progressively atrophy, and the host thymus is acute progressive atrophy after inoculation of cancer cells, cell proliferation is blocked, and the volume is significantly reduced, **thus revealing: It must find ways to prevent thymus atrophy, promote thymic hyperplasia, and boost immunity.(method, medicine, technology, basic theory)**

3) The results of animal experiment research results: The experimental results

confirmed that **the first immunosuppression**, and then easy to have the occurrence and development of cancer, **if no immune function decline, it is not easy to vaccinate successfully.** The experimental results suggest that improving and maintaining good immune function, maintaining a good central immune organ thymus is one of the important measures to prevent cancer. Another experimental result in our laboratory suggests that metastasis is associated with immunity, low immune function, or the use of immunosuppressive agents to promote tumor metastasis. **Thus the revelation: It must find the way to immune reconstruction of cancer patients(method, medicine, technology, basic theory)**

4) through our proposed new concept of cancer metastasis treatment, the new theory of understanding: The key to cancer treatment is anti-metastasis, how to eliminate cancer cells on the way to transfer. **It must find the way to eliminate cancer cells on the way to transfer(method, medicine, technology, basic theory)**

Through the above research results: We found the way to take the immune regulation and control method, and established the XZ-C immunomodulation therapy to treat cancer.

In the past 30 years, we have initially embarked on a new way of using Chinese medicine immune regulation and control, regulating immune activity, preventing thymus atrophy, promoting thymic hyperplasia, protecting bone marrow hematopoietic function, improving immune surveillance, and combining Western medicine at the molecular level to overcome cancer.

3). Footprint (scientific research footprint)

(1) Anti-cancer, anti-cancer metastasis research, scientific research achievements, scientific and technological innovation series

The following arguments in the XZ-C (XU ZE-China) series are the first to be presented internationally, all of which are original papers.

1. "Thymus atrophy, low immune function is one of the causes and pathogenesis of cancer"

   ——New findings on experimental research on the etiology and pathogenesis of cancer

   - See the monograph "New Concepts and New Methods of Cancer Treatment" P.13

2. "XZ-C immunomodulation treatment" "thoracic chest lift" theoretical basis and experimental basis

   ——Proposed the theoretical basis and experimental basis of cancer immune regulation therapy

——Because of the new enlightenment discovered by the above experimental research, the treatment principle must be to prevent progressive atrophy of the thymus, promote thymic hyperplasia, protect bone marrow hematopoietic function, improve immune surveillance, and control immune escape of malignant cells.

- See the monograph "New Concepts and New Methods of Cancer Treatment" P.17

3. "Cancer treatment should change the concept and establish a comprehensive treatment concept"

- propose a new concept of cancer treatment principles

——The target or target of cancer treatment must establish a comprehensive treatment concept for both tumor and host

—— Should overcome the one-sided treatment concept of simply killing cancer cells

- See the monograph "New Concepts and New Methods for Cancer Treatment" P.28

4. "New Combination of Multidisciplinary Treatment of Cancer"

- Proposing a new concept of a combination of cancer treatment models

- The new model of multidisciplinary treatment is:

Long-term treatment mainly: surgery + biological treatment + immunotherapy + Chinese medicine, Chinese and Western combined treatment

Short-course treatment is supplemented: radiotherapy, chemotherapy, not long-range, not excessive

- See the monograph "New Concepts and New Methods for Cancer Treatment" P33

5. "Analysis, evaluation and questioning of systemic intravenous chemotherapy for solid tumors and four evaluations"

——Analysis of the problems and drawbacks of systemic intravenous chemotherapy for solid cancer

——Question and evaluation of systemic intravenous chemotherapy for solid tumors, calculation of drug volume, evaluation of efficacy

- See the monograph "New Concepts and New Methods of Cancer Treatment" P.57

6. "Initiative systemic intravenous chemotherapy for abdominal solid tumors should be reformed as intra-target chemotherapy for target organs, and reform initiatives for traditional chemotherapy for cancer"

——Because systemic intravenous chemotherapy cytotoxic drugs cannot directly reach the portal system by the superior vena cava administration, the vena cava system and the portal system are generally incompatible, and it is difficult to reach the portal vein by the superior vena cava.

——What are the cancer cells of abdominal solid tumors (stomach, colorectal, liver, gallbladder, pancreas, spleen, abdominal cavity, etc.)? Mainly in the portal system, postoperative adjuvant chemotherapy from the venous vein to the vena cava is unreasonable, does not meet the anatomy, physiology and pathology, because it can not directly enter the portal system

- Therefore, the route of administration should be changed to the endovascular treatment of target organs

- See the monograph "New Concepts and New Methods of Cancer Treatment" P.63

7. "There are three main forms of cancer in the human body"

——Proposed theoretical innovation of new concept of cancer metastasis treatment

——This third manifestation is proposed to be a group of cancer cells on the way to metastasis. The treatment target of cancer should be directed to the above three forms of existence, especially for cancer cells on the way to metastasis.

- See the monograph "New Concepts and New Methods for Cancer Treatment" P.38

8. "Two Points and One Line" in the Whole Process of Cancer Development

——Proposed theoretical innovation of cancer metastasis treatment

- One of the purposes of cancer treatment is to prevent metastasis

The whole process of cancer metastasis development can be summarized as "two points and one line"

——Traditional cancer treatment only pays attention to "two points" and ignores "first line"

The new concept believes that both "two points" should be emphasized, and that "one line" should be cut off.

- See the monograph "New Concepts and New Methods for Cancer Treatment" P.43

9. "Three Steps of Anticancer Metastasis Treatment"

——Proposed theoretical innovation of cancer metastasis treatment

——Incorporate the "eight steps" of cancer cell transfer into "three stages" and try to break each transfer step.

- See the monograph "New Concepts and New Methods for Cancer Treatment" P.47

10. "Developing the third field of anti-cancer metastasis"

——Proposed the theoretical innovation of the new concept of cancer metastasis treatment, and found and proposed the third field of human anti-cancer metastasis

——The circulatory system has a large number of immune surveillance cells, and the "main battlefield" of cancer cells on the way to annihilation is in the blood circulation.

4). Proposed "conquer cancer and launch the general attack to cancer" is unprecedented work

(1).It is first proposed internationally "XZ-C Scientific Research Plan for conquering cancer and launch the General Attack to Cancer" including :

a. The overall strategic reform and development of cancer treatment in China;
b. Avoid talk, work hard, start to go
c. No matter how far the road to cancer is, it should always start to go.
d. Proposed to conquer cancer and launch the general attack to cancer, this is unprecedented work

(2).For the first time in the world proposed the "Necessity and Feasibility Report on conquering cancer and launch the General Attack of Cancer"
Including :

a. The overall strategic reform of cancer treatment in China will focus on treatment and turn to prevention and treatment.
b. XZ-C proposes the general idea and design of conquering cancer
c. What is the total attack on cancer and the goal of the total attack?
d. XU ZE proposes ideas, strategies, plans, blueprints to overcome cancer and launch a general attack

(3) For the first time in the world proposed "Providing the construction of cancer prevention and development, prevention and treatment of hospitals"
(Global demonstration cancer prevention and treatment hospital)

a. The current problems in the hospital hospital hospital model
b. How to overcome the road of cancer is to study the establishment of prevention and treatment hospitals for the whole process of cancer occurrence and development, and reform the current mode of hospitalization for re-treatment and light defense.

c. XU ZE's strategic thinking, planning sketch, prevention and treatment of cancer occurrence and development

(4) For the first time in the world proposed the "The General Plan for Overcoming Cancer and the Basic Design of Science City"

a. Equivalent to designing an overall framework for Chinese characteristics to overcome cancer design
b. How to set up the basic idea and design to overcome the general attack of cancer
c. How to overcome cancer? The Cancer Animal Experimental Center and Innovative Molecular Oncology Medical College and Multidisciplinary Research Institute must be established.
d. Cancer and Multidisciplinary Research Institute
e. How to overcome cancer? It is necessary to "set up the science base of the medical, teaching, research to overcome cancer and launch the general attack of cancer – The Science City"

(5) The cancer research papers reported at the American Society of International Oncology, and research papers go international

a. Received an invitation letter from the American Association for Cancer Research AACR to Xu Ze, who reported "XZ-C immunomodulation anticancer therapy" at the International Cancer Society in Washington, USA in September 2013, which has attracted extensive attention from the international oncology community. And highly valued.
b. From October 27 to 30, 2013, the author attended the 12th International Conference on Cancer Research at the American Association for Cancer Research (AACR) in Washington, DC, which attracted great attention from the oncology community.
c. On February 14, 2014, Dr. Bin Wu gave a lecture on "The thymus atrophy and immunocompromised cancer is one of the causes and mechanisms of cancer" in the academic lecture hall of the Hopehouse University Library Building in Washington. The report, as well as the "protection of the chest" (protecting the thymus to improve immunity), the academic report of the theoretical basis and experimental basis for the treatment principle of "protecting the marrow to produce blood" (protecting bone marrow hematopoietic stem cells) was warmly welcomed and highly valued by the participants.

d. World-class tumor immunoscientists such as Stanford University School of Medicine, University of California, San Francisco, and Harvard Medical School fully affirmed Professor Xu Ze's research results and agreed that the immune system can enhance the anti-recurrence and metastasis of cancer patients themselves. It is agreed that the immune system can enhance the anti-recurrence and metastasis immunity of cancer patients by immune regulation, and can fully improve the quality of life of patients with advanced cancer. It is the most effective anti-cancer pathway after surgery, radiotherapy and chemotherapy.

(6) Visiting the Stirling Cancer Institute in Houston, USA

In order to strengthen the exchanges and cooperation between international scientific and technological organizations, on December 10, 2009, we were invited to visit the Stirling Cancer Institute in the United States. We were warmly welcomed and warmly welcomed by the colleagues of the Institute. The 86-year-old professor and A number of professors, researchers, nude animal model laboratories and anti-cancer drug analysis laboratories participated in the discussion and exchanges, and reported the latest scientific research results with slides.

We presented a color map of the Institute of Cancer Metastasis and Recurrence in our Institute to the Institute of Oncology, and introduced the research on tumor-free technology in radical surgery and the experiment of removing thymus to produce cancer-bearing animal models. Research, and the exclusive development of ZC immunomodulation of anti-cancer, anti-metastatic Chinese medicine series Z-C1-10. I also presented the monograph "New Concepts and New Methods for Cancer Metastasis Treatment" published by me. It is the three hundred original books that won the book award in China, and was warmly welcomed and appreciated by the researchers.

(7) The basic planning and design of XZ-C launching the general attack

Professor Xu Ze (XU ZE) proposed the overall design of the Science City to conquer cancer and to launch the general attack to cancer

<u>Dawning Scientific Research Spirit</u>

<u>Hard work and Strive</u>

↓ **30** years of cold windows and hard effort

Retrospective reflection and review

416

Follow-up, summarizing successful treatment experience (typical cases in the second monograph); rethinking the lessons of treatment failure (the first monograph failed to prevent recurrence and failed to prevent metastasis).

Development and Innovation

48 kinds of Chinese herbal medications with good inhibition rate screened from 200 chinese herbal medications, XZ-C immunomodulation Chinese medication series preparations. After 30 years of clinical testing and verification, it is realized or understood and rises up to the theoretical knowledge and the new concepts and new models.

Facing the Future-oriented medicine

Recognizing the shortcomings and problems of traditional therapy in the 20th century, and recognizing the striving direction of the 21st century.

Looking forward to watch

Recommendations:

- Establish an innovative molecular oncology hospital – to train senior oncology researchers for the country.
- Establish innovative molecular cancer onset, develop and prevent hospitals (combined with Western medicine at the molecular level) – benefiting more cancer patients and serving more cancer patients.
- Establishing an Innovative Molecular Oncology Institute – researching cells to begin malignant transformation – to CT can be found for a significant period of time to reach the three-early target, "target" metastasis, cancer lesions, and precancerous conditions.
- Establish an innovative molecular oncology drug factory – stepping out of a new path to overcome cancer with Chinese characteristics.
- Establish an environmental protection and cancer prevention research institute and carry out anti-cancer system engineering

(8) The theoretical system of XZ-C immunomodulation and cancer treatment has been initially formed.

In the book "New Concepts and New Methods of Cancer Treatment", Professor Xu Ze published a series of research papers on basic and clinical research results with 30 years of self-reliance and hard work.

This book has formed the theoretical system of XZ-C immune regulation and control for the treatment of cancer, which are the theory basis and the experiment foundation of cancer treatment and they are being undergone the clinical application observation and verification.

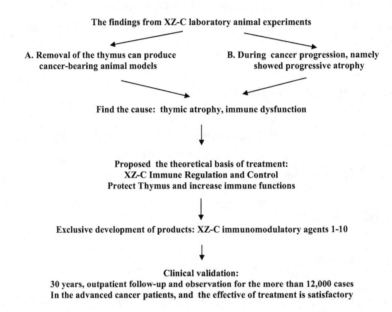

The findings from XZ-C laboratory animal experiments

A. Removal of the thymus can produce cancer-bearing animal models

B. During cancer progression, namely showed progressive atrophy

Find the cause: thymic atrophy, immune dysfunction

**Proposed the theoretical basis of treatment:
XZ-C Immune Regulation and Control
Protect Thymus and increase immune functions**

Exclusive development of products: XZ-C immunomodulatory agents 1-10

**Clinical validation:
30 years, outpatient follow-up and observation for the more than 12,000 cases
In the advanced cancer patients, and the effective of treatment is satisfactory**

Theoretical System of XZ-C immune regulate and control of cancer therapy

(7).The Exclusive research and development products: a series of XZ-C immune regulation and control anti-cancer Chinese medication products

(introduction)

The self-developed XZ-C (Xu Ze China) immune regulation anti-cancer series of traditional Chinese medicine preparations, from experimental research to clinical verification, applied to clinical practice on the basis of the success of animal experiments, after more than 12,000 clinical cases in 20 years, Significant effect. Clinical application can improve symptoms, good spirits, good appetite, significantly improve the quality of life, and significantly prolong the survival period. It is independent innovation and independent intellectual property rights.

To search for and screen new anti-cancer and anti-metastatic drugs from traditional Chinese medicine:

The purpose is to screen out the anti-cancer, anti-metastatic and anti-recurrent immunomodulatory Chinese medicine XZ-C1-10 which has no drug resistance, no toxic side effects, high selectivity and long-term oral administration. (XZ-C immunomodulation series of Chinese medicine products, see the first volume, the eighth volume)

A. The 83-year-old year (April 2016) proposed to advance moving together with the "Cancer Moon Shot", because since 2013, Xu Ze has proposed "the necessity and feasibility of conquering cancer and launch the general attack to cancer" and <<the report about "conquer cancer and launch the General Attack to Cancer and Preparing to set up the science city of Conquer Cancer Science City>> which is being planned and designed. "New Moon Plan" (US) and Dawning C Plan (middle)

Are moving forward together, heading for the science hall to overcome cancer.

1. **"Introduction to the Cancer Moon Shot"**

   On January 12, 2016, US President Barack Obama announced a national plan to overcome cancer in his State of the Union address:

   Plan Name: "New Moon Plan"

   Goal: Conquer cancer

   Nature: National plan to overcome cancer

   Announcer: President Obama

   The person in charge of the plan: Vice President Biden

   Announced: January 12, 2016

   The specific plan of the plan: unknown

2. **Dawning C-type plan introduction**

   a. Before January 12, 2016, the progress of the XZ-C Scientific Research Plan for Overcoming the General Attack of Cancer Attack was put forward.

   b. Before January 12, 2016, we have carried out research results in the field of cancer research, technology innovation series

   c. Dawning C-type plan (developed in July 2015)

   I "Overcome the general attack of cancer"

   II "Preparation of the whole process of prevention and treatment of hospitals"

   III "Preparing to build a cancer science city"

   IV "Forming a Multidisciplinary Research Group"

   V "The vaccine is the hope of mankind"

   VI "The prospect of immunomodulatory drugs is gratifying"

3. **situation analysis**
   a, analyze their respective technological advantages
   b. Analyze the current status quo
   c. Analyze the next research prospects
   d, "Dawning C-type plan" technology innovation realization outline
   e. How to implement this unprecedented event in human history?
   f, expected results

(8) Conducting anti-cancer metastasis research is an urgent need

1. Conducting anti-cancer and anti-cancer metastasis research is an urgent need for the development of oncology. "Oncology" is one of the most backward disciplines in medical science. Its "name" is not yet unified. Some people write it as "tumor" and " Cancer, "cancer", "malignant tumor", "new organism". Because a disease name is defined, its cause and pathogenesis must be clarified. Because the etiology, pathogenesis, and pathophysiology of oncology are not well understood, the oncology discipline is still a scientific virgin for scientific research, and it needs a lot of basic scientific research.

2. Anti-cancer metastasis, recurrence, basic research must be carried out on animal models of cancer-bearing animals. Currently, many large hospitals have not established laboratories and cannot conduct basic research on cancer. It is necessary to establish various cancer metastasis animal models in nude mice to study cancer cell metastasis. The law and mechanism (the author's laboratory uses pure Kunming mice to make cancer-bearing animal models about 10,000 times), because without the breakthrough of basic research, the clinical efficacy is difficult to improve.

3. Research on anti-cancer and anti-cancer metastasis focuses on the study of unknown knowledge. Researchers should look ahead and face the science of the future. Science is the end of the world. Researchers must surpass the old knowledge and constantly update with a developmental perspective. Constantly surpassing, constantly developing and moving forward.

(9) How to innovate in science and technology? How to leave a scientific research footprint?

An old cement road, with hundreds of people walking every day, will not leave footprints, only a new cement road, every step will leave eternal footprints, so scientific research must have innovative thinking, must be innovative Results.

In the past 30 years (1985-), our research history, cancer research work, scientific research series of scientific research achievements in animal experiments, clinical basic research and clinical verification work, only the results catalogue (scientific research footprint) is listed here, and each research result is Belonging to original innovation or independent innovation, it is every eternal scientific research footprint.

(10) In his 85-year-old year, he published the medical monograph "Condense Wisdom and Conquering Cancer - Benefiting Mankind", XZ-C: How to overcome cancer? How can I prevent cancer? I see how to cure cancer.

Professor Xu Ze proposed the engineering planning diagram for how to overcome cancer.

This medical monograph is a practical, applied, research-oriented, implementation of how to overcome the outline of cancer. This set of scientific research programs, scientific research design, scientific research planning, and blueprints can be used by countries, provinces, and states to implement the vision of cancer and benefit humanity.

The main project of this implementation outline is to conquer cancer and to launch the general attack to cancer with cancer prevention and cancer control and cancer treatment at the same attention and at the same time and to create a scientific research base for multidisciplinary and cancer-related research - Science City

The two-wing project is:

A wing - how to prevent cancer? To reduce the incidence of cancer

B wing - how to treat cancer? To improve cancer cure rate

aims:

A: Reduce the incidence of cancer

B: Improve cancer cure rate, prolong patient survival and improve quality of life

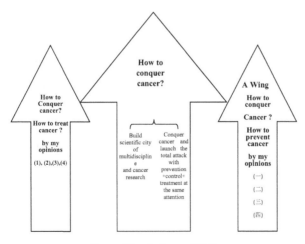

Figure . Schematic diagram of XZ-C

3. The Sunset Glows like a Morning Sun

Dawning into the air, calling the dawn

(1) Sunset is not necessarily lower Dawning

The sunset may not be too late as Dawning. "The evening glow may not be lower than the morning." Many celebrities in ancient and modern China and abroad still maintain a strong vitality in their later years, and they are eager to continue to contribute to society.

When Marx was 51 years old, I began to study Russian in the Russian calendar. Due to his diligence, he could read Russian originals only half a year.

Engels mastered more than 20 languages in his life, and he began to study Norwegian in his 70s. In the last few years of his life, he also worked hard to study medicine.

The Russian writer Lev Tolstoy wrote a novel titled "I Can't Silence" at the age of 82.

Indian literary master Tagore began to learn painting in his 70s, and has painted more than 1,500 paintings. He has performed personal exhibitions in many parts of the world.

Italian sculptor, painter, architect and poet Michelangelo designed the St. Mary's Church at the age of 88.

When the British playwright Shaw Bernard was 93, he wrote a script called "Fables of the Fellowship."

The Spanish painter Picasso painted 165 paintings at the age of 88. He was still engaged in engraving work when he was 90 years old.

American Adolf Zucker was the chairman of the Hollywood Film Studio at the age of 91.

At the age of 82, Winsler Churchill wrote a four-volume work titled "History of the English-speaking People."

American comedian George Burns made an outstanding performance in "Sunshine Kids" at the age of 80 and won the first prize.

Huang Gongwang is one of the painters in the history of Chinese painting called "Yuan Sijia". When he was an 80-year-old man, he still went out to sketch and created a huge painting "Fuchun Mountain Residence" with a length of three feet. Become an immortal work.

Li Shu, an outstanding thinker of the era, wrote the famous book "Book Collection" at the age of 73.

Liang Zhang, a famous literary scholar of the Qing Dynasty, wrote the first syllabary of the "Yuanlian Conghua" in China.

When Xu Teli was in his 70s, he studied the classics of Marxism-Leninism, copied the incisive statements in the book and put them on the wall, and read them repeatedly every day until they could recite them.

Qi Baishi took the motto of "Heavenly Reward" and painted more than 800 paintings at the age of 93.

Feng Yuxiang was hardworking all his life. When he went to the United States in 1948, he was an old man in his 60s, but he still studied English with tenacious perseverance. Six months later, he gave a speech to the Americans in English.

When the photography master Lang Jingshan was 100 years old, he held the "Old Age 100 Works Exhibition" in Beijing, which won high praise from the audience.

When the famous painter Zhu Qizhan was 95 years old, he was invited to lecture in New York, Houston and other places in the United States. He was also invited to Singapore to hold a personal exhibition.

(According to "The People's Railway", Meiyun / Wen)

(2) Publishing the monographs on cancer research

Professor Xu Ze continued to research after he retired, and Science has continued to achieve the following series of scientific research results and published a series of cancer research monographs.

In 1996, I was 63 years old and I was retired. After I retired, I have been living in a small building for 20 years. I have been working alone and fighting alone. I have continued a series of experimental studies and clinical verification observations. I have achieved the following series of scientific research results. The following monographs have been published: **Three monographs, Chinese version, domestic issue and six monographs, English edition, Washington publication, international distribution. These nine monographs are the result of the scientific research of the four different stages, four different levels of mountain, which are difficult to trek, hard to climb, one step at a scientific research footprint.**

A.67-year-old flower year published the first monograph "New understanding and new model of cancer treatment" Hubei Science and Technology Press, Xu Ze, January 2001

B.73-year-old ancient rare year published the second monograph "New Concepts and New Methods for Cancer Metastasis Treatment"
Published by Beijing People's Military Medical Press, Xu Ze, January 2006

In April 2007, the People's Republic of China Publishing Office issued the "Three One Hundred" original book certificate.

C.78-year-old Quaint Year published the third monograph "New Concepts and New Methods for Cancer Treatment"
Published by Beijing People's Military Medical Press, Xu Ze, Xu Jie/, October 2011
Later, the American medical doctor Dr. Bin Wu and others translated into English, and the English version was published in Washington, DC on March 26, 2013.

D.80-year-old published the third monograph in English, New Concept and New Way Of Treatment of Cancer, published in Washington, March 2013, in English, internationally

E.82 years old published the fifth monograph "On Innovation of Treatment of Cancer" - "On Cancer Treatment Innovation"
Published in Washington, December 2015, full English, globally distributed

F. At the age of 83, he published the sixth monograph "New Concept and New Way of Treatment of Cancer Metastais"
- "New Concepts and New Methods for Cancer Metastasis Treatment"
In August 2016, Washington published the full English version and released it worldwide.

G. At the age of 83, he published the seventh monograph "The Road To Over Come Cancer"
- Conquer the road to cancer
Published in Washington, DC in December 2016, full English, globally distributed

H. At the age of 86, he published the eighth monograph "Condens Wisdom and Conquer Cancer for the Benefit of Mankind" - "Gathering Wisdom, Conquering Cancer - Benefiting Mankind"

Volume: How to overcome cancer? How to prevent cancer? December 2017

Published in Washington in English and globally distributed

Volume 2: How to overcome cancer? How to treat cancer? February 2018

4. The pictures of all of the monographs

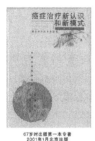

67岁时出版第一本专著
2001年1月北京出版

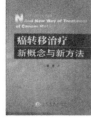

73岁时出版第二本专著
2006年1月北京出版

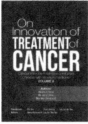

62岁时出版《癌症治疗创新论》
2015年12月华盛顿出版
全英文版，全球发行

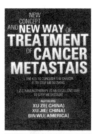

83岁时出版《癌转移治疗的新概念与新方法》
2016年8月华盛顿出版
全英文版，全球发行

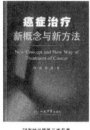

78岁时出版第三本专著
2011年10月北京出版

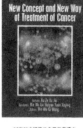

80岁时出版第三专著的英译本
2013年3月华盛顿出版(英文版)国际发行

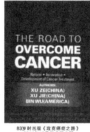

83岁时出版《攻克癌症之路》
2016年12月华盛顿出版
全英文版，全球发行

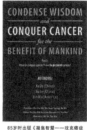

65岁时出版《凝集智慧——攻克癌症
为人类造福》上册
2017年12月华盛顿出版
全英文版，全球发行

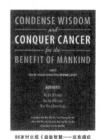

86岁时出版《凝集智慧——攻克癌症
为人类造福》下册
2018年2月华盛顿出版
全英文版，全球发行

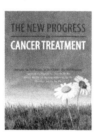

Visiting the Sterling Cancer Institute in the United States in 2009
Published at the age of 86, "New Progress in Cancer Therapy"
Presenting the research results and experimental research of our institute
Published in Washington, June 2018, full English version
Color albums and monographs worldwide

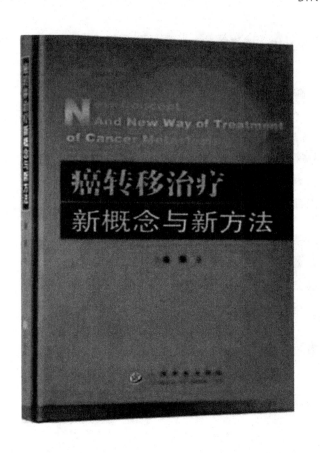

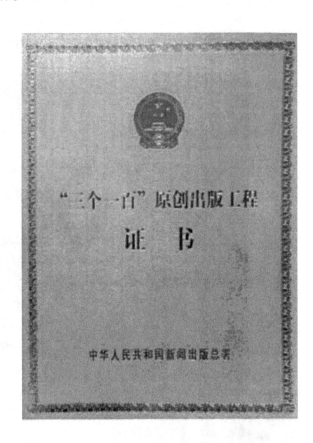

The Chinese Poem with the pictures:

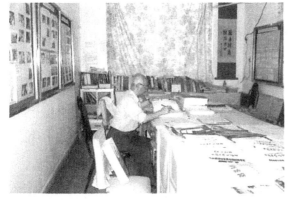

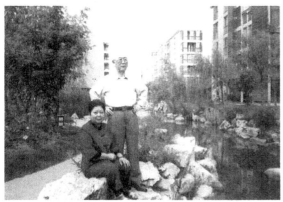

徐泽别名子久

医学教授

七旬之后

医研之余

吟以自娱

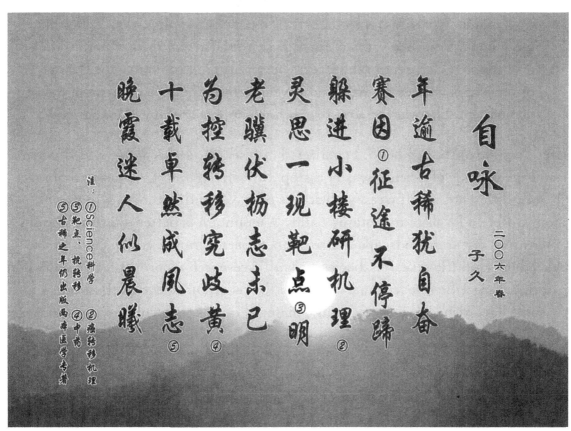

自咏

子久

二〇〇六年春

年逾古稀犹自奋

赛因①征途不停蹄

躲进小楼研机理②

灵思一现靶点③明

老骥伏枥志末已

为控转移究歧黄④

十载卓然成凤志⑤

晚霞迷人似晨曦

注：
①Science科学
②癌转移机理
③靶点、抗转移
④中药
⑤古稀之年仍出版高亦医学专著

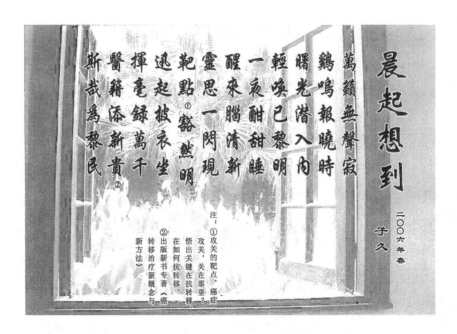

5. Postscript

Where did these 8 medical monographs come from? Some of the first drafts came from the original record of "Morning in the morning" and then compiled into a manuscript. I sent it to the street to copy the typing room and put it into a book. From the years of the flower, to the age of the ancient, to the year of the shackles, sent to the street copying typing room to type hundreds of times. Sometimes my wife and I went to the typing room to print the manuscript. She was the first reader and supporter of my "Monograph".

After I retired at the age of 63, I continued to research, self-reliance, self-financing, and the journey of Science was non-stop. Still struggling, arduously climbing, four different scientific research stages of one scientific research footprint, four different levels of mountain results. A mountain is better than a mountain scientific research landscape. Perseverance, perseverance. Since 1980, I have insisted on scientific research diaries, scientific research records, the accumulation of these scientific research materials and the record of scientific thinking, and some have also been selected as the material of this series of "monographs".

I read five years of private school in my childhood (then in the early 1930s, there was only one elementary school in a county, and the villages were mostly private). I loved the ancient books and poems. In addition to medical research, you can enjoy yourself.

晨起想到

二〇〇六年春

万籁无声寂
鸡鸣报晓时
曙光潜入内
轻唤已黎明
一夜酣甜睡
醒来脑清新
灵思一闪现
靶点豁然明
迅起披衣坐
挥毫录万千
医籍添新贵
斯哉为黎民

自　咏

二〇〇六年春

年逾古稀犹自奋
赛因征途不停蹄
躲进小楼研机理
灵思一现靶点明
老骥伏枥志未已
为控转移究歧黄
十栽卓然成夙志
晚霞迷人似晟曦

Printed in the United States
By Bookmasters